Fighting for Life

The Twelve Battles That Made Our NHS,
and the Struggle for Its Future

ISABEL HARDMAN

VIKING
an imprint of
PENGUIN BOOKS

VIKING

UK | USA | Canada | Ireland | Australia
India | New Zealand | South Africa

Viking is part of the Penguin Random House group of companies
whose addresses can be found at global.penguinrandomhouse.com.

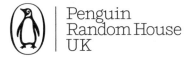

First published 2023
001

Copyright © Isabel Hardman, 2023

The moral right of the author has been asserted

Extracts from 'The Building' and 'Annus Mirabilis' taken from
The Complete Poems of Philip Larkin © Estate of Philip Larkin.
Reprinted by permission of Faber and Faber Ltd

Set in 12/14.75pt Bembo Book MT Pro
Typeset by Jouve (UK), Milton Keynes
Printed and bound in Great Britain by Clays Ltd, Elcograf S.p.A.

The authorised representative in the EEA is Penguin Random House Ireland,
Morrison Chambers, 32 Nassau Street, Dublin D02 YH68

A CIP catalogue record for this book is available from the British Library

ISBN: 978-0-241-50434-5

www.greenpenguin.co.uk

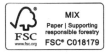

Contents

1. Holding on for something new

They called her Aneira, Nye for short. For her whole life she was going to celebrate two birthdays: her own, and that of the health system she was born under. Both have lived to an age that few would have taken for granted at the time she took her first breath. And at the time she took that breath, one minute past midnight, it was the start of her life – and that of the National Health Service.

Aneira Thomas was the first baby born into a system of healthcare which meant her mother wasn't going to have to pay the doctors and midwives for assisting her labour in a small Welsh cottage hospital. It meant that she would benefit from free vaccinations and free medicines for all the normal childhood illnesses that would come along and which had, in the past, often signalled the end to a short life. For her mother, it meant proper healthcare, too, at a time when women tended to see their middle age as the start of a decline due to poor eyesight, bad teeth and devastating untreated injuries sustained in childbirth – if they made it through labour at all. But the National Health Service has come to mean more than 'just' free healthcare, transformative though that has been. It is part of our modern British story. Of all the threads making up the welfare state, this is the one we have chosen to cling on to most tightly. It is the one we boast about to visitors from overseas – often with little regard for what their health system is like by comparison, because it is our automatic assumption that our NHS is the best in the world. We like to use that possessive pronoun too: *our* NHS. Politicians can scarcely get through a week without praising it, just in case someone doubts their commitment to *our* NHS.

Within our NHS there are nearly 2 million people working across the UK; there are countries smaller than our health system. There are the nurses who held the hands of the Covid patients who died alone, watching their families say goodbye over FaceTime as the ventilators kept them going. There are the doctors who made a point of examining their AIDS patients without gloves – and the princess who helped them – to make a point about this devastating and misunderstood illness. There are the porters who, along with perhaps the chief executive, are the only people who really know their way around the entire hospital, and who have wheeled mothers clutching the tiny wrinkled hands of their newborns before taking the body of a ninety-year-old to the mortuary. Just as we are all either going to get cancer or have someone close to us who will have it, so we all either know someone who works in the health service or are ourselves a part of this small nation. Most of us entered the world in an NHS hospital; most of us will die under the system's care, too. We know the sacrifices NHS workers make in their personal lives, in their own health, even with their very lives – to the extent that in the middle of the coronavirus pandemic, we took to the streets to applaud them once a week. Yet it is not just the individual stories of those workers, doctors, nurses, managers, porters, paramedics, cleaners and receptionists that make us feel emotional and possessive about *our* NHS. Health workers are venerated in many countries, but we are exceptional in our love of the *system*. Or, at least, in our love of what it stands for.

Aneira's birth wasn't the start of that story, but it was a symbol of the fights that had brought the NHS into being on 5 July 1948. Her mother, Edna, was engaged in her own fight that night: the fight to slow down her labour. Normally when the nurse calls the doctor to say there's a head visible in the labour room, the first thing they tell the mother is that it is time to start pushing. But at three minutes to midnight on 4 July 1948, this doctor said something else: 'Edna. You need to wait. It's not long now. Don't push. Just hold on, Edna.'

When the hand on the clock moved past midnight, he let her get going. It had been the doctor's idea to keep Edna back. It was his idea to name the baby Aneira. 'She should be named for the man who made this possible,' he suggested to Edna as she looked for her newborn in the nursery. 'After the man who allowed her to be born here, for free. After Nye Bevan. Call her Aneira.'

Aneira was the first person born under the National Health Service and the first person to enjoy an entire lifetime of its free care. In her book *Hold On Edna!* she writes about what healthcare meant to her mother: 'If my father had been injured, just a year before my birth, we'd have starved. And if one of my siblings had fallen seriously, critically ill, they mostly likely would have succumbed to their sickness. Edna has lived with this knowledge all her life: hearing the stories of limbs withering away, cancers left untreated, hacking coughs slowly turning into something more sinister until, one day, they'd stop and there'd be silence.'[1] That changed for everyone in 1948, and so many decades later, it is still not something many British people take for granted.

This is the story of the National Health Service. Like all life stories, there are a fair few ups and downs. Aneira herself has had good times and bad, saying the NHS has saved her own life repeatedly. The health service hasn't had an easy life, and has needed intensive care over the years, too. We love what it stands for just as we admire the principles of our friends, but we do also know that even the best people fall short of their own standards sometimes. To understand a life properly, you can't gloss over those bits in the way other treasured national institutions like *Desert Island Discs* can politely sidestep failed marriages that the interviewee doesn't want to discuss. So this is a biography, not a hagiography. There will be chapters with scandals, false starts and embarrassing moments. There will also be heroism, quiet determination, and extraordinary triumphs against the odds. It is the combination of these two aspects of a character that makes a life, and examining both will help us understand not just how we got to where we are today in the twenty-first-century NHS, but also who we are as a society and what we have come through.

Each chapter is based around a key fight that shaped the health service, and often British society more widely. There are periods that the book won't cover in a great deal of detail, just as most lives have spells lasting months or even years where things just plod along unremarkably and it is quite difficult to remember what one was doing on a particular Tuesday afternoon. This book also explores the intertwined stories of the services that started in all four nations of the

UK on 5 July 1948. They have progressively uncoupled, particularly from the turn of the century onwards, due to devolution: the world-famous blue lozenge NHS logo only officially applies to England. Scotland has its own logo, which is a pair of caring hands raised to the sky, and its own particular way of organising its NHS. The Welsh NHS similarly has taken its own path. In Northern Ireland, there has never actually been an NHS: it is Health and Social Care. HSC is free at the point of access, like the NHS in the rest of the UK, and was created at the same time.

You will find that much of this narrative focuses on NHS England, with explanations of what happened in Scotland and Wales at the same time. By the end we will have answered the big questions that apply to the NHS across Britain. These include why we have such an emotional attachment to the health service – one that goes far deeper than our feelings about free schooling, or the benefits system, or even the homes that the state provides for some of us to live in. What is the nature of that emotional attachment: is it really, as Nigel Lawson – who was Chancellor of the Exchequer when the health service was going through a severe funding squeeze in the 1980s – claims, the closest thing the British have to a national religion? Why is the system funded in the way it is, and structured in the way it is – and is that because it is the ideal design or just what was possible? To what extent can we say that advances in life expectancy, treatment outcomes and medical science are thanks to the NHS, or has it been more of an observer than we care to admit? Why are there repeated scandals, often featuring the same mistakes and bad cultures, in areas such as maternity? Why has mental health been the poor relation of physical health from the start right up to the present day? Has there ever been a time when there was enough money for the NHS? Or is it really what Chancellors like Lawson, and indeed his Labour counterparts doing the same bean-counting, often end up regarding as a plughole down which a government can pour money with precious little evidence of where it then goes? And, as it approaches a lifespan that in 1948 would have looked like a good innings, what is the future of the health service?

★

To answer these questions and to understand why we love the NHS, and why it was even necessary, we have to go back into Edna's own lifetime. She was thirty-nine when she gave birth to Aneira, her seventh child. Just two years after Edna was born, the National Insurance Act 1911 was passed, which laid some of the foundations of the NHS. It meant that workers aged 16–70 earning less than £160 a year and all manual workers had to have health insurance, with contributions from their employers. The model for this came from the first welfare state in the world, created in Germany by Prussian Chancellor Otto von Bismarck. That involved a compulsory social insurance model to cover healthcare costs. The National Health Insurance system in Britain, introduced by the Liberal government with David Lloyd George as its Chancellor, meant the working men who were covered were eligible for basic healthcare from a 'panel doctor' – a general practitioner who worked privately from their own surgery. Panel patients didn't provide the doctors with sufficient income, though, and so they would compete to provide care for the uninsured family members of these workers. They worked in hospitals, made and dispensed their own medicines, and even sold cigarettes in their practices. The panel patients themselves were only covered for basic care, not hospital treatment.

Hospitals had been around in various shapes and forms since the Norman conquest. One of the most famous in the world, St Bartholomew's Hospital in Smithfield, London, was built in 1123 for the sick poor and was part of the Priory of St Bartholomew. Barts survived the dissolution of the monasteries, which led to a decoupling of the religious institution from healthcare provision. By 1911, there was a patchwork of voluntary and municipal hospitals. The first were funded by philanthropy, and had grown in the eighteenth century. Some of the country's biggest institutions – including Westminster Hospital, the Foundling Hospital for abandoned infants, and the Bristol Royal Infirmary – were founded on this basis in the 1700s. It wasn't easy to get admitted to these hospitals, even when your life was in danger: you needed a letter from a hospital governor. In 1827, William Marsden, a surgeon working in London, came across a young girl who was starving and dying on the steps of St Andrew's

Church, Holborn. He searched in vain for a hospital to treat her, and she died two days later. Marsden was appalled by the way the donors of these hospitals controlled admissions, and decided to set up his own institution. He founded the London General Institution for the Gratuitous Cure of Malignant Diseases in Hatton Garden. It would admit anyone who needed treatment, including cholera patients – which no other hospital did. It gained a royal charter in 1837, and was renamed the Royal Free. It is still one of the world's best-known hospitals, and today towers over Hampstead in North London. It was where I was born on the NHS in 1986.

Then there were municipal hospitals: the successors of the workhouses. These hospitals were often known as infirmaries, and funded through the rates – taxes on property. They tended to be places where the chronically ill went for the rest of their lives, until they left in a coffin. Doctors were also setting up cottage hospitals: small buildings with twenty or so beds, often in rural areas, where they could treat patients for a charge.

Alongside the foundation of the big hospitals like the Royal Free was a growing interest in the importance of public health, and the role of the state in this. Previously health had been a private concern, addressed by charitable institutions, not the very small state. But the discovery that illnesses like cholera spread in insanitary conditions, which could only be addressed by government, started to change this. In 1847, the first medical officer for health was appointed in Liverpool following sanitary legislation, and others followed in cities including London the year after. The Vaccination Act 1853 made it compulsory for parents to vaccinate their children against smallpox within the first three months of their lives. Two-thirds of babies had received these vaccinations by the 1860s – though then, as now, there was an anti-vaccination movement, which responded to (valid) concerns about the safety of some of the vaccines used. The Crimean War and the work of Florence Nightingale, the name always on the tips of our tongues after the word 'nurse', underlined the importance of disease prevention and infection control. Legislators were beginning to feel that these kinds of policies were not unnecessary intrusions into people's lives, but the duty of a responsible state.

Several pieces of public health legislation were passed in the ensuing years, culminating in the creation in 1919 of a Ministry of Health. The phrase 'National Health Service' had entered the lexicon from Dr Benjamin Moore, who wrote about the need for proper organisation of healthcare in his book *The Dawn of the Health Age* in 1911, and also helped found the State Medical Service Association in 1912. Moore was a Liverpool physician, which has led that city to join the many places, organisations and individuals in the UK who claim to have 'started the NHS'.

Now we are well into Edna's childhood. She was ten years old when the government created a dedicated department for health. Her family, like so many in Britain, had been used to seeing illness as the sure sign that death was near: children dead of typhus in a workhouse, a mother found dead at home having avoided the doctor for fear of the cost. Edna's father was a miner, and had a welfare scheme and medical room at his colliery. But serious injuries down the pit or infections caught from small cuts were harder to treat, not covered by the welfare scheme, and often led to the man of the house becoming unable to work and the family falling into destitution. Women weren't covered, and as is the instinct of most mothers, they would put their children and husbands first when it came to health and food. Edna herself had lost friends to illnesses with names we can barely spell today because they are so uncommon, including typhus. Her mother died at home of stomach cancer, which went untreated because there was no money for a doctor. Edna herself considered a backstreet abortion when she became pregnant with a fourth child in 1937. She visited a woman who 'made unwanted babies disappear', but decided against the procedure in the end.[2]

In that time, though, the health of the nation generally had been improving. Infant mortality was falling as a result of improved diets, as were deaths from tuberculosis, a disease so virulent that many of the hospitals across the country were for the isolation and treatment of patients infected by it. Maternal deaths were falling. By the inter-war period, British healthcare was among the best in the world: it was not a scandal of quality of care or medicine that was the driver for the NHS. The problem was who could access it. Not all areas had decent numbers of hospitals or GPs – charities did what they could but there was no national planning for where they set up, while doctors worked where they wanted, not where need was greatest. As we have seen, insurance coverage was patchy, and non-existent for children and for women who kept home rather than working. The middle classes, meanwhile, resented the amount they had to pay in fees or membership of contributory schemes.

It is not right to say that the creation of the NHS marked the moment at which proper healthcare in Britain began, nor is it the point or organisation to which all improvements in the nation's health can be traced. The country was already heading towards a better standard of health. But it was the Second World War which made a state-planned, free health service seem both possible and necessary. Why was this?

The war had an effect on a number of parts of government and society – and on certain key individuals – which would open a window, and a very brief one at that, for a national health service of some kind. As war loomed, the government prepared to take over the hospitals so that it could organise the treatment of people injured in air raids. The Ministry of Health appointed regional hospital officers to plan hospital services, whether it be for the casualties of bomb blasts in danger zones or for mothers giving birth in hospitals in outer areas.

Bristol was one of those danger areas, and the fear was that the city simply didn't have enough space for the casualties that would ensue. On the outskirts, in a quiet village called Frenchay, was a children's sanatorium in a stately home, surrounded by seventy acres of parkland. Here, the government ordered construction of an emergency services hospital with sixteen wards in one-storey brick huts. Those huts remained throughout the site's life as an NHS hospital, all the way until it closed in 2014. For other hospitals, particularly the voluntary institutions which were facing financial crises and had gone into the war trying to obtain state grants in order to keep operating, the Emergency Medical Service was a chance to survive. It was also the first time that voluntary hospitals, normally in competition with one another, were working together as part of a wider collective effort. It was this wider collective effort that not only paved the way for a system such as the NHS, but also created the ethos underlying that health service that gives it such an emotional tug today. The instruction in the Covid-19 pandemic to 'protect the NHS' had strong echoes of the communications during the Second World War about 'careless talk costs lives': people were encouraged to behave with the collective good in mind.

Those who had been campaigning for better healthcare for a while sensed their political opportunity. Among them was an extraordinary woman who is – as is so often the case for female trailblazers of her time – little known today. Edith Summerskill was a trailblazer in two fields, in fact. She was a doctor, which was unusual enough for a woman when she qualified in 1924. She then became an MP aged thirty-two – also highly unusual. She described the moment she became a socialist thus:

> It was the suffering of a woman which finally drew me into the political world. One wet cold night many years ago, at the age of 22, a newly qualified doctor, I went to attend my first confinement. Very nervous, I arrived with my new black bag. My knock was answered by the young husband, pallid and shabby, with the familiar signs of long unemployment upon him.
>
> He took me upstairs to a room stripped of all but the bare necessities of life. There lay the patient on a mattress, covered by a threadbare blanket, a girl of my own age, in labour with her second child. By the bed stood a cot and standing grasping the wooden bars was a child with bulging forehead and crooked legs. The classic picture of rickets, a disease of undernourishment. The young mother clutched my hand with her own moist bony fingers, on which she wore a greenish brass wedding ring, twisted round with cotton to prevent it falling off. In that room that night I became a socialist and I joined in the fight, not against a class but against a system.[3]

Summerskill went along to a meeting of the newly formed Socialist Medical Association. This was the idea of Charles Wortham Brook, a GP who had trained at Barts. Brook was corresponding regularly with a Berlin dentist named Dr Ewald Fabian, who explained to him that, in Germany, socialist doctors were organising into large campaigning groups to get their views heard by a wider audience. Fabian visited Brook in London, and found the 'set-up of the British voluntary hospital system seemed quite incomprehensible to him'. He wrote to the secretary of every Labour Party in the country, asking for the names of doctors 'who were known to be members of the Party or thought to be sympathisers', and in September 1930 a group of such doctors met in the National Labour Club in Tufton Street, Westminster.[4] The SMA's three main objectives were 'to work for a Socialised Medical Service both preventive and curative, free and open to all; to secure for the people the highest possible standard of health; to disseminate the principles of socialism within the medical and allied services'.[5] By 1934, the SMA had its first big victory: the Labour Party's official policy was now for a free medical service managed by local government.

Come the war, the members of the SMA started to make the case from whatever platform they could find for a national hospital service that would continue after the war. In his speech to the 1940 annual general meeting of the association, Brook argued: 'The present Emergency Medical Service, despite its serious shortcomings, might well constitute the basis of a permanent coordinated National Hospital Service in the immediate post-war period.'[6] Many of his points in this speech did not go down well with fellow doctors: he suggested that the government could pay GPs a basic salary and capitation (a payment per patient) – and indeed that question became a matter of great contention for those who did set up the NHS. Summerskill, meanwhile, spoke in a debate in the Commons in October 1940:

> In a few weeks a tremendous change has been taking place in the medical service. Here we have a demand, on the one hand coming from sick people who not only need free medical advice but deserve it, and on the other, doctors with nothing to do, with their practices gone, longing to provide that service. The Right Hon. Gentleman's predecessor admitted, when I said that the time had come for a State medical service, that the next step in our social services was to

introduce some form of State medical service, but he thought public opinion and the medical profession were not ready for it. I believe that the times have changed.

During the last seven weeks, not only have doctors' houses been bombed, but with this material destruction the prejudices of generations have been destroyed. The time has arrived for action, and I ask the Minister to make his name as well known as that of Chadwick [the public health reformer Edwin Chadwick, who uncovered the link between poor sanitation and disease in the 1840s], and to take this opportunity to introduce this service so that after the war we may at least say that out of all this destruction and misery there has come some good.[7]

Socialists arguing for a state medical system: hardly the Pope arguing in favour of the Reformation. But what was striking – and what they would see as the war went on – was that others were also coming to agree.

One of the most important of those in agreement was William Beveridge. At this stage in a narrative, we normally introduce a character by some of their attributes. The problem with Beveridge is that you could use any adjective to describe him, even a long chain of directly contradicting ones, and they would be correct. His own biographer José Harris wrote that 'he has been described to me personally as a man who wouldn't give a penny to a blind beggar and as one of the kindest men who ever walked the Earth'.[8] Most who knew him seem to agree he was a vain man. Most also agree he was one of the most talented people they had ever met.

Perhaps it is better for us to look at Beveridge's CV running up to the Second World War. He was educated at public school and Oxford, and started his career at Toynbee Hall in East London. Toynbee Hall was a late Victorian-era institution, which carried out a charitable form of social work. In the few years he was there, the young graduate studied the causes and consequences of poverty – or what he later described as 'want'. He saw, too, what unemployment, or 'idleness', did to a family. Beveridge also met some of the men who would shape the left in years to come: George Lansbury and

Ramsay MacDonald, who both went on to lead the Labour Party, and Beatrice Webb, a secretary to one of the leading socialists at the time – Clement Attlee.

A few years later, in 1907, Beveridge travelled to Germany to study the Bismarck model of social insurance as a means of protecting those suffering from the misery of untreated disease. The following year, he was working as a civil servant for the Board of Trade, appointed by Winston Churchill to work on, among other things, the Lloyd George insurance scheme. During the First World War he worked in the Ministry of Munitions and the Ministry of Food, where he became permanent secretary. He was a key figure in the move from the state leaving people to get on with it towards the sense that it was part of the role of government to protect those people. He had a spell back in academia, before returning to politics in 1936 to work on the preparations for rationing in the looming war. So it was that, in 1941, Beveridge had what the biographer of the welfare state Nicholas Timmins calls 'a knowledge of the origins and scope of social services in Britain that was probably unequalled'.[9]

This status did not lead to a job that the civil servant felt was equal to him, though. In a meeting with Arthur Greenwood, the Minister for Reconstruction, he was offered something that brought him to tears: to chair an interdepartmental committee on the coordination of social insurance. He was bitterly disappointed – not thrilled – by this, seeing it as a 'kicking upstairs'. He had been writing to key figures in the wartime coalition government, including Churchill, Attlee, Ernest Bevin and Herbert Morrison. Timmins says baldly that 'none wanted the awkward and arrogant ex-permanent secretary around'. Bevin, though, saw an opportunity for getting him out of the way, by giving him the task of reforming sickness and disability schemes. No one was particularly interested in this job – indeed Beveridge seems to have struggled to muster the motivation himself for a little while after accepting it. But what he then started to produce changed the course of Britain for ever.

He wrote in a paper in July 1941 that the 'time has now come to consider social insurance as a whole, as a contribution to a better new world after the war'.[10] A few months later, he still managed to surprise those ministers with another paper, which laid the foundations of his plan. This document, entitled 'Heads of a Scheme for Social Security', argued that 'no satisfactory scheme of social security can be devised' without 'a national health service for prevention and comprehensive treatment . . . available to all members of the community; universal children's allowances for all children up to 14 or if in full-time education up to 16; full use of powers of the state to maintain employment and to reduce unemployment to seasonal, cyclical and interval unemployment, that is to say to unemployment suitable for treatment by cash allowances'.[11]

At this point, the fighting began. Greenwood was horrified that this random committee he'd set up was now advocating a free national health service, comprehensive benefits for children, and full employment. This was not what dusty committees with annoying and awkward chairs were supposed to do. In the early months of 1942, he asked Beveridge to withdraw his plans, and after he repeatedly refused, came up with a compromise: this report was going to be published as Beveridge's 'own report' and not government policy. Beveridge continued to plug away, making his case in public as well. In March 1942, he wrote in *The Times* that the government 'should set in hand preparation of plans whereby the evils of peace – poverty, squalor, preventible [*sic*] disease, inequality of opportunity, waste of abilities – may be abolished after it has abolished the evils of war'.[12] That July marked thirty years since the introduction of national health insurance. The *Times* correspondent analysed the scheme as 'palpably inadequate' for the present day, pointing out that: 'Statutory medical benefit includes only the services of general practitioners, which in view of the rapid advance in medical science is often totally inadequate for quick restoration to health.' The paper's editorial added that it hoped the Beveridge Committee on Social Insurance and Allied Services would 'offer a well-considered plan of development enabling this generation to fulfil the promise of the great experiments in social legislation with which Sir William Beveridge himself was associated thirty years ago'.[13]

Beveridge was indeed planning to go much further. In December 1942, he published his final report, entitled *Social Insurance and Allied*

Services. What a suitably dusty name for a report that was really supposed to be an answer to an internal government personnel issue. But the reception to Beveridge's writing went rather further than a few interested civil servants. It became an unlikely bestseller.

Beveridge broadcast the report on the nine o'clock news that night. He told listeners that his plan hadn't 'yet been considered by government or Parliament' and was 'simply proposals that I have made'. Those proposals included an 'all-in scheme of medical treatment'. He urged people to buy the full report to get all the details. As a demonstration perhaps of the scale of the want that the civil servant, now in his sixties, was proposing to address, there were queues outside His Majesty's Stationery Office of people wanting to buy their own copy. HMSO is not normally deluged like Wimbledon is during the tennis. Within a month, it had sold 100,000 copies. *Social Insurance and Allied Services* was vividly written in parts. Copies were dropped into areas of Europe occupied by the Nazis, to the extent that Hitler was provided with a briefing on the details of the Beveridge proposals.[14] It was an international and domestic sensation. But it was also long – 200,000 words long. The author himself conceded that 'you'll find it rather a long document' and suggested readers only bother with the first part and part six.[15]

The most memorable passages of the report include the 'five giants' that Beveridge felt the state should tackle. He set out three guiding principles for his recommendations. The first was that this was a time for big change, not small solutions influenced by sectional interests: 'Now, when the war is abolishing landmarks of every kind, is the opportunity for using experience in a clear field. A revolutionary moment in the world's history is a time for revolutions, not for patching.' The second contained one of the most vivid and enduring images of the lengthy tome: 'Organisation of social insurance should be treated as one part only of a comprehensive policy of social progress. Social insurance fully developed may provide income security; it is an attack upon Want. But Want is one only of five giants on the road of reconstruction and in some ways the easiest to attack. The others are Disease, Ignorance, Squalor and Idleness.' The final principle was that social security was a partnership between the state and the individual: 'The State in organising security should not stifle incentive, opportunity, responsibility; in establishing a national minimum, it should leave room and encouragement for voluntary action by each individual to provide more than that minimum for himself and his family.'[16]

The report was not a detailed exposition of how a health service should be financed or run, but it did contain the assumption that there would be a national health service, and that treatment would be free. There was no detail on organisational matters: Beveridge did not make the case for a nationalised hospital service or anything of that level of detail. At the press conference following the publication of the report, he was asked whether voluntary hospitals would be able to continue. He replied: 'It does not affect them one way or the other. Out of the contribution of 4s 3d a sum of 10d is set aside for medical services. This would produce about £40,000,000 a year, and it would be a matter of departmental responsibility as to how the money is allotted. The voluntary hospital service can be left alive. It was not possible to discuss the question with the medical authorities, so I have left the question open.'[17] Beveridge was impatient. He wanted this to be part of the post-war reconstruction, not something to aim for in the future.

The Times described the report as 'remarkable both for its imaginative treatment of a complex subject and for the common sense way in which it deals with practical issues. It is comprehensive in its sweep without losing grip on the economic and administrative realities on which any forward policy must be based if it is to succeed.' The paper also said that: 'Sir William Beveridge and his colleagues have put the nation deeply in their debt, not merely for a confident assurance that the poor need not always be with us, but for a masterly exposition of the ways and means whereby the fact and the fear of involuntary poverty can be speedily abolished altogether.'[18]

Meanwhile, in the left-wing magazine *Tribune*, its founder wrote: 'Sir William has described the conditions in which the tears might be taken out of capitalism.'[19] That writer was the Labour MP Aneurin Bevan, who saw that in the report written by a man who would – briefly – be a Liberal MP lay an opportunity for the Labour Party.

Bevan already had a very high profile in British politics. This was a result of his often-controversial stance not just on the Second World War itself, but also on the way the wartime coalition government was going about trying to protect the country and the population. He was one of the most consistent voices of opposition against the curbs on civil liberties that the government imposed on the country. This, his biographer Nick Thomas-Symonds argues, was in part because he scorned the way in which the official leaders of the opposition to the coalition government merely performed that role in order to ensure business got through the Commons, and also because he felt the people worst hit by the restrictions were those who had the least power. Thomas-Symonds says: 'His whole argument about civil liberties in wartime was an expression of his desire to argue for the plight of the underprivileged, for those who lacked power.'[20] Not everyone felt so sympathetic towards the way Bevan exercised these principles: his wife, Jennie Lee, often opened post addressed to the couple containing hate mail or even excrement.[21]

When the war began, Bevan had been MP for Ebbw Vale, a constituency of Welsh mining towns and villages, for a decade. His political life was about gaining power and making the most of it for the people he had been born among and had worked among in his early years. When he was thirteen, he started working in his local pit. He was hard-working, but a nightmare employee, as he constantly frustrated what he saw as the attempts by colliery bosses to cut corners and endanger lives, or require more from the workers than was fair. He rose through the levels of politics from local to national, but in between he worked with a local society in Tredegar, which was to have as much of an influence on him – and therefore on the NHS – as the bestselling Beveridge Report did.

The Tredegar Medical Aid Society was one of many attempts by workers to improve the quality of the healthcare that they were entitled to through the 'poundage' schemes – the panel doctor arrangements – that they were enrolled in through their employment. It was founded in 1890, with each member paying a contribution in return for free healthcare which went much further than the very basic treatment they'd previously been able to access: doctors and nurses, opticians and dentistry, as well as transport to a hospital of their choice. The society set up its own hospital in the town, and by the time Bevan was MP for the area, nearly everyone in the town was a member. It was a universal local health service. It wasn't the only one: Llanelli, which was fifty miles away in another South Wales valley, had set up similar, and there were pioneering attempts to expand healthcare provision in other parts of the country such as Peckham. But Tredegar was the collective free healthcare that Bevan himself knew. It was also the subject of a novel written by its secretary, Dr A. J. Cronin: *The Citadel*. In Cronin's book, the doctors, indeed the wider medical system, are complicated heroes, often led astray by their desire to make money – the novel's protagonist Andrew Manson included. *The Citadel* attracted a great deal of attention, largely because of the way it attacked the greed of many doctors.[22] When it was adapted into a film, the chief censor, J. C. Hanna, was worried about its effect on the 'confidence of the nation in the medical profession'.

It is often claimed – including on the cover of its latest edition – that *The Citadel* was the novel that inspired the NHS. Similarly, Tredegar is often described as the model for the NHS. The reality is a little more complicated: Cronin was preaching to the converted, as his largely middle-class audience were already fed up with the insurance they were paying, and told pollsters they wanted hospitals to be a public service.[23] The system as it was had few fans. But the novel does not make the case for another system specifically. Manson himself muses on the solutions to a system that does not reward any doctor trying to practise honourably: 'There ought to be some better scheme, a chance for everybody – say, oh, say State control! Then he groaned, remembering Doctor Bigsby and the MFB. No, damn it, that's hopeless; bureaucracy chokes individual effort – it would suffocate me.' What it did do was become part of the popular consensus that the current situation was unsustainable.

There is also the line from Bevan about his desire to 'Tredegarise' the country: 'All I am doing is extending to the entire population of Britain the benefits we had in Tredegar for a generation or more. We are going to "Tredegarise" you.' Bevan was responsible for closing the Tredegar scheme, too: when he was setting up the NHS. The committee had hoped to be able to continue alongside or in some way within the NHS. But Bevan wrote: 'You have shown us the way and by your very efficiency you have brought about your own cessation.'[24]

The glaring difference between the Tredegar Medical Aid Society and the NHS that Bevan founded, of course, is that our national health system is not funded through personal contributions but through general taxation. For Bevan, healthcare was a right that was automatic for every citizen, not acquired through membership.

But there are two important legacies from Tredegar that we can see in the NHS, even today. The first is, of course, the principle of decent healthcare that is free at the point of access. The second is harder to pin down, but explains a great deal about why this country doesn't have a merely transactional relationship with what could quite easily be dismissed as just one of many ways of paying for healthcare. This system was a collective piece of work by people who, in their time, were often too easily ignored and ridden rough-shod over by those who were more powerful. It represented a society coming together and saying that those people deserved better. Even though most people today only really come together for the NHS by paying their taxes, that spirit has still managed to linger.

For Bevan, the Beveridge Report came at a time when, aside from the undeniable force of his arguments, he was without power: a backbencher, not a minister. He and his socialist colleagues were delighted that this document had committed to a national health service, but they had to watch as the Conservative-led coalition government made its own response as to what that might look like. They also watched as the medical profession started to set the scene for the battles to come.

A common part of the creation myth around the NHS is that the Tories opposed it, and so did the doctors. I have a rather faded coffee mug on my desk with an old Labour campaign poster on it that makes the former claim, while the latter is wheeled out today whenever the British Medical Association is objecting to some new reforms in the health service. Both are true, but it is also true that there was going to be *a* national health service after the war. The question was what sort.

In government, the anxiety that started with Greenwood's intervention back in July had been building ever since. A few weeks before Beveridge published his report, the Chancellor of the Exchequer Sir Kingsley Wood wrote to Churchill to complain it was about to propose 'an impracticable financial commitment' and would hike taxes by a third. The prime minister had reportedly refused to meet Beveridge and had disliked the level of publicity and the urgency of the report. Churchill was also reluctant to commit to it without an election giving him a mandate to do so, and merely agreed, after some Cabinet infighting between the two parties, to prepare the legislation enabling the proposals.[25]

When MPs finally got the chance to debate the report in February 1943, they found the government was still in a highly non-committal mood. The Commons debate was precipitated by the government withdrawing summarised copies of the report from circulation to the armed forces, on the grounds that it was too political. A Labour MP, John Dugdale, took issue with this and, waving a copy of the banned pamphlet, mockingly quoted from it the lines he thought had particularly upset ministers: 'This does not alter three facts: that the purpose of victory is to live into a better world than the old world; that each individual citizen is more likely to concentrate upon his war effort if he feels that his Government will be ready in time with plans for that better world; that, if these plans are to be ready in time, they must be made now.'[26] His implication was that the government was dragging its feet, and trying to cover that up.

The press had enthusiastically followed that line, too. The *Sunday Pictorial* – later renamed the *Sunday Mirror*, reported on 14 February that 'there is a conspiracy afoot to torpedo the Beveridge Plan and MPs of all parties are taking part in it'. It claimed that a 'slaughter of Beveridge's New Deal for the common people' was planned in the form of a 'monstrous motion' that would include only 'pious resolution of welcome' in Parliament, rather than one committing the government to it. 'That motion, if carried, does not mean that the

Government has to accept the Plan or do anything about it. It will merely have to "bear it in Mind" in planning the future. In fact, once the debate is over if MPs accept the motion, Beveridge can be decently buried and forgotten.' The motion that was tabled by ministers was indeed insipid: 'That this House welcomes the Report of Sir William Beveridge on Social Insurance and Allied Services as a comprehensive review of the present provisions in this sphere and as a valuable aid in determining the lines on which developments and legislation should be pursued as part of the Government's policy of post-war reconstruction.'[27]

Greenwood himself opened the debate, but made it clear that he wanted the plan implemented 'without a day's unnecessary delay'. It then fell to Sir John Anderson, who held the position of Lord President of the Council (better known today as Leader of the House of Commons), to give such a dry speech about the government's position (or lack thereof) that Bevan repeatedly intervened to complain that 'it is not much use listening to him'. Bevan was, as he had been when a miner, a bit of a pain throughout the session, repeatedly interrupting others on points of order about amendments and how much time MPs were being given for this discussion. He didn't give a speech of his own. The debate closed with Herbert Morrison, the Labour Home Secretary who was already a foe of Bevan's, giving a speech in which he was very careful to underline the areas the government very definitely did support. 'We are going to have a big comprehensive health service,' he told MPs, 'and that is a very big change to which subject to reservations the Government have committed themselves.' One of those reservations was that the government was not going to 'destroy the institution of voluntary hospitals', though he mused that 'they could all be taken over by the municipality'.[28] Morrison was speaking from experience here. He had been leader of London County Council between 1934 and 1940, and had considered taking over the voluntary hospitals there but had postponed it on the grounds of cost. His commitment to local authorities running hospitals was to become one of the big Cabinet clashes over the design of the health service. Morrison only managed to reassure the would-be Tory rebels, and the amendment calling for the 'early implementation' of Beveridge still attracted 132 votes from across the House: a significant revolt against the government in any time, let alone during the war.

Finally, Churchill gave a broadcast on life after the war on 21 March 1943 in which he promised a 'Four Years' Plan', which would 'cover five or six large measures of a practical character which must all have been the subject of prolonged, careful, energetic preparation beforehand and which fit together into a general scheme'. It would be subject to the test of a general election, he promised. He boasted about his own involvement in 'all these schemes of national, compulsory organised thrift', mentioning along the way that he'd brought 'my friend' Beveridge into public service and that he was Lloyd George's 'lieutenant'. 'The time is now ripe,' the prime minister said, 'for another great advance' – and he and his colleagues were 'strong partisans of national compulsory insurance from the cradle to the grave'. He set up a committee to consider implementing the proposals. The welfare state was on its way, and it now had a slogan from Churchill: 'From the cradle to the grave.'

Meanwhile the Labour Party was busily producing its own policy paper on the health service. A month after Churchill's broadcast, the party published a pamphlet called *National Service for Health: The Labour Party's Post-War Policy*.[29] This set as Labour's aim something it called 'full health', and argued that the only body capable of achieving this was the government. 'The full health that we aim at is to a great extent a consequence of good government. No agency less universal in its authority than Government can secure for the whole people the conditions necessary for health; and no ill-health in any part of the population can be a matter of indifference to the people's Government.' And that would require a medical service. This needed to be 'planned as a whole, so that there are no gaps in it'; 'preventive as well as curative'; 'complete, covering all kinds of treatment required'; 'open to all, irrespective of means or social position'; 'efficient and up to date'; 'accessible to the public'; 'preserve confidence between doctor and patient', including the ability of patients to change their doctors if dissatisfied; 'equitable for the medical profession', including no tolerance for 'sweating or overwork of doctors, nurses, or other health workers'; and 'so organised as to enable the medical profession to pull its weight effectively in all those tasks of democratic government which affect the nation's health'.

It argued that the Ministry of Health should 'be in a position to plan the lay-out of the nation's hospitals, doctoring, etc., according to the nation's need', but also that local authorities must be given 'wide powers' for securing a 'comprehensive hospital service' – as opposed to the current patchy provision across different parts of the country. The party wanted health centres and general hospitals within each region, the latter containing around 1,000 beds and 'treating all kinds of cases except infectious cases or mental disease of certain kinds'. And the doctors needed to be 'organised as a national, full-time, salaried, pensionable service'. 'National Service for Health is a service honourable enough for any recruit,' the paper argued, clearly anticipating that not all doctors were going to leap for joy at this proposal. 'It should be a service well enough paid and protected to meet the needs of every doctor in a democratic Britain.'

This was the political reaction. But what of the people working in healthcare at the time? Even though health is so much more than medics, the reaction of the doctors was what attracted the most attention, and not just because of their prominent and respected role in society.

The British Medical Association is, as you'd expect from a trade union of doctors, rather august in appearance. It operates from an imposing red-brick and columned building designed by Sir Edwin Lutyens in Tavistock Square, London. That appearance disguises what is essentially an organisation of well-dressed street fighters. It has long struggled with whether it is a union or not. It was founded in 1832, initially as the Provincial Medical and Surgical Association – which shared medical knowledge, particularly in relation to the cholera outbreak that was under way at the time. It quickly became a political organisation, though, and rebranded to the BMA. But still it disliked the term 'union', because such a term was 'derogatory to its dignity'.[30] It had long campaigned for its members' interests, like all good unions – and it opposed the Poor Law on the grounds that the pay for doctors was 'as insulting and degrading to the character of the medical profession as they were unjust and injurious to the poor'.[31] It also opposed Lloyd George's insurance reforms. Because of the nature of doctors' work, it has always been the case that the BMA doesn't just respond to policies on pay, but on the wider principles of health-care. This makes it a very potent organisation, and the character and education of its membership make it even more so. It is hard to find a Health Secretary in the entire history of the health service who has finished their time fond of the BMA. It is hard to find many reforms, whether the design of the NHS or making changes to it since, that the BMA has supported.

But it is not right to say – as some do – that the BMA *opposed the NHS*. As we shall see, it fervently and furiously opposed some aspects of it, often with foul language. But it had in fact accepted that there should be some better-organised way of funding and providing healthcare. The fights weren't about the principle. They were all about *how* to realise it.

By the time the Beveridge Report published, having opposed the national health insurance initially the BMA was now pushing for it to be extended to cover other services, including consultants, and to cover dependents of the insured worker. It wanted a 'general medical service for the nation'. It had even set up its own Medical Planning Commission ahead of Beveridge getting his unwelcome job offer, which reported in June 1942 and proposed that doctors choose between being full- or part-time workers in a new insurance-based system covering the whole population. Hospitals would be run by regional councils, and GPs would be paid a basic salary, capitation, and money for other services on top of that.

The report in the *British Medical Journal* of the meeting of the BMA's council in February 1943 accepted that there was going to be a national health service of some kind, and argued that the union shouldn't oppose the compulsory insurance scheme proposed because to do so would be to lose sympathy from the general population for its more important fight in determining the 'conditions and terms of service' – in other words, it wanted to focus on the pay and who would be in charge of doctors. It added: 'The Council advises co-operation, with the important proviso that the character, terms, and conditions of the services must be negotiated with and agreed by the doctors of this country. And the doctors of this country do not believe that it is in the public interest that the medical profession should be turned into a whole-time salaried civil service, with the doctor the servant of the State. The doctor must be the servant of his patient.'[32]

This was not an unreasonable objection: it wasn't that long ago that the state had very little to do with medical care, and there was still considerable unease about the idea of doctors being directed by politicians – in the same way that those in other lines of work, including journalists, resist the meddling of MPs. Perhaps this suspicion of the state provided the gunpowder for the explosions that the trade union was about to set off, as the government started to consider how to set up a national health service.

One of the loudest noises in these explosions was from Dr Charles Hill. He was one of the first celebrity medics – there are too many to count now, but in his day it was unusual for doctors to take to the airwaves, and illegal for them to advertise their services. Known very well to the population as 'the Radio Doctor', Hill had been broadcasting health advice on the BBC during the war as part of the Ministry of Health's *Kitchen Front* programme every morning. He had a rich, rolling and soothing voice. He was also secretary of the BMA, and had to negotiate a compromise between the need for more medics to join the armed forces and the necessity of keeping some at home to treat everyone else. In 1943, he joined a BBC debate on the Beveridge proposals in which he expressed concern about the implications of a full-time salaried state medical service, saying it would 'bring doctors into the civil service'.[33] He continued this opposition to making doctors into a 'branch of the local government services' when Ernest Brown, now the Liberal Minister of Health, started the negotiations on a health service by suggesting doctors could become employees of local authorities. Hill primed doctors to be 'ready for a fight'. 'Fight' is a rather mild term, though, for what happened next, because even though Hill and his BMA colleagues did not oppose the entire principle of the NHS, they very nearly derailed it anyway.

In February 1944, Henry Willink, a Conservative, was the Minister of Health who published the government's White Paper *A National Health Service*.[34] This made clear the government's commitment to a 'comprehensive health service for everybody in this country'. Even at this stage, though, Churchill was anxious about the proposals it contained, and on the eve of publication he expressed a desire not to publish. He was told in a memo from Lord Woolton, the Minister for Reconstruction, that his anxiety was misplaced: 'This is a compromise scheme, but it is a compromise which is very much more favourable to the Conservatives than to Labour Ministers and when it is published, I should expect more criticism from the Left than from Conservative circles.' He warned that if Churchill withdrew the paper and tried to start again, 'the Labour Ministers may withdraw their support of the scheme and stand out for something more drastic which would be far more repugnant to Conservative feeling'.[35] Woolton was eventually right in his predictions of what the Labour Party would do differently if given the choice, but on this occasion Churchill agreed and the compromise document was published.

The White Paper also argued that this was 'not a completely new' idea, and that 'the stage has been reached, in the Government's view, at which the single comprehensive service for all should be regarded as the natural next development'. It also made clear that the question before the House wasn't that healthcare in Britain was bad – it was that not everyone could access it. 'The record of this country in its health and medical services is a good one . . . the main reason for change is that the Government believes that, at this stage of social development, the care of personal health should be put on a new footing and be made available to everybody as a publicly sponsored service.' The plan in this paper was for GPs to be salaried, and a new body would oversee them from the centre. Joint authorities of local councils would take over the municipal hospitals, and would provide services using contracts with voluntary hospitals. It praised the history and heritage of the voluntaries: 'The voluntary hospital movement not only represents the oldest established hospital system of the country, but it attracts the active personal interest and support of a large number of people who believe in it as a social organisation and who wish to see it maintained side by side with the hospitals which are directly provided out of public funds . . . It is certainly not the wish of the Government to destroy or diminish a system which is so well rooted in the goodwill of its supporters.' This was in keeping with what Beveridge envisaged, allowing the voluntary hospitals to get on with things in their own way. But the voluntary hospitals themselves didn't feel they would have much of a chance of being able to get on with it; surely their donors would see little point in supporting them financially now the government was removing their reason to exist?

The voluntary hospitals weren't the only ones who were unhappy with the White Paper. In fact, it was hard to find anyone who finished reading it with much satisfaction. Even the clergy got involved, with the Archbishop of Westminster complaining that it would curtail doctors' liberty. Willink wrote him a rather hurt and lengthy letter insisting he had misunderstood the paper.

Willink was forced into further compromises over the ensuing year, culminating in an updated White Paper, which he finished in June 1945 but never published. John Pater, then a civil servant in the Ministry of Health, describes it in his book *The Making of the National Health Service*:

> Briefly, it can be said that these modifications consisted of a series of concessions intended to mollify medical and voluntary hospital criticisms of the original White Paper. And they might well have done so, as both the negotiating committee and the BMA had unofficially indicated. But the price paid included not only the abandonment of important elements, such as controls on the distribution of doctors, the rapid development of health centres, and the cardinal principle of combining planning and execution in the same local hands, but also the creation of a planning and administrative system of almost unworkable complexity.[36]

It didn't survive the ensuing general election. By the end of July 1945, the Labour Party had won a landslide majority of 145 seats. It was the party's first majority government since its formation. It changed Britain.

Bevan was now going to go from a pain-in-the-backbenches to a key national figure of government. But it wasn't pre-ordained that he would end up at Health. In fact, Clement Attlee had pencilled him in for Education, and 'Red Ellen' Wilkinson at Health and Housing, before changing his mind.

Now, with a stonking majority and a country eager to enjoy the new Britain it had longed for throughout the long years of war and rationing, it was time to set upon Labour's vision for a national health service. The party's 1943 paper provided the basis for that, along with its election manifesto – which promised 'that the best health services should be available free for all' – and, of course, Bevan had his own influences, as detailed above. But foremost in Bevan's mind was his vision for his office. On arrival in the Ministry of Health and Housing, the new Cabinet minister sat down in his desk chair and complained: 'This won't do. It drains all the blood from the head and explains a lot about my predecessors.'[37] He was about to engage in a full-blooded fight, after all – the battle lines having already been drawn by the medical profession in the preceding years.

Once he'd got a chair to his liking, he set to work quickly on what to do about a national health service. By October, he had a memo before Cabinet asking one 'big question of principle' before he set out his general plans.[38] It was a big question about a big change: Bevan wanted to nationalise all the hospitals and combine them into a 'single hospital service' overseen by the Minister of Health and with responsibility delegated to 'new regional and local bodies'. It would also involve 'the centralising of the whole finance of the country's hospital system, taking it right out of local rating and local government'. He put his finger on the problem that had dogged Willink's White Paper, which was that in trying to keep voluntary hospitals happy by leaving them be, he was in effect leaving them to wither on the vine – or else forcing the state to finance them anyway. 'I do not see how we could possibly be justified in doing what the White Paper proposed and leaving the hospitals under the independent management which they have now,' he wrote. 'I believe strongly that we must insist on the principle of public control accompanying the public financing of the hospitals, broadly in proportion to the extent of that financing.' He was also not that impressed by the voluntary system as a whole, making a distinction between the large teaching hospitals and the majority, which were 'mediocre': 'I think the system has outlived its usefulness, and the time has come to leave it behind.' The municipal hospitals fared little better in his judgement: 'Nor has the record of the local authorities in this field been very encouraging. Although they run many more hospital beds than the voluntary hospitals, nearly half of their ordinary hospital accommodation is still run by them in the general surroundings and atmosphere of the old Poor Law system, and their general hospital service as a whole is of questionable efficiency.' What this meant was that 'neither of the present hospital systems is the right one, and we have to look for something new in place of both'.

Bevan acknowledged that he didn't know the position of the doctors on this, but anticipated there would be an 'outcry' from some of them when they found out he wanted to nationalise the voluntaries. But that wasn't the immediate fight on his hands. Into the fray came Herbert Morrison, someone he had long clashed with politically (but paradoxically had supported in a failed leadership bid against Attlee a few months earlier, straight after the party won the election and before it formed a government). Morrison was a local-government man, and disliked this proposal to take all the hospitals away from local authorities. He wrote his own memo, which described Bevan's piece as a 'brilliant and imaginative paper' before warning that it risked 'major damage to the fabric of local government'.

Bevan responded a few days later that Morrison's fears could be 'overcome', and repeated his arguments about the problem of state funding without state control, and the quality of the two existing hospital systems. He rejected Morrison's plan to return to the Joint Hospital Boards that Willink's White Paper had proposed, arguing that the scheme had the 'grave disadvantage of splitting the health service in half' and 'left the voluntary hospitals under independent management'. The pair continued to scrap for a couple more months, but Bevan ultimately won. Morrison never forgave him for that, referring to the NHS as 'Nye's precious health service'.[39]

In December, Bevan presented his general proposals to colleagues. This was his full vision for a national health service.[40]

Most of the health service was going to be free of charge, funded by the Exchequer and through local rates. Everyone would be entitled to a family doctor of their own choice; access to a 'full range of hospital, sanatorium, convalescent and rehabilitation services', along with 'a full range of specialist "second opinions" and care, in the hospitals, in the Health Centres and at . . . home'; nursing at home when needed; dental and eye services; a full maternity service; health visiting; child welfare; vaccination; and supplementary care and after-care in sickness.

It was highly centralised. The health service would be organised across a 'tripartite system' of hospitals, GPs and local authorities. The Minister of Health would have direct responsibility for hospital and specialist services, but would delegate the administration to regional and local bodies. The country was to be divided into 'around 20' regional hospital boards, which would work on the organisation of services in their area, and oversee the day-to-day running of the hospitals. General practitioners would not be nationalised, but would become independent contractors of primary care services – that is, providing the basic care that most people would need and acting as a conduit to the other branches of the system. They would work, when possible, from new health centres in publicly provided premises, but until those were developed they could join the health service from their own surgeries. 'This will be so arranged that everyone can be assured of a family doctor from the outset,' Bevan explained. Finally, local authorities would be responsible for community health, including health visiting, vaccinations and midwifery. Councils would have a duty to provide ambulance services. At the centre, the minister would get further advice from a Central Health Services Council staffed by representatives from the medical profession, local government and lay figures.

In January 1946, Bevan was back before the Cabinet, asking now for their approval for the National Health Service bill. Bevan wrote in a memo to colleagues that he felt the bill itself would have a reasonably easy passage, once the 'emotional stages' about nationalising hospitals had been discussed at second reading. He was referring to the reaction of Conservatives to the state taking control of healthcare, though some Labour colleagues also felt the local authorities would be better placed to administer hospitals than central government would. Where the difficulty would lie would be in the 'detailed arrangements of the new service, which can be left to subsequent regulations and which will involve close negotiations with the professional and other interests'.[41] He was right about the parliamentary stages of the legislation. When the bill came before Parliament, it passed with Labour's huge majority – but the Conservatives did vote against it at every stage. They had been supportive in principle of some kind of national health service. But not this one. That was the argument their spokesman, Richard Law, used when he responded to Bevan in the Chamber during the second reading (which is the debate between MPs about the principles rather than the details of a piece of legislation) arguing that the health minister had missed a 'great opportunity' with the legislation of 'bringing to the House of Commons proposals which would have been warmly welcomed by every party in the House and by every section of opinion, lay or medical, outside. Instead, he has preferred to bring to the House these proposals which are in fact feared and distrusted by the great majority of those who will be called upon to make them effective.' He added that 'I am anxious to make clear our position on these benches in regard to the principle of a national, comprehensive, 100 per cent, health service. Of course we accept that principle today, as we accepted it in 1944, when the Coalition White Paper was published.' His main complaint was the nationalisation of the voluntary hospitals, the decision to cut local government out of their oversight, and the proposals – as he saw them – to 'impose upon the medical profession a form of discipline which, in our view and theirs, is totally unsuited to the practice of medicine'.[42]

All those objections were not unreasonable. But it is also the habit of opposition parties to seize on not unreasonable points to cover what is in fact their dislike of something that is popular. It is much easier to claim 'we would do this better' and stand against it – and don't forget that Churchill had been extremely anxious throughout the Beveridge process about what he was committing his party to. That is the reading of the Labour Party throughout the years since:

that the Tories never really wanted *any* health service, let alone the one the country ended up with. It is also why the Conservatives have never really managed to cut loose the NHS albatross from around their neck: not only did they vote against this NHS, they were also never really sure about how to do it themselves had they got the opportunity. What they ended up with was what Lord Woolton had feared: a service that was far more repugnant to Conservative feeling than the one Churchill had panicked over.

It was also a departure from the war years of the parties working together for the good of the country. Obviously the 1945 election had changed that, not least because Churchill was so shocked that the country wasn't thanking him for his war-hero leadership. But perhaps Bevan himself was also a factor in Conservative opposition to his legislation. After all, *he* had never worked with the other parties during the war, even when the national spirit expected it. He had been a thorn in their flesh throughout the conflict. Now it was their turn to behave in exactly the same way.

In this same second reading debate, Bevan used the phrase, often repeated, that 'we should universalise the best', suggesting that he too felt there were aspects of British healthcare that were already working extremely well – and that this was not going to be a bog-standard system to fall back on, but one everyone would want to be a part of. But it also reminds us that the National Health Service was created as a solution to a problem of access, not of quality. British healthcare was – for those who could get it – very good already.

Either way, Parliament wasn't where the action was. The legislation passed all its parliamentary stages and became an Act of Parliament in November 1946. Outside Westminster, Bevan had been busily courting the institutions of the medical world to try to win their favour. He made it his mission to strike up friendships with the presidents of the Royal Colleges of surgeons, physicians and obstetricians. It was the support of these organisations of doctors that was to prove vital in getting the NHS off the ground and running – another contradiction of the lazy claim that the doctors opposed the NHS. Bevan had already given major concessions to the remuneration and freedoms of consultants as a result of his discussions. They would be able to continue in private practice in 'pay beds' that were situated in NHS hospitals for ease of access. They could also receive 'merit awards' of cash on top of their basic earnings if they were deemed sufficiently impressive by colleagues. It was these concessions that sparked one of the most famous remarks by Bevan about the health service: 'I stuffed their mouths with gold,' he said a decade after the formation of the NHS. He had accepted that this was the only way to ensure the hospital consultants signed up to the NHS at all – as, without them, the service wouldn't work. But the stuffing with gold was a relatively easy exercise in comparison to the fight over GPs. The BMA was a different matter. It had to wait for the March 1946 publication of the White Paper to get going. And when it did, it had two main objections.

The first was about the independence of doctors – the civil servant problem that Charles Hill had warned about back in 1943. The Labour Party paper of that year had argued for a full-salaried service, and members of the Socialist Medical Association were still pushing for it now. Given that Bevan was planning to nationalise the hospitals, the threat of some kind of state control of doctors in which they would be forced to become full-time salaried government workers was not one entirely concocted by the BMA to frighten its membership. The second objection was about money, which had the effect of frightening the most over-represented part of the union's membership – the GPs. Bevan's plan was that they would be paid a basic salary and receive capitation fees – something the BMA had itself proposed only a few years before. There would also be limits on GPs entering areas where there were already too many doctors, which in the health minister's view was crucial to ensuring the service was truly nationwide, rather than concentrated in towns and cities and leafy areas, where GPs liked to live.

The initial response of the BMA to the White Paper was that it was 'willing and anxious to co-operate with the Government in evolving this service' and that 'for a quarter of a century the medical profession has stressed the need for a complete health service'. But it was 'opposed to any form of service which leads directly or indirectly to the profession as a whole becoming full-time salaried servants of the State or local authorities'. Part of the freedom the association demanded was that 'doctors should, like other workers, be free to choose the form, place, and type of work they prefer without governmental or other direction'.[43] The journal's leading article reflected elsewhere that 'no one can regard with equanimity the proposal that these places of learning should become State hospitals owned by the Minister of Health'.[44] This was all set out in restrained, official-sounding language. The reactions of the BMA doctors at large were rather different.

Alfred Cox, a former secretary of the BMA, wrote to *The Times* complaining in extraordinary language about the bill. That newspaper rejected his letter, so he sent it to the *British Medical Journal* instead. It isn't hard to see why *The Times* might have had some qualms about the content of this missive. Cox wrote: 'I have examined the Bill and it looks to me uncommonly like the first step, and a big one, towards National Socialism as practised in Germany. The medical service there was early put under the dictatorship of a "Medical Fuhrer". This Bill will establish the Minister of Health in that capacity.' The signs for this were that the minister was responsible for all hospital, medical and nursing services; that he could control all appointments to the regional hospital boards that were to administer the service locally; and that he could stop any new GPs setting up in oversubscribed areas.

'If I am right in my belief that the provisions of this Bill indicate that the medical profession is in future to be under what amounts to a dictatorship, what is to prevent other professions and trades being similarly dealt with?' Cox asked. 'I call it a dictatorship because the reading of the Bill convinces me that the Minister, unless this Bill is radically altered, can, in future, do anything he likes with the doctors (and through them with their patients) except leave them alone. Did the electorate really think that this is what we fought for?'[45]

It was extraordinary language given the evils the country had just emerged from fighting – and which were still being detailed in the press – though perhaps Churchill's line during the election campaign the previous year that the Labour Party was 'some form of a Gestapo' had made such language seem more acceptable. Cox's letter sparked a round of correspondence in which other doctors debated just what sort of Hitler the Minister of Health might be. Douglas Robertson argued that 'the minister will become, in fact, a complete dictator, little different from Hitler in National-Socialist Germany. Actually the Minister is, by inference, so mentioned no fewer than 53 times in the short White Paper summary.'[46] G. H. Urquhart wrote: 'Little more than a year ago we fought for our very existence against a country which had yielded up its freedom to political power-seekers. With this terrible example before our eyes are we, like they, going to walk into this cunningly devised trap of "National Socialism", a gilded cage of bondage from which there can be no return to freedom? Belsens and Buchenwalds are the logical outcome of dictator-made laws when resistance or protests run counter to the whims or fancies of "dictator-ministers".' Kenneth Macleod, meanwhile, accused Edith Summerskill of 'not a little trace of the doctrines of Nazism', adding: 'Perhaps she does not see the dangerous road along which her socialistic beliefs are driving her'. He was upset that 'we are in a trap from which there is no escape'.[47]

In the 1990s, Mike Godwin came up with a rule that the longer an online discussion, the more likely someone will end up comparing something about the subject to the Nazis or Hitler. It is perhaps comforting to learn that the originators of what is now known as Godwin's law were in fact respectably dressed doctors writing in the country's leading medical journal in the 1940s, not unkempt dropouts tapping away at a computer keyboard in their mother's basement.

The BMA, with Hill leading the charge, continued to press for the legislation to be amended to prevent doctors from being forced into a salaried service. The association was also deeply worried about the ownership of GP practices, and the right of doctors to appeal to a court if they were struck off from practising. Bevan's initial approach when the negotiations started was to be aggressive, attacking the BMA for its case document, which criticised his legislation as being 'in places so obscure that to bring it into force as it stands will create chaotic conditions'. He questioned the state of mind of the committee – and asked whether it was even a proper negotiating committee. On the second day of the negotiations, though, Thomas-Symonds describes his tone as having 'altered', now full of 'reassurance and conciliation'. It didn't make much difference: the BMA dug in. It held repeated polls of its members, including a crucial one in January 1948 on which the support of the BMA for joining the NHS or not hinged. A vast majority – 86 per cent – were against joining. Hill had once again been prominent in all this, even appearing on a newsreel in January in which he warned the public that 'the doctor should be your servant, not the State's servant. You should choose him, or change him'. He claimed that the 'real issue is not whether you want a better health service (everyone wants that) but whether you want your doctor to be your doctor or the state's doctor'. Of course, the Act wasn't making the doctor into a salaried officer of the state, as Hill claimed. But the insinuation worked a treat on BMA members.

Bevan was, by now, livid. He complained bitterly to Cabinet colleagues in January about the attitude of the BMA, describing their actions as an 'attempt not merely to seek detailed improvements of the Act but completely to sabotage it and prevent its ever coming into operation'. He was particularly angry with Hill, who he reminded colleagues was 'the accepted Conservative candidate for Luton, and it would be a feather in his cap to try to enter Parliament as the Conservative who stopped a major social measure to this Government'.[48]

That Bevan was seriously fed up with the BMA was again clear in the statement he gave to the Commons on 6 February 1948. He was also cross with the Conservative Party and supporting newspapers for their 'grave misrepresentation of the nature of the Health Service and of the conditions under which the medical profession are asked to enter the Health Service'. But far worse was the 'campaign of personal abuse, from a small body of spokesmen who have consistently misled the great profession to which they are supposed to belong'. He drove his criticism home: 'I make a distinction . . . between the hardworking doctors who have little or no time to give to these matters, and the small body of raucous voiced people who are alleged to represent the profession as a whole.' He found it 'frightening' to talk to doctors and discover the extent to which the BMA had misled them. 'From the very beginning, this small body of politically poisoned people have decided to fight the Health Act itself and to stir up as much emotion as they can in the profession.' He listed the Ministers of Health with whom the BMA had clashed: all of them, from all parties. 'I am very conscious of my limitations. But it can hardly be suggested that conflict between the British Medical Association and the Minister of the day is a consequence of any deficiencies that I possess, because we have never been able yet to appoint a Minister of Health with whom the BMA agreed.' Writing seventy-five years on, there is still some difficulty in finding this agreeable Minister of Health from the considerably longer list today.

Was the National Health Service even going to happen? Both sides were refusing to back down. In the end, it was those Royal Colleges whom Bevan had studiously courted in the early days that saved the day. Lord Moran, the president of the Royal College of Physicians, suggested an amendment to the Act, which would make clear in statute that a full-time salaried service could only be introduced by a further Act of Parliament. Bevan made conciliatory noises as he conceded this in the Commons, saying: 'It seems clear that more than my spoken assurance is needed, and I am certainly quite willing to do anything to banish this apprehension for good.' He added: 'I trust that what I have said will finally free doctors from any fears that they are to be turned in some way into salaried civil servants. I look forward now to a future of active and friendly cooperation with the profession in putting into operation next July a great social measure, which can be made a turning point in the social history of this country and an example to the world.'

He was speaking in April 1948. Just three months later, Aneira Thomas was born – and with her, the National Health Service.

2. Bills, bills, bills

The first day of the National Health Service was a strange mix of the familiar and the altogether new. Aneira Thomas was not born into a new hospital with new staff. It was the system underpinning everything that had changed: the modern high-quality health service that Bevan wanted to create didn't appear overnight. And 5 July 1948, known as the Appointed Day, was in many ways not momentous: there weren't NHS street parties or people clapping by their front doors at the advent of this new service. Local papers – at this time commanding huge and faithful readerships – warned that the scheme might not be ready. The *Hull Daily Mail* complained that 'there is more than a danger that lack of adequate preparation will produce something approaching chaos for a considerable time, and rosy optimism should be tempered with a realisation that acute disappointment may be in store for large sections of the public; medical services, already heavily taxed, will undoubtedly suffer further strain'.[1] The Ministry of Health suggested that people could help out by not rushing the new service.[2] In the end, the chaos did not ensue immediately: because this was a British health service, there wasn't a crush of would-be patients hammering on the doors of their doctors' practices, but polite, orderly and quite short queues of people waiting for treatment.

Bevan received a report of how the first day had gone via the teleprinter networks set up to communicate bombings and other wartime emergencies. 'It was satisfactory; no major hitches; no big strain on the new organisation, though a few doctors were rushed,' reported the *Daily Herald* a couple of days later.[3]

On 5 July, the minister himself visited Park Hospital in Trafford, and was greeted with a guard of honour, with nurses lining the driveway. He handed over the 'keys to the NHS' at the hospital – formerly a voluntary which had, like many others, been struggling for funds for years. He met there another first: the first 'nationalised' NHS patient. Sylvia Beckingham, thirteen, had been in Park Hospital for three weeks with a liver condition, and found herself surrounded not just by nurses but also by the Minister of Health, photographers and reporters. She told the waiting press: 'Mr Bevan asked me if I understood the significance of the occasion and told me that it was a milestone in history – the most civilised step any country had ever taken. I had earwigged at adults' conversations and I knew this was a great change that was coming about and that most people could hardly believe this was happening.'[4]

The build-up to the Appointed Day had been a big one. Every household had been sent a booklet explaining what the National Health Service would mean for them. It opened:

> Your new National Health Service begins on 5th July. What is it? How do you get it?
>
> It will provide you with all medical, dental, and nursing care. Everyone – rich or poor, man, woman, or child – can use it or any part of it. There are no charges, except for a few special items. There are no insurance qualifications. But it is not a 'charity'. You are all paying for it, mainly as taxpayers, and it will relieve your money worries in time of illness.

There is so much in that opening page that sets the tone for the way the British public have related to their health service ever since. Firstly, the idea that it was 'your' health service: nowadays, *our* NHS. The language was not about state control, but about something people would feel belonged to them. And, most powerfully, it would stop people worrying about the cost of being ill. Many of us today have been through times where money is so tight that it feels as though it is throttling you with fear, where it's not clear if the cash machine will give out the £10 you've asked for, or there's a possibility your rent cheque will bounce. That fear was even more visceral in 1940s Britain, as we saw from Edna's story: she and her family would dread illness and even pregnancy as something they simply could not afford. Bevan himself captured this perfectly in his 1952 book *In Place of Fear*. That giddy rush of relief for people who could now go to the doctor about that cough, that pain, that rash, must have been intoxicating at the time. It still bubbles up in people today, who often thank the NHS for giving them all the treatment they've needed in hospital 'for free'. Curmudgeons will point out that in fact they have already paid. Curmudgeons, as so often, miss the emotional reaction that people have to matters of their health.

The leaflet went on to instruct people to 'choose your doctor now', reassuring those who might have been a little upset by Hill's broadcasts about the state getting involved in the doctor–patient relationship that 'your dealings with your doctor will remain as they are now: personal and confidential'. The difference, it added, was that 'the doctor will be paid by the Government, out of funds provided by everybody'. It then ran through the other services – medicines, drugs, appliances, dentistry and eye care, hearing, home health services and so on – that all patients were now entitled to, largely for free.

Another emotional description of the forthcoming health service came from Edith Summerskill. She was now serving as Parliamentary Secretary to the Ministry of Food, but recorded a party political broadcast on the BBC in which she told the story relayed in the previous chapter about her socialist awakening as a doctor, before explaining how the new health service would work. Attlee himself did a broadcast on the eve of the Appointed Day, predicting that some patience would be needed: 'There are bound to be early difficulties with staff, accommodation, and so on. In a great plan like this there must be some rough edges, but these will be overcome with patience and goodwill. Owing to the war there are great arrears to be made up in the provision of hospitals and in the reinforcement of medical and nursing staffs. We shall have to be a bit lenient with the service at first.'[5] There had been more than a few grumbles about sticking to 5 July as the Appointed Day, not least because Bevan had still been trying to get the doctors' agreement just weeks before the whole thing was due to get going.

Bevan also sent a charming message to the medical profession ahead of the launch, representing an attempt to draw a line under things:

On 5 July we start, together, the new National Health Service. It has not had an altogether trouble-free gestation! There have been understandable anxieties, inevitable in so great and novel an undertaking. Nor will there be overnight any miraculous removal of our more serious shortages of nurses and others and of modern replanned buildings and equipment. But the sooner we start, the sooner we can try together to see to these things and to secure the improvements we all want . . . My job is to give you all the facilities, resources and help I can, and then to leave you alone as professional men and women to use your skill and judgement without hindrance. Let us try to develop that partnership from now on.[6]

He had been rather less charming about one of his other opponents – the Conservatives – the night before the Appointed Day, when Labour held a party rally to celebrate the anniversary of the party winning power and also the founding of the NHS the following day. Bevan spoke. Recalling a period of three years in which he had been unemployed and had to rely on the earnings of his sister, he said: 'No amount of cajolery, and no attempts at ethical or social seduction, can eradicate from my heart a deep burning hatred for the Tory Party that inflicted those bitter experiences on me. So far as I am concerned, they are lower than vermin. They condemned millions of people to semi-starvation . . . I warn you young men and women, do not listen to what they are saying now. Do not listen to the seductions of Lord Woolton . . . They have not changed, or if they have they are slightly worse than they were.'[7]

Bevan did actually have friends who were Conservative MPs, and enjoyed being part of a social and debating circle organised by the wealthy Beaverbook family. In private, he enjoyed the finer things in life, to the extent that he had been accused by friends of being a champagne socialist (he did reportedly retort that the quality of the drink he was swilling made him no better than a 'Bollinger Bolshevik', but you get the point).[8] Someone daubed 'Vermin Villa, Home of a loud-mouthed rat' across the white stucco façade of Bevan's home in the hours after reports of the vermin comment emerged.[9] Some Tories saw this as a badge of honour, and jokingly formed a

'Vermin Club'. Others felt it soured both the launch of the health service and the political discourse more widely: the deputy matron at Park Hospital admitted she had to 'Shanghai a few people to go down the drive: it was because of that unfortunate speech he'd made the weekend before about anybody who voted Tory was vermin, and it did rise a few hackles, you know'.[10] Churchill's retort hardly raised the level of debate, with the former prime minister saying, 'I can think of no better step to signalise the inauguration of the National Health Service than that a person who so obviously needs psychiatrical attention should be among the first of its patients.'[11]

What the 'vermin' remark did tap into was something the Labour Party has exploited right up to the present day: that you can't trust the Tories with the NHS. Even though the Conservatives had been making their own preparations for some kind of free-at-the-point-of-use health service, they had opposed *this* health service, and their votes were on the parliamentary record. It has meant that for the rest of the lifetime of the NHS, however long or short, the Conservative Party will never have the full political permission to do as it pleases with the health service in the way that it would like. Alan Milburn, one of the party's health secretaries in the New Labour era, reflects that 'when it comes to NHS reform, the right has the volition, but it doesn't have the permission. The left has the permission, but then it lacks the volition.'[12]

Labour's satisfaction was justified, but has not always been healthy, either. The left has at times retreated to an ideal of the NHS that has never existed: Bevan set it up with concessions to consultants and GPs that allowed the former to treat private patients in 'pay beds' in NHS hospitals, and the latter to remain independent contractors. He did not achieve the model that the Socialist Medical Association had campaigned for of a full-salaried state-run medical service with the banning of private practice.

The SMA likes to insert itself into the development of the NHS along with *The Citadel* and Tredegar, and it deserves a place in that tradition. Some of its members went further than that: Edith Summerskill seriously upset Bevan's wife during the 1951 general election campaign when she claimed that it was the Socialist Medical

Association that was responsible for the National Health Service. Bevan, she told an audience in Brixton, was only the 'midwife' appointed by Attlee to bring it to being, but 'some of us, who, as founder members of the Socialist Medical Association, were responsible for planning the National Health Service twenty years ago, strongly resent any individual or group asserting for their own private political purposes that they are sole defenders of the National Health Service'.[13] In truth, people like Summerskill making the case for a state medical service – and fleshing it out in policy documents – was an important part of a push that had been going on for much longer towards a health service. Given Bevan also retained some parts of the Willink White Paper, though, that Conservative might also lay claim to being one of the people responsible for the creation of the NHS.

Not everyone was part of the rush to claim that they had been one of the key ingredients in the health service, though. For some, 5 July 1948 represented the start of a dark era for healthcare, which has only got worse as the adulation of the NHS has grown. The arguments from such writers and politicians – generally on the right of politics – tend to run along the lines that people have been so emotionally caught up in the ideal of a free NHS that they do not notice it is not in fact the envy of the world, that it has very poor outcomes on many measures, that there are other state-enabled systems around the world which produce better results and cost less, and that its hospitals are often poor quality and dirty. The reader today will be very familiar with the opinion piece that runs thus: 'The British are so religious about the NHS that they can't accept its faults.' But the arguments of the 'NHS as a religion' crowd fail to acknowledge that the survival of the health service has never been guaranteed, even if the affection of the British people has been. In the first decade, it wasn't clear how long it would last – Bevan himself had appealed to the medical profession to give it a go and see how it went as part of his negotiations, and described it as the 'biggest single experiment in social service that the world has ever seen'. Throughout its existence, broadcasters and writers have asked how much time the NHS has got left, and whether its day has been and gone. Indeed, the history of the NHS has been one of existential crisis, catching breath, and then another potentially terminal threat. Such is the fear that things could topple over and the consent for the service be lost at any moment, that the reaction to criticism from within the service can hurt its ability to address even valid points for improvement.

But alongside this fear of an existential crisis, which is always part of our relationship to the NHS – rather like Tinkerbell needing to be told children believe in fairies – is a memory, whether personal or folk, of the difference that the health service made in those early days. In place of fear came treatment. And this is what it looked like.

By the Appointed Day, more than 21,300 doctors had applied to take part in the new health service, and nearly 36 million patients had joined these doctors' lists – of which nearly 15 million were new patients. These were patients who had either had to pay upfront for any healthcare they received, or had received very little attention from the medical world at all. Chief among the second group were women. Largely uninsured, women had become accustomed to a long decline in their later years. One GP remarked: 'Although the men have been insured, the women and children have never been able to get medical treatment before. The women just got slower and duller and falling asleep in the evening, and it was just expected as their personality, and, you know, you could suddenly change that.'[14] A newly qualified doctor later recalled: 'There was abuse – because suddenly it was all free. But the other side was the colossal amount of very real unmet need that just poured in needing treatment. There were women with prolapsed uteruses literally wobbling down between their legs that had been held in place with cup and stem pessaries – like a big penis with a cup on it. It was the same with hernias. You would have men walking round with trusses holding these colossal hernias in. And they were all like that because they couldn't afford to have it done. They couldn't afford to consult a doctor, let alone have an operation.'[15]

Dr Elinor Corfan had been a doctor for just four years when the NHS began. She described what life had been like for many before: 'Like their mothers, it was also the children of the poor who suffered most. In the 1930s and 1940s, when, except for smallpox, there was no immunisation, infectious diseases were widespread and were the scourge of childhood.' She also said she had been 'much too busy to notice the famous appointed day' but that she could see the difference within two years: 'Coming into general practice in 1950 was a heartening experience. I could see how the new regime was working and patients were touchingly grateful. Long gone was the feeling of hopelessness, of being impotent. We could prescribe freely. If I was worried about patients, I could make as many home visits as necessary without having to consider whether they could afford it.' Elinor also saw the 'certainty of a profitable market in the NHS' for pharmaceutical companies as one of the causes of great leaps in treatment over the ensuing years. 'In the 1950s, I visited an elderly man with advanced Parkinson's who had been bed-ridden for years, nursed by a devoted wife. I prescribed the new costly drugs, which slowly became effective. It caused quite a sensation in the neighbourhood when he first walked out of his door. I felt exhilarated by this freedom to fulfil my obligations as a doctor.'[16]

There was also, though, confusion about what the new service meant, and quite how much would be free. Doctors in Liverpool reported that their surgeries were crammed with patients asking how the scheme worked rather than seeking treatment, while chemists in the city had to refuse requests for free brilliantine and toothpaste.[17] All this unmet need – and all these free teeth and spectacles – meant that, come the first anniversary of the service, there was a problem. And not a small one, either. It was a big, costly problem. In its first year alone, the health service had given out 27,000 hearing aids, 4.5 million pairs of glasses, and 164,000 surgical and medical appliances. At a news conference in October 1949, Bevan tried to justify the costs of these and the service more widely, saying: 'One of the chief sources of our troubles here in Britain – and not only here in Britain but in other parts of the world – is the increasing demand made upon hospital facilities by the aged sick, one of the great problems of modern civilisation.' He tried to reassure the public that he recognised it would 'take some years for the scheme to bed itself in' and that 'more facilities will be needed before criticism will die down'. But he added:

Have you realised, if I may, that most of the shortcomings which had been revealed by the British health service are not the result of the intrinsic defects of the service itself, but because of the overwhelming volume of need that the service itself has revealed. This will happen, I venture to say, in other nations when they start the same kind of service, that there has gone on in the past a vast amount of silent suffering, a vast amount of remediable pain, and what a national health service does is to first of all make it articulate, and to the extent that it makes it articulate, men are driven to address it, and I believe in Great Britain, we have made a great start.[18]

It was a great start on an emotional level, but economically it was proving to be too costly. Bevan found himself doing what all health ministers have done ever since he set up the service: he kept having to go cap in hand to the Treasury to ask for more cash to keep the thing going.

These regular requests for money – in March 1950 he was demanding an extra £100 million – made Bevan unpopular with Cabinet colleagues and Treasury ministers. The former weren't getting anything like the same spending boosts for their departments at a time of huge need across the country – for better housing, transport and so on. The first nine months of the NHS cost £208 million – noticeably more than the estimated £132 million. Then, in 1949–50, it was £358 million. It was too much. Morrison, still peeved about the way Bevan had won his battle on local authorities and hospitals, was now even more annoyed with the way his colleague seemed to think he was entitled to be extravagant with public money. But he wasn't the only one. 'Nye is getting away with murder was the general feeling of my colleagues,' Morrison reflected in his autobiography. 'It was not so much a selfish attitude to the problems of his fellow ministers as Bevan's unquestioning regard for dogma. The original plan was that the medical services should provide everybody with everything needed for nothing and nothing must alter that.'[19]

Within a year, Bevan was having to introduce the amendments to the National Health Service Act which would safeguard the freedom of doctors to treat private patients. He'd promised this to get the service over the line, but within that piece of legislation was a bigger change: prescriptions would no longer be free; they would be capped at one shilling per prescription issued. Both Bevan and Attlee had been alarmed by reports of patients demanding more than they really needed – and of doctors being only too happy to oblige, with the former saying, 'I shudder to think of the ceaseless cascade of medicine which is pouring down British throats at the present time,' and the latter announcing 'there has been some excessive and unnecessary resort to doctors for prescriptions'.

But Bevan still found himself under pressure from Chancellor Stafford Cripps to cut spending, agreeing in 1950 to a Cabinet committee which would monitor the money on a monthly basis. He was resentful of this, but was quickly diverted by a new battle with Cripps's junior, Hugh Gaitskell. The pair ended up snipping away at one another over dinners organised by the Chancellor for ministers with high-spending portfolios, with Gaitskell developing what Harold Wilson later told Bevan's biographer Michael Foot was 'a mission or an obsession' with NHS charges.[20] Bevan, for his part, seemed to feel Gaitskell was 'cold and lacking empathy',[21] and so the difference between the pair was not just political but also personal.

In 1951, with Labour now on a tiny majority of just five in Parliament, following an election where Bevan was repeatedly jeered for his 'vermin' comments, he moved to become Minister of Labour – but only on the agreement with Attlee that 'no health charges would be imposed'. That was what his wife Jennie Lee thought had been discussed between the two men, at least, but it quickly proved that either Bevan had misunderstood their conversation, or that Attlee was prepared to double-cross his difficult minister.

On 9 April, the Cabinet met as usual in the morning. It was going to be a long day. Morrison was in the chair as Attlee was unwell. Gaitskell, now Chancellor, was ready with his plan for the Treasury to get the rampagingly expensive National Health Service under control. He argued that to keep spending within the £400-million limit already agreed by ministers, he would be introducing charges for dentures and spectacles to raise £13 million in the coming year and even more in the long term. Bevan quickly interjected, even though Health was no longer his brief. He had 'always been opposed to the introduction of charges for dentures and spectacles', he argued,

because it would be 'undesirable in principle, and politically dangerous, for the Labour Party thus to abandon the conception of a free
Health Service'. More than that, it wasn't even financially necessary,
not least because £13 million was 'so small a sum' – and he was 'disturbed' by Gaitskell's plan to allocate the saved money to Defence.
'Such charges', he reminded his colleagues, 'could not be imposed
without fresh legislation', and he therefore threatened to resign
because he could not vote for such a bill.[22]

The Cabinet minutes from this meeting say delicately that 'a long
discussion ensued' – civil service code for a flaming big row. Bevan,
backed by Harold Wilson, argued that it was going to be difficult to
persuade Labour backbenchers to vote for a departure from a free
health service. Their opponents mocked this argument, pointing out
that 'the principle of a free Health Service had already been breached
by the National Health Service (Amendment) Act 1949, which
authorised the imposition of a shilling charge for prescriptions'.[23]
They pointed out that Bevan was the very minister who had introduced that, and he hadn't encountered much opposition in the
Commons – though the charges had then been paused. Others
expressed concern about the political effect of Bevan resigning,
warning that it could lead to the government falling.

Back and forth the argument went, with Bevan suggesting increasing National Insurance contributions or cutting the surplus that
Gaitskell's Budget had planned for in order to keep away from
charges, and the Chancellor retorting that this would be inflationary
and the money could be better spent.

Morrison could see that a huge and potentially dangerous split had
opened up in Cabinet, and suggested they meet again that evening.
In the meantime, he would visit Attlee in hospital – where he was
being treated for a duodenal ulcer – and get his view.

They all came trundling back to meet that evening at 6.30, this time
in the prime minister's Commons offices. Morrison and the chief
whip had been to see Attlee in hospital and had a read-out of their
conversation, which amounted to a public dressing-down for Bevan.
'First, he had pointed out that in all Cabinet discussions of Budget
proposals there must be a substantial measure of give and take between

Ministers. The Chancellor of the Exchequer had particular responsibility for the national finances; and no other Minister ought to claim that any particular estimate should be treated as sacrosanct. It would be a most unusual thing for a Minister to resign on a Budget issue: so far as he was aware, the only Minister who had ever taken this step was Lord Randolph Churchill, whose political fortunes had never recovered thereafter.'[24] In other words, Bevan should stay in his lane.

In fact, Attlee had added more warnings: that resigning would damage the Labour Party now and in the future, that it would provoke a political crisis when 'there could hardly be a worse moment for a General Election', and that if there were to be an election, the government would lose it. 'If the situation arose, the responsibility for bringing it about would rest with any Ministers who resigned from the Government at the present juncture.' And so Attlee was instructing Cabinet colleagues to support Gaitskell.

Bevan's response was angry and bitter. He was not surprised to hear that the prime minister took this view, but Attlee did know that he, Bevan, could not abide by the collective responsibility required for a decision 'to abandon the conception of a free Health Service'. Underlining Morrison's earlier complaint about this being 'Nye's precious health service', he continued that 'he had given five years to building up the Health Service; he had proclaimed it on many public platforms as one of the outstanding achievements of the Labour Party in office: he had, in particular, upheld the conception of a free Service as the embodiment of Socialist principles'.[25] He could not vote for the charges. He added that he had recently realised he could bring more influence to bear on government policy from outside the Cabinet anyway, and so it was time for him to go.

Now it was Wilson's turn. He stuck to his position of supporting Bevan, warning that he too would resign. George Tomlinson, the Minister of Education, also indicated that he would quit. Another long discussion ensued, in which ministers panicked about the split in the party and the likely general election that would follow. Bevan refused to accept responsibility for such consequences. He sourly pointed out that he wasn't the one who had created this split by proposing charges. Gaitskell refused to agree to any mitigations suggested by colleagues such as delaying the charges until Attlee was better. Eventually, it became clear that there was no compromise. The Cabinet split, with Bevan making clear that he would be resigning the next day and making a personal statement in the Commons shortly after. Colleagues continued to beg him not to resign as the meeting closed.

In the event, it took him a little longer to quit: on 14 April, Ernest Bevin died of a heart attack while still a Cabinet minister, sending the party into a period of mourning. Attlee wrote to Bevan pleading with him to try to 'forget' his differences with colleagues and stay in the Cabinet. On 21 April, Bevan sent Attlee a resignation letter. On 24 April, he quit the government, along with Wilson and the Minister of Supply, John Freeman. In his resignation speech, Bevan annoyed even the left of his party by talking about 'my health service'. Later that year, Labour lost the general election that ensued, and Winston Churchill was back in power.

Churchill had opposed the National Health Service when it was going through the Commons. But by the time he returned to the premiership, he could see that the service wasn't going anywhere. Perhaps as a result of it no longer being a big battleground, the Ministry of Health under the Conservatives became a political backwater for the next few years, with multiple personnel changes and little interest in it. This was in part because there wasn't a big beast like Bevan at the helm any more. It was also because there wasn't much to fight over in public. Now, the Minister of Health was having to answer questions about bedpans being dropped in hospitals he only a decade ago had little to do with.

Iain Macleod was one of those ministers. He was a 'One Nation' Tory, the son of a Yorkshire GP, and a welfare state convert. He had campaigned for social security for all, along the lines of the Beveridge Report, when he stood in the Western Isles in 1945. Unsurprisingly he failed to win that seat, but was eventually elected for Enfield West in 1950. He wrote pamphlets with his colleague Enoch Powell on social services, and with other colleagues on what One Nation Toryism meant. His commitment to the welfare state, though, did not make him a Bevan fan; in fact, when he spoke as a backbencher in a debate about National Health Service charges in March 1952, he made it very clear that he felt quite the opposite about the man who'd set up the service.

Bevan spent much of the debate chuntering away at the Tories for, in his view, trying to destroy the NHS. He also warned the Conservatives that they would be 'decisively defeated' if they had an election that week 'because the people were beginning to take a decent sense of pride in the fact that every person in this country had access to the best that medical knowledge could provide without let or hindrance of cash. That was something of which everybody, including the Conservatives, were beginning to be proud. Now the Conservatives are proceeding to pull it down. Where it will stop, I do not know.'

It is not hard to see in these words the beginnings of the anxiety on the left that the NHS is just a stop away from being pulled apart altogether by the Conservatives. That anxiety has taken many forms over the years, including over introducing charges or cutting resources for the service – or in more recent years the spectre of privatisation. It started only a few years after the service had begun, so it is reasonable to assume that feeling will always be with us. Macleod didn't have much truck with it, though. He spoke directly after Bevan, and told the House he had just listened to a 'vulgar, crude and intemperate speech', adding later that 'to have a debate on the National Health Service without [Bevan] would be like putting on Hamlet with no one in the part of the First Gravedigger'.[26] He reminded Bevan of the origins of charges in the health service (Bevan's own 1949 Act), and quoted back the former minister's own words about profligate prescribing by doctors. Sitting in the debate was Churchill, who was so impressed by this backbencher whose name he didn't know that he summoned him to Downing Street and appointed him Minister of Health a couple of months later, in May 1952. By now charges were a part of the NHS landscape – and both Labour and Tory fingerprints could be found on them.

In a sense, Bevan's final battle over the NHS (and one of his final political battles too, as he died of stomach cancer aged just sixty-two in July 1960) helped the Conservatives as well as the health service. Alan Milburn's line about the left having the permission to change the NHS that the right lack applied to the charges: if the Tories had been the party to introduce charges, it would have provoked a much bigger political backlash. As it was, they had been a major feature of the 1951 election – but Labour was divided on it. Edith Summerskill's 'midwife' comment about Bevan came as she defended the charges during the campaign, pointing out that he had no problem with the 1949 Act that ended the free-for-all anyway. She didn't have a problem with charging for teeth and spectacles, she insisted, and ignored the heckles of her party colleagues to demand that they 'forget it. Close your ranks. Remember the real enemies are the Tories.'[27] Labour is always a party that has needed reminding of that last point. Anyway, the charges were there, and it was Labour's fault. But what was also still there, and from now on impossible to remove, was the National Health Service. So Churchill and his ministers needed to get on with it.

The former Conservative Cabinet minister Michael Portillo offered an interesting analysis from the right of why the NHS is such an emotive part of British politics:

> The 1945–51 Labour government, despite all its reforms, was a disappointment to the Labour Party itself. The government lost momentum and compromised more than its zealots would have wished. Following the split in the party Labour mythology built up the NHS as the outstanding socialist achievement. The effects of that mythology have been with us ever since. The principle of a free health service has not since been breached any more deeply than it was by the cabinet that founded the NHS. Charges to patients today make up less than 3.5 per cent of NHS revenue. By his political martyrdom, Bevan made the NHS sacred in the form he had created it.[28]

Macleod was one of the figures who articulated from the Conservative side that the NHS was now sacred. In 1958, the year the health service turned ten, he wrote: 'The National Health Service, with the exception of recurring spasms about charges, is out of party politics.'[29] Rudolf Klein describes quite how fervent the sentiment about the health service was at this time: 'as an institution, the NHS ranked next to the monarchy as an unchallenged landmark in the political landscape of Britain. Public opinion polls consistently showed a high degree of enthusiasm for the NHS, with 90 per cent or more of the respondents declaring themselves to be satisfied with the service. More surprisingly, perhaps, two-thirds of the medical profession declared that – given a chance to go back ten years and to decide whether or not the NHS should be started – they would support the creation of the service.'[30] Already, there wasn't room for questioning its principles or indeed its overarching design.

It was getting harder to question the expenditure, too. In 1956, an influential inquiry into the cost of the health service reported back after four years of work. Chaired by Cambridge economist C. W. Guillebaud (Macleod's former tutor), the inquiry surprised many, particularly in the Treasury, when it found that the cost of the NHS was in fact falling as a share of gross national product. NHS historian Charles Webster describes this as 'a shock and a disappointment to the government, which was expecting to use the Guillebaud Report as an instrument for imposing a regime of even tighter retrenchment'. It became, in Webster's words, 'a classic defence of welfare-state expenditure',[31] frightening off successive governments from setting up similarly independent inquiries into the NHS ever since. The Guillebaud Inquiry is viewed in many health circles as having saved the NHS, not just at the point it reported but for many years hence. It did make things difficult for the Treasury – but it did not change the impression, forged in that institution within a year of the NHS beginning, that this public service was a new black hole down which ministers would pour money with precious little reward.

One of the reasons doctors were so surprisingly happy with the health service was that it now gave them certainty about their income, a steady supply of patients, and the freedom to start to innovate. This was also an era in which pharmaceutical companies found a large state-organised health service very handy as a market for their new drugs. The history of innovation in the NHS is a mixed one, as we shall see, but the first few decades brought many big advances in treatment.

The 1960s saw a complete change in the lives of people with kidney failure. Dr John Hopewell started working as a consultant surgeon at the Royal Free Hospital in 1957, when there was pretty much no treatment at all for patients suffering from end-stage renal failure. He later recalled: 'As a medical student I had seen patients with acute renal failure from crush injury resulting from the air raids on London, for whom little could be done except to call in the consultant from Hammersmith Hospital to advise on fluid and electrolyte balance.'[32] But within a decade, there was a unit in every region providing treatment – and a dramatic shift in the way it was administered.

An 'artificial kidney' had already been built by the Dutch inventor Willem Johan Kolff, which cleaned the blood of patients whose kidneys couldn't do it for them. He had managed to hide these machines from the occupying forces during the Second World War, and once the war was over, Dr Eric Bywaters from the Hammersmith Hospital travelled to Amsterdam to collect one. But it wasn't an easy 'kidney' to operate, and the doctors using it weren't initially all that impressed with its results. It was all but abandoned until 1957, when Professor Ralph Shackman – also a pioneer in kidney transplantation – turned it back on again and started to develop dialysis that worked for doctors and patients. At the same time, a dialysis unit at Leeds General Hospital was being established by surgeon Leslie Pyrah. Hopewell described 'something less than grudging support from the medical establishment in England' for it, but within years not only were patients able to have dialysis in hospital, they were increasingly able to have the machines installed at home. Doctors were handing over operation of the dialysis machines to nurses, which changed the power dynamic onwards. Health policy historian Sally Sheard describes this as 'the beginning of a radical shift within the health service that had been raised on "doctor knows best".'[33]

Technology was changing patients' lives and the working relationships within the NHS. In some instances, the NHS was providing the opportunities for that technology to be developed, too. Sir John Charnley was working as an orthopaedic surgeon at Park Hospital on the day Bevan visited it in July 1948. A decade later, now at the Wrightington Hospital in Lancashire, he decided to turn his hand to a long-term problem: how to give people with painful hips a new life.

The hip replacement – or arthroplasty – was something surgeons had been working on for more than fifty years, trying various materials including glass, Vitallium and Bakelite to replicate the worn joint. Antibiotics had made operations safer to do, and gave hospitals more beds to play with because patients could be discharged more quickly. In 1951, George McKee had carried out a primary hip replacement on a patient in the Norfolk and Norwich Hospital. McKee started using chrome and cobalt in his replacements, and though these were much more successful than previous attempts, patients were still in pain.

Charnley described the problem he came across: 'If you replaced only the ball of a hip joint, then you left the living socket, and the living socket was painful, and so this concept of putting in two artificial parts in the rubbing surfaces was a very obvious way.' He treated a patient who had come to him with a hip implant that worked, but which squeaked when he moved. His wife, Jill, described the effect: 'This patient came to John because the squeak upset his wife so much. When they were having a meal together and he leaned forward to get the salt, it squeaked and it made her feel sick. That started Charnley on thinking about what was going on in the joint.'[34] He realised that the important thing to do was to create as little friction as possible between the ball and socket of the hip implant, and he set about designing not just the implant but also the method of inserting it.

Charnley experimented with Teflon cups and pink dental cement to hold the parts of the joint in place. The problem with Teflon – something we know better as the coating on non-stick cooking pans – was that it started to fall apart once in a patient's body. He had carried out 300 operations with these initial attempts at replacement joints. Now, he was faced with 300 patients whose failing joints he needed to repair. He did this himself. But he also didn't want to give up on finding a hip replacement that would work. His workshop assistant, Harry Craven, had come across polyethylene plastic, and despite being instructed by a now-weary Charnley to throw it away, had ignored him and got on with building a new model. When

Craven tested that, he found it could last for about seventy years. 'He couldn't believe it. Oh, you'd better get some made,' recalled Craven.[35] Charnley is now widely regarded as the father of modern hip replacements. All his work took place with NHS patients, on NHS premises.

Science was also advancing in less convenient ways. By the 1960s, it was undeniable that smoking, previously promoted by both doctors and government as a healthy pastime, was in fact deadly. By 1949 in the UK, 81 per cent of men were smokers, and 39 per cent of women.[36] The government was also coining it in from tobacco taxes, to the extent that Harold Macmillan remarked in his diary in 1956 when he was Chancellor of the Exchequer that 'if people really think they will get cancer of the lung from smoking, it is the end of the Budget'.[37] But by the point Macmillan was writing this, the link between smoking and lung cancer was clear to policymakers. What wasn't clear was whether they were going to do anything about it.

In February 1954, Iain Macleod gave a press conference in which he warned of the dangers of 'excessive' smoking. As a measure of how worried he was, the minister smoked throughout this meeting. Most of the journalists did, too – and at this stage the vast majority of doctors were puffing away as well. Even Sir Austin Bradford Hill, the smoking researcher who had done so much to establish the link, still offered cigarettes to his visitors because 'it would be impolite not to'.[38] Smoking had become part of British culture, and it was going to be a hard habit to kick. It was also going to be very hard for the Treasury to let go: by the 1960s, the revenue from tobacco to the government could cover the cost not just of the NHS but also of the roads.

Macmillan's diary entry was written after a long Cabinet meeting, which had concluded with a discussion about lung cancer. The Minister of Health, Robert Turton, warned colleagues that deaths from cancer of the lung had risen from 1,880 in 1931 to over 17,000 in 1955, and that since ministers had last discussed this matter two years ago, further evidence had emerged showing a statistical connection between smoking and lung cancer. Soon, he predicted, scientific research would establish a causal connection, too. Turton was under pressure from his advisers to make a statement warning the public. It would be, he said, 'restrained rather than alarmist'. The prime minister, Anthony Eden, made a sort-of decision in that he wanted the government to decide what its attitude was and set up a committee.

Doubtless many of the members of that committee were smoking as they worked on it, too. One figure who wasn't lighting up was George Godber, then the Deputy Chief Medical Officer. He was not only convinced of the dangers of smoking, but was horrified that neither the politicians nor his boss, Chief Medical Officer Sir John Charles, were taking this seriously. He started to canvass his friends in the medical world – and, over a lunch with physician and epidemiologist Charles Fletcher, hatched a plan. Fletcher later recalled:

> We thought of various things like trying to stop smoking in trains, trying to put posters up, and various things we thought about. But none of them seemed very likely. And at the time the Chief Medical Officer, Sir John Charles, was obviously frightened of doing anything about it . . . Well, at the end of our lunch I said to George Godber, 'Do you think it would help if our College were to produce a report on the evidence about this?' He said, 'Yes, I think that would be very helpful, it might stimulate my minister to do something about it.'[39]

Fletcher and colleagues at the Royal College of Physicians set to work, and in 1962 they published a report, *Smoking and Health*, which was 'intended to give to doctors and others evidence on the hazards of smoking so that they may decide what should be done'. The report warned that not only did smoking cause lung cancer, it also caused diseases such as bronchitis and contributed to coronary failure. The report demanded public education, restrictions on sales to children, curbs on smoking in public places, and anti-smoking clinics.

The doctors held the first-ever press conference of the RCP. Their report had an initial print run of 5,000. But the response was, in Fletcher's words, 'absolutely staggering', with their press conference plastered all over the front page of every newspaper. The report sold 33,000 copies in just over a year. The one group of people who seemed inert, though, were ministers. 'There was tremendous publicity. But the government did nothing, except say that they would instruct the local authorities, who were responsible then for health education, to do some health education. And it really was extremely depressing, the, the way the government just shelved us off – "No, nothing to do with us. We can't do anything."'[40]

The National Health Service, though, did start to take some action. It set up a number of anti-smoking clinics run by psychologists, to help people learn to avoid smoking.[41] There wasn't, however, a medical response. Virginia Berridge, an expert in the way governments have dealt with substances such as tobacco and alcohol, says the focus tended to be on 'abstinence through self-control' rather than medicine itself. It wasn't until the 1980s, when nicotine replacement therapy started to become available, that kicking the habit was something doctors were concerned with. The NHS became increasingly involved in trying to get people to stop, not least because of the cost of treating the consequences of not stopping – in the form of lung cancer. Alongside this, anti-smoking advertising placed by health education agencies started to appear. One memorable one in 1980 featured boxer Jim Watt, who broke off from training with a punch bag to tell viewers 'you won't catch me smoking', while a message appeared along the bottom of the screen reading 'cigarettes are for losers'.[42]

By the turn of the twenty-first century, the UK government was spending millions on smoking cessation services and on advertising to encourage people to stop. The 'Don't give up giving up' campaign featured a cigarette moulded into a looped memorial ribbon, along with advice and stories from real smokers who had quit. In the 1960s, though, the focus was less on emotions and more on the raw calculation about protecting public finances, whether it be from the revenue hit of a weakened tobacco industry, or the spending black hole of the NHS. Mind you, not much has changed: not only is the NHS still regularly seen as a Whitehall spending black hole, but as late as the 1980s Ken Clarke was happily lighting up cigars in the Health Secretary's office.

3.   Making the modern health service

The first decade of the NHS had dramatically changed the British public's health, and its relationship with doctors. But patients were, by and large, still pitching up at hospitals that looked and worked suspiciously like pre-NHS services. They were crumbling, cold and outdated. Some were former workhouses. Hundreds of them were 'cottage hospitals', serving a limited local area from a small building of thirty beds or even fewer. Isolation hospitals for tuberculosis were emptying as modern treatments caused illness to retreat from society. And there was no room for the fancy new equipment that doctors were wheeling into their buildings.

A fifth of these hospitals had been built before 1861, 45 per cent before 1891.[1] They were in bad shape when the NHS was created: some due to bombing in the Second World War, some because local authorities had put off maintenance as they waited for the health service to take shape.[2] One junior doctor at the time, now the historian Dr Geoffrey Rivett, recalled Salford doctors wheeling patients from the ward to theatre with an umbrella over the trolley, because there were so many bombed-out gaps on the site.[3] Ten years later, not much had changed. Only one new hospital had been built. There hadn't been enough money for a building programme as Britain recovered from post-war austerity. There hadn't been enough money for the funding of the health service itself, let alone a new physical home for it. Hospitals lost out to housebuilding, in terms of both money and the scarce materials needed to construct anything. New Towns such as Harlow, Stevenage and Crawley sprang up, with no hospital to serve them.

This meant that, by 1960, doctors and nurses were working in buildings that were ill-suited to modern healthcare. Some would lose hours each day just walking from one wing of an ornate but chilly Victorian hospital to the other. The culture inside these hospitals reflected their aged walls, too. Nurses were expected to report for duty with stiffly starched uniforms and pure white caps. The cap didn't simply have to fit. It had to be perfect. One nurse at the time recalled: 'If the cap was not folded in a way that it looked like the bakers' hat, you would be asked to remove it from your head and then the sister would re-fold it.'[4] In some hospitals, nurses were expected to attend church daily, or at least on Sunday; sisters were not allowed to be married and the matron reigned supreme. They sat in the dining rooms according to rank, and had strict curfews at night.

If this seems a punishing regime, spare a thought for the poor patients in these hospitals. Being sick was not a restful experience at all. In fact, for some patients a spell in hospital was about as comfortable as life in the workhouses that these old buildings had once been. Their days would often start at 5 a.m. with the nurses waking them to take their temperatures and other readings, before washing them and making their beds. Lights went out at 10 p.m., by which time the patient was probably grateful for the break as the day was packed with activities, largely centred around making sure the wards were as immaculate as the caps on the nurses' heads. In fact, a report on 'the pattern of the inpatient's day' said it was 'no longer unusual to hear of patients talking about "going home for a rest".' It added that 'the patient is called upon to endure a marathon beginning far too early in the morning and lasting until late in the evening'.[5]

It was time for the service to shape up. Everyone agreed on that, whether they'd supported the NHS from its inception or they were still sceptics. A hospital building programme seemed inevitable, as did new ways of working inside the buildings. You won't be surprised to learn that. But what might shake the modern reader a little is the name of the man who led much of that change.

Enoch Powell was not, when he became health minister, known for the things – or to be precise, one *thing* – that we associate him with today. At the time, his political reputation was as a purse-pincher: he had resigned from Harold Macmillan's government because he objected to what he saw as inflationary spending policies. Even before then he was something of a loner, struggling to fit in from the very beginning of his academic career, and waking early each day – the same time as many contemporary NHS patients, as it happens – to work on his translation of Herodotus. He was born John Enoch Powell but switched to using Enoch as his first name as a teenager, when he realised there was already one classical scholar known as J. Powell.[6] He became a professor of Greek, cherished an ambition to be Viceroy of India, and when that plan failed, returned disappointed to Britain to enter politics there instead.

He was a formal man, a tall, slightly hulking figure, who always wore a black jacket and striped trousers when speaking in the Commons.[7] And when he spoke, everyone listened. His oratory was powerful – electrifying, even. He put his gifts to good use when he objected to Britain's treatment of prisoners of war in Kenya. In March 1959, eleven Mau Mau detainees were beaten to death by their guards in the Hola prison camp. Later that year, Powell gave a furious, emotional speech in which he objected not just to the incident but to the way other MPs had dismissed the dead as being 'sub-human'. It was 1.15 in the morning. But it was such a fine speech that it shook the Commons awake. Even MPs who would later become fierce critics of Powell wrote to him congratulating him on his arguments. It wasn't long before he joined the government – and not much longer still that he resigned over the government's refusal to cut spending.

But in July 1960 Powell was back as a minister. He hadn't expected to be sent to the Ministry of Health, nor had he taken much interest in the NHS up to that point: he told one interviewer he had gone into politics because he was 'concerned with the coherence of the British Empire' and had paid no more attention to health 'than any normal constituency member would'. But government reshuffles are often lotteries, and Powell, at the time at least, still felt that he'd won something. He saw that 'for the first time since the war, a major block of capital had been promised in the preceding election of 1959 for the National Health Service and therefore I entered a department which was busy thinking about how it would avoid wasting, how it would best apply this massive injection of capital which meant a virtual rebuilding and refashioning of the hospital equipment of England and Wales'. It was, he said 'a promising intellectual job'.[8]

Powell was an intense character. He was also a curious Conservative because, unlike many of his free-market fellow travellers, he wasn't bothered by the intellectual debate about the NHS. He thought the debate was in fact over. Voters liked the NHS, they wanted it to continue, and so the most efficient use of time was to get on with making it better. He told the *Daily Express* that 'if the people have willed a National Health Service, it is because they desire it and are prepared to pay for it'.[9] His biographer Simon Heffer writes: 'His officials soon worked out that, for all the emphasis Powell had put on free markets and limiting the role of the state, he regarded the NHS as an essential social service and not as an economic good.'[10]

That said, Powell was determined to get health service spending in check. A few months after his appointment, he wrote a memo to Macmillan in which he argued that 'substantial reductions' to spending were needed. 'If no brake is placed now on the increase in expenditure on the Health Services, a halt may later have to be called in circumstances of embarrassment and possibly a crisis,' he warned.[11] Cabinet minutes from October 1960 show that Powell's colleagues agreed with his suggestion that the weekly health service contribution must rise by one shilling. Over the months that followed, Powell returned to the coffin-shaped Cabinet table to make the case for putting up prescription charges, too. On a chilly January morning in 1961, the Cabinet agreed that while this increase would be 'politically unwelcome' and might not even save that much money, it should go ahead anyway.

Powell got a chilly reception in the Commons when he confirmed these increases. He sold the raised charges as necessary so the government could 'continue their policy of developing the Health Service and, in particular, to carry through a long-term programme of modernising our hospitals'. These were at risk of not happening at all if spending kept rising, he argued. To angry shouts of 'Shame!' and 'Disgraceful!' Powell confirmed that prescription charges would rise to two shillings an item the following month. When he added that the National Health Service contribution would rise by one shilling a week for workers, he was heckled once again, with an opposition MP turning back Macmillan's own phrase 'they've never had it so good' on the minister. His shadow minister, Kenneth Robinson, condemned it as 'the biggest single assault on the whole principle underlying the National Health Service since it was conceived', and suggested Powell should have resigned again on principle rather than introduce such charges.[12] He didn't, and the following year he delighted Labour once more by pitching into a furious fight with nurses over their pay. Powell became convinced that nurses were asking for the impossible, and his discussions with some matrons didn't help that: 'It actually happened to me that I was being told by the matron of a hospital which I remember but will not specify, that there was a shortage of nurses and I said, "Well, what would you be able to do which you are not doing now if you had more nurses?" And she actually said "there would be more polishing". I hardly believed my ears!'[13]

One of the reasons Powell wanted to be parsimonious with day-to-day spending on the NHS was that he was keen to force the Treasury into agreeing a long-term approach to capital money so that, finally, the health service could start to have some buildings that suited it. Essentially, he was the minister responsible for the creation of the modern hospital. Many of us are still being treated in the district generals that started life under Powell.

He did not, though, create the modern hospital himself. That was largely down to a man who became Powell's friend and is one of the giants of the NHS, Sir George Godber. Godber was by now Chief Medical Officer. A substantial figure who wore a monocle, he too was an unusual fellow in that he had turned his back on clinical medicine after a few years of practising in order to work in public health, which wasn't the done thing for an ambitious young doctor – and his superiors often reminded him of that. But Godber felt uncomfortable with the prospect of charging patients for their treatment, and had seen that 'we would have a national health service sooner rather than later, and I wanted to get to the place where it was going to be promoted and run from'. Even before he had qualified, Godber was planning to get on the staff at the Ministry of Health. He had to wait five years before he could – only because the government wouldn't take people any sooner after qualifying. So while he waited, he worked as a junior doctor in London, where he came to see a national health service as one which could tackle many of the disturbing things he encountered. Running an evening surgery in Limehouse to cover some of his bills, he saw 'what it was like to be sick and poor' and later said, 'I will never forget some of the things that I did see in households there at that time.' That included children dying of communicable diseases such as measles and whooping cough.[14]

Once in the ministry, Godber found himself responsible for moving maternity services into the suburbs of London for people evacuated from the Blitz. The hospitals there were already struggling desperately under the weight of civilian casualties from bombings and the increased local population. Like hospitals everywhere else in the country, they hadn't been fit for purpose for a while anyway. This experience, and his work surveying hospitals in the East Midlands and Sheffield as part of preparations for the NHS, left a deep impression on Godber. What the survey found, in his words, was that 'it wasn't a hospital service. [The survey] was intensely critical of the fact there wasn't a real service, there was simply a patchwork. And all the surveys said this in effect.'[15]

Godber saw the NHS change what it meant to be sick and poor in its first decade, but he was still waiting for the service to change what a hospital meant. By then, everyone agreed that new hospitals were urgently needed. The *British Medical Journal* had marked the tenth anniversary of the NHS with a special supplement in which it complained that 'it is humiliating to see the up-to-date new buildings being built in many other countries less materially well-off than Great Britain, and to reflect that we have not been able to afford new buildings for nearly ten years.'[16] Politicians agreed. The 1959 Tory manifesto promised 'a big programme of hospital building'. So, too, did the Labour offer, which complained that the Tories had 'starved the Service of money' and completed only one new hospital. It pledged £50 million a year on hospital development.

Neither party offered much of an idea of what these new hospitals would be like. The politicians were leaving that largely to the people in and around the NHS. Godber wanted to replace the scrappy patchwork with an efficient system of 'district general hospitals', which would serve a set number of people, with a set number of beds and a focus on the different parts of the hospital working better together. He saw the models for these new buildings in Scandinavian countries, which had built new hospitals on a regional basis after they were devastated in the Second World War.[17]

The Nuffield Provincial Hospitals Trust produced a series of highly influential reports which examined what modern hospitals needed to be able to do. The researchers turned to the US, Denmark, Sweden and other European countries for ideas – given there were few to be found in Britain at the time. They looked at the big principles of design, and the small details that make a hospital hum. Those details included working out how much space was needed between beds so nurses could change patients and give them treatments. They filmed nurses carrying out these chores in two hospitals, reporting that 'the nurses invited to take part in the filming were not the very slimmest' in order to offer a realistic sense of how much space was necessary.[18]

The Nuffield work signalled the end of long, high-ceilinged Nightingale wards of around thirty beds and little in the way of privacy, personal space or toilets. One design proposal split the ward in half, with sixteen beds and a nurses' station in each room, split again into smaller bays of three or four beds. Godber was enthusiastic about the Nuffield proposals and the Ministry of Health set up its own Hospital Buildings Division, which continued the work.

Building new hospitals wasn't just a chance to get the NHS running better. It was also an opportunity to say something about this new service. New buildings would send a message that this was an evolving, modern system. And quite quickly, a form of design emerged which seemed to send that message very loudly indeed: the tower block.

Architects in the 1960s liked designing towers: they showed that a building was new and forward-thinking – part of the future rather than a homage to the past. Where better to do that than in the medical world, which was already advancing so fast? They were particularly charmed by a specific tower design, which sat on top of a fatter, horizontal base. It was known as the 'matchbox on a muffin' in the hospital world. The wards rose into the sky in a neat stack in the tower; the ancillary services sat beneath it. This meant equipment was sterilised and food prepared at the bottom of the hospital, before being sent up to the wards and theatres in lifts. This set-up had a number of attractions, not least that it didn't take up much space on the ground compared to the older, low-rise hospital buildings. And it dominated the skyline in many towns and cities. The local matchbox on a muffin would become a landmark, and part of the identity of an area. Philip Larkin wrote a poem, 'The Building', about a hospital in Hull. Scholars aren't sure if he meant the new Hull Royal Infirmary, a matchbox on a muffin designed by Yorke Rosenberg Mardall and opened by the Queen in 1967, or the city's general hospital, a former workhouse. Larkin's lines suggest the former: 'Higher than the handsomest hotel / The lucent comb shows up for miles, but see / All round it close-ribbed streets rise and fall . . .' and later, 'It must be error of a serious sort / For see how many floors it needs, how tall / It's grown by now, and how much money goes / In trying to correct it.'

Together with the recently appointed permanent secretary at the ministry, Bruce Fraser, Powell and Godber put together a White Paper for a ten-year building programme, which the Treasury, remarkably, signed off. It culminated in the *Hospital Plan for England and Wales*, which Powell presented to the Commons in January 1962. He later called it 'my magnum opus'.[19] An equivalent plan for Scotland followed shortly after. The English and Welsh plan envisaged a £500 million programme which would build 90 new hospitals and overhaul 134 existing ones, as well as make hundreds of major improvements. These new district general hospitals would each cover a population of around 100,000, with 600–800 beds, and would be close to the town or city centre of the area they served. They would include an accident and emergency unit, a maternity unit, geriatric wards, short-stay psychiatric units, and isolation wards for infectious diseases. They would also have most specialties within their wards, apart from radiotherapy, neurosurgery, plastic surgery and thoracic surgery, which needed larger catchment areas.

This was the first time an off-the-peg model of a hospital had been offered in the UK. It would mean many areas getting eye-catching new hospitals, which was a source of great excitement to patients and healthcare workers – and their MPs. But it also meant a lot of hospital closures. The Hospital Plan didn't envisage this being a particular problem for the workforce. It predicted: 'Many existing hospitals will cease to be needed, and will be closed, but it will be rare for difficulty to arise in finding posts elsewhere in the Service for staff who want them.'[20] As we shall see later in this chapter, it's not as though the NHS was enjoying a glut of staff. But what the plan didn't take into account was how upset people would be when their old and obsolete local hospital had to close.

Things started moving quickly. Some hospitals were already being built. And just three years after the Hospital Plan was published, sixty-six new or near-new hospitals had been built, and ninety-five major works completed. Powell was promoted to the Cabinet a few months after he presented the plan – up to this point he had merely made occasional visits to discuss his brief. Macmillan felt the Cabinet table needed a little restructure of its own, though. He instructed the Secretary to the Cabinet to move Powell's chair, which was directly opposite his, to another position, because 'I can't bear those mad eyes staring at me a moment longer!'[21]

The Minister for Health soon found himself having to stare down protestors who wanted to keep their local cottage hospitals, despite his insistence that the new district generals would give them better treatment. In Bovey Tracey in Devon, more than 300 people attended a 'Save Our Hospital' meeting to protest the closure of their local hospital, which had only eighteen beds. *The Times* reported local doctors arguing it would take too long to get to Exeter from the village, especially when tourists were clogging up the local bypass. One told the reporter: 'You could say this is one of the many issues where the centre hasn't the faintest idea of what the edges feel.' A month later, the paper criticised Powell for suggesting he had received no complaints at all about the closure of cottage hospitals across the country. The paper's leader writer did concede that 'a sense of proportion should all the same be kept' because: 'The case for the hospital plan is far from confined to the economies it may bring. More important is the fact that it promises in general a better service. The comprehensive district hospital, carefully sited, should be able to provide treatment of an order which makes well worth while some small inconvenience in reaching it on the part of some patients and their visitors.'[22]

Powell found MPs no more reasonable. He reflected many years later that they were 'addicted to the institutions in their own constituencies' and would protest furiously when a 'raddled old institution was being rendered unnecessary'. One MP, he claimed, had 'bitterly opposed' his plans to close the local hospital, but changed his stance when his own son died in such a place. 'To go to the wrong hospital is the most dangerous thing that can happen to you,' Powell argued. 'Now this isn't easy to explain to a member of parliament with a well-loved hospital who do wonderful work.'[23] It is unlikely that any of the health ministers who followed him would disagree with that observation.

Many of those successors, though, might have asked Powell to tweak or even overhaul large aspects of his magnum opus. Even once local opposition was quelled and the new hospitals were in place, things didn't always go to plan. The buildings themselves were more expensive than expected, and some had far shorter lifespans than originally envisioned. A number developed a problem known as 'concrete cancer'. This was a chemical reaction, which caused large reinforced concrete slabs to disintegrate. The Princess Margaret Hospital in Swindon was one such cancer patient. Designed in 1959 by top modernist architects Philip Powell and John Hidalgo Moya, it was one of the first general hospitals to be finished, with the *Architectural Review* writing a gushing piece in 1965 that it was 'a measure of the popularity of this most distinguished building that it is not unknown for people to visit for a Sunday afternoon's outing'.[24] But just over thirty years later, *Building* magazine reported: 'Concrete cancer, windows that cause overheating in the summer, and health and fire safety difficulties are blamed on the design of Princess Margaret Hospital and the speed at which it was built.'[25] It complained that the building was 'not visually appealing', which shows the rapid switch in taste from the 1960s excitement about these modern tower blocks to a general consensus that they were in fact eyesores. Less superficially, the design of the Princess Margaret didn't stand the test of time for its patients and the nurses looking after them. In 1998 the *Health Service Journal* reported that 'the wards are unsuitable for modern nursing . . . and the layout can't change because of concrete dividing walls.'[26]

Powell and Moya designed other hospitals too: Wexham Park and High Wycombe were both matchboxes on muffins. Praise at the time for the former went far beyond the trade press. In *Country Life*, Michael Webb wrote: 'In essence, this is not a building but a miniature town.' He called the layout 'lucid and coherent', and his paean included this glorious paragraph: 'A handsome faceted concrete vault – resembling a pineapple skin – expresses the distribution of the load, from the peripheral precast columns between the floor slabs, to the four main columns. Floor slabs project and the wood-framed windows are recessed. This gives a sculptural quality to the façades, provides emergency access terraces (which lead into proper terraces slotted in between the rooms) and prevents the feeling of vertigo engineered by sheer-sided towers.'[27] By the 1990s, though, the chair of the hospital was complaining that 'the main entrance of the hospital looked like the entrance to a scruffy benefit office'.[28]

A more immediate concern for Enoch Powell than the future of sheer-sided towers was that the costs of the building programme soon spiralled out of control. This was partly down to naivety across the board about how expensive a modern hospital really was to build. Many of the hospitals promised never appeared – or weren't built until the 1980s, when they popped up as 'nucleus' hospitals, which were cheaper because of their standardised design. By 1966, it was impossible for the now-Labour government to pretend that everything was on track. The Ministry of Health published a revised 'Hospital Programme', which asked the regions to keep their own building schemes in budget – and warned that those costing more wouldn't get any extra funding. Some of the smaller hospitals the public were so keen to hold on to would stay open for longer. The spiralling costs led to a new district general hospital design in the late 1960s known as the 'best buy' hospital, built in Frimley in Surrey and Bury St Edmunds. Sold as 'two for the price of one', this design didn't work in many locations because they were low-rise and therefore needed a fair bit of land. So the government then settled on a 'harness' standard model, which was only four storeys, centred around a main corridor for staff to use to move between departments easily, and was originally intended for seventy new hospitals. In the end, though, only two true harness hospitals were built, because the government once again ran out of money.

Had it not been for Powell, though, the Hospital Plan might never have started at all. Kenneth Robinson became Minister of Health when Labour won the 1964 election, and believed Powell, whom he had sparred with constantly but respectfully in the Commons, was the only person who could have got it off the ground. He later told Nicholas Timmins that the hospital programme was Powell's 'great achievement', and 'one that possibly only he as an ex-Treasury minister with a "dry" reputation could have achieved'.[29]

Powell was also generally concerned that the way a patient experienced a hospital was often an afterthought to the way doctors and nurses needed to move around in it. He gave a speech in October 1962 specifically on 'humanisation of the hospital service'. This wasn't about big building projects, but little things like realising that patients shouldn't be made to wait for a long time on 'long wooden benches like the forms in a workhouse refectory'. It was also about attitude. He told his audience: 'Believe me, there is a world of difference between the departments where the patients feel "this department's old and overcrowded, but they have done their best to make it best for us" and the department where the patients feel "this hasn't changed since the Poor Law, and they make us about as welcome as paupers". Believe me, too, the difference does not depend on money.' He covered food, visiting hours, and the need to change those unkind waking hours patients were subjected to.[30]

But Powell's real passion lay not in the district general hospital buildings, but in another set of reforms that he failed to realise in his time in front-line politics. In March 1961, he gave a speech which stunned his unsuspecting audience (no, not *that* speech, which we shall come to shortly). It was, in a way, about buildings, too: towers, in fact. These towers belonged to mental institutions.

*

On 9 March 1961, Powell made the short walk from Parliament over to Church House in Westminster, where the annual conference of the National Association for Mental Health was getting under way. As Minister for Health, it was his job to give the opening remarks, and the audience had settled in for what they'd expected to be a run-of-the-mill speech from a politician. Instead, they were jolted wide awake.

First, Powell told them he expected there to be about 'half as many places in hospitals for mental illness as there are today' – a cut of around 75,000 beds. And those remaining would largely be in general hospitals, rather than 'great isolated institutions'. Just to make sure everyone listening – and by now everyone was listening – had got the point, Powell added:

> Now look and see what are the implications of these bold words. They imply nothing less than the elimination of by far the greater part of the country's mental hospitals as they exist today. This is a colossal undertaking, not so much in the new physical provision which it involves, as in the sheer inertia of mind and matter which it requires to be overcome. There they stand, isolated, majestic, imperious, brooded-over by the gigantic water-tower and chimney combined, rising unmistakable and daunting out of the countryside – the asylums which our forefathers built with such immense solidity to express the notions of their day. Do not for a moment underestimate their powers of resistance to our assault. Let me describe some of the defences which we have to storm.[31]

Asylums had been built to be self-contained: the water tower was a symbol of their isolation from the rest of society. Many of these towers were ornate and did indeed brood over the institutions for which they provided drinking water and an emergency supply of water for firefighting. The purpose of the asylums' isolation was ostensibly to keep communities safe from the patients – and the patients safe from the difficulties of the outside world. But the outside world had changed a lot since their construction.

The two world wars had a profound effect on society's attitude to mental illness, as well as the approach that psychiatrists took. There was an influx of patients who were fit, healthy young men suffering from 'shell shock' – first dismissed as malingering cowardice best cured by returning to the front line as soon as possible. By 1948, the idea that a mental breakdown was caused by personal failings and weaknesses was largely regarded as outdated in the psychiatric world. Soldiers weren't ostracised from society like other mentally ill people. The question of whether anyone should be locked away began to creep into the wider debate. By 1959, the government was committed to moving care for the mentally ill and elderly out of institutions and into the community.

Powell had, like most men of his generation, fought in a war. He was clearly keen for another. He didn't just want to move mentally ill patients out of asylums; he wanted those buildings demolished. Even buildings the government had spent money upgrading and improving 'must be swept away' because 'the very improvement of existing facilities militates powerfully against their supersession by something different and better'. He said non-hospital services in the community would need 'progressively to accept responsibility for more and more of that care of patients which today is given inside the hospitals'.[32] This was the start of what became known as 'care in the community'.

The *Lancet* reported one member of the audience's astonishment at what they'd just heard: 'We all sat up, looked at each other and wondered what had happened, because we'd been struggling for years to get the idea of community care and the eventual closure of mental hospitals on the map, and here it was offered to us on a plate.' Not everyone was delighted: Timmins reports a 'mix of enthusiastic backing and of horror at what he proposed'.[33]

Anyone who recognises the phrase 'care in the community' today will know it rarely conjures up thoughts of a magnum opus. But why does it have such a bad reputation? Powell might argue that those around him and who came after him never had the same commitment to the reform of mental institutions as he did. Bruce Fraser felt the only way local authorities would stick with this kind of reform would be if the government produced a ten-year plan for health and welfare services in the same way as it had produced the Hospital Plan.

This didn't just cover mental health but also care of the elderly and the physically disabled. When Powell launched the *Health and Welfare* White Paper in 1963, it was more of a commentary on what local authorities were planning to do, and did not contain much in the way of helping those authorities realise their plans. A Nuffield Trust analysis concluded that the Ministry of Health 'had done little research in this area and had insufficient time or, indeed, experience to undertake any before the date set for the plan's release'. It also lacked power as a department to influence local decisions.[34] Councils often had other priorities for their money.

It turned out that the 'immense solidity' of the asylums Powell had wanted to eliminate was far greater than even the rhetoric of his 'water towers' speech allowed. The first full closure of a mental hospital did not come until 1986. By this time, 'care in the community' had taken on sinister connotations. In 1984, a young social worker named Isabel Schwarz was stabbed to death in her office in Bexley by one of her former clients, Sharon Campbell. After it became clear that a number of warning signs about Campbell's condition had been missed, the government set up an inquiry into community care, led by Roy Griffiths. There were calls to stop further planned closures until there was sufficient community care for the seriously ill patients who were due to be discharged. Towards the end of the Conservative government, in 1996, health ministers were conceding that mental health remained a 'major exposure', with ten homicide inquiry reports involving mentally ill people due in just three months of that year.[35] Even later than that, in 1999, the Minister of State for Health, John Hutton, told the Commons that 'for too many patients, care in the community has become "couldn't care less in the community"' because mental health remained at the margins on the NHS. Powell hadn't stormed the defences of the asylums. He was the first minister to take the opportunity to change the way mental health was treated by the still relatively new health service. He didn't win this battle. And neither did any of his successors. The fight to treat mental illness with anything like the same standard, speed and gravity as physical conditions continues in the NHS today.

★

Powell's 'water towers' speech is little known outside health circles. That's not just because it ultimately didn't have the impact he intended – or at least not for a few decades. It is largely because this Conservative politician is remembered for another speech on a very different topic.

This speech was also written to make its audience sit up sharp in shock. Its argument was made using classical references and forceful language. Unlike the 'water towers' speech, it had a profound impact on British society.

For one of the most infamous speeches of the twentieth century, it had a remarkably small audience: a meeting of the Conservative Political Centre in Birmingham on 20 April 1968. By now Labour was in government and Powell was shadow Secretary of State for Defence. But on this day Powell was freelancing, speaking off-brief and without Tory leader Ted Heath or his shadow frontbench colleagues or the party's Central Office knowing what was going on. He knew that what he would say would have far greater reach than the small audience in the Midland Hotel. He told his friend Clement Jones: 'I'm going to make a speech at the weekend and it's going to go up "fizz" like a rocket; but whereas all rockets fall to earth, this one is going to stay up.' He tipped off local broadcasters, and a camera crew was waiting for Powell when he spoke.

The broadcast clips of what quickly became known as the 'Rivers of Blood' speech certainly went up like a rocket. Westminster exploded. Members of the shadow Cabinet threatened to resign; Heath sacked him the next day. *The Times* described the speech as 'evil'.

His target wasn't, as many have come to believe, immigration per se, but the Race Relations Act introduced by the Labour government. This legislation, he argued, risked 'throwing a match on to gunpowder'. But he also complained that the country must be 'mad, literally mad' to be allowing so many children and spouses of immigrants to enter the country. 'It is like watching a nation busily engaged in heaping up its own funeral pyre,' he said. Powell warned that integration of immigrants was difficult, especially when there were marked differences such as those of colour. Some of the worst lines included what he later argued was merely a quotation from a woman he said he had met (but who could never be tracked down by the press), who had complained that when she went to the shops she was 'followed by children, charming, wide-grinning picaninnies. They cannot speak English, but one word they know. "Racialist," they chant. When the new Race Relations Bill is passed, this woman is convinced she will go to prison. And is she so wrong? I begin to wonder.'

His peroration lent the speech its popular name. He quoted Virgil's *Aeneid*: 'As I look ahead, I am filled with foreboding. Like the Roman, I seem to see "the River Tiber foaming with much blood".'

Powell was long gone from the Health brief, but he referenced the NHS in the speech. It formed both an illustration of the pressure of immigration on public services and also a distinction between those he saw as being immigrants and people who were something else. The existing population of Britain found themselves 'strangers in their own country', he claimed, including finding 'their wives unable to obtain hospital beds in childbirth'. In the rows that followed, Powell seemed unable to produce any evidence to back this assertion up. But he stood by the claim for decades. In 1989, he had this exchange with Sue Lawley on the BBC's *Desert Island Discs*:

Lawley: 'It's perhaps not surprising [Heath] didn't like the tone. You talked about the indigenous population not being able to find hospital beds to give birth to their children . . .'

Powell: 'I didn't say that. You're not quoting me. You're saying what you think I said. You will not find that.'

Lawley: ' "They found their wives unable to obtain hospital beds in childbirth, their children unable to obtain school places, their homes and neighbourhoods changed beyond recognition, their plans and prospects for the future defeated." '

Powell: 'Yes I'll stand by all that. It was a description of the circumstances in which many hundreds of thousands of people were already living and many more hundreds of thousands were shortly to find themselves living.'[36]

Powell himself seemed to have a distorted memory of what he had said, never mind what others thought he had said. There was also a strange contradiction between his allegations about immigrants crowding out spaces in maternity beds and his assertion that Commonwealth citizens who came here as doctors weren't immigrants anyway. Indeed, he praised them, saying: 'This has nothing to do with the entry of Commonwealth citizens, any more than of aliens, into this country, for the purposes of study or of improving their qualifications, like (for instance) the Commonwealth doctors who, to the advantage of their own countries, have enabled our hospital service to be expanded faster than would otherwise have been possible. These are not, and never have been, immigrants.' He had discovered as health minister that the number of beds in a hospital was entirely meaningless: it was the number of staff that mattered.[37]

And it is for this reason that Powell's 'Rivers of Blood' speech (he always referred to it as the 'Birmingham speech') is worth including in a book about the NHS. As Powell's critics at the time and in years to come pointed out, he presided over a great deal of what he clearly saw as useful immigration of doctors and nurses to work in the NHS.

Indeed, the history of the NHS is one of immigration. We have already seen that as a service it was started without the money it needed, and indeed without the buildings. But it was also clear from the start that there weren't the staff. Nationally, there was a labour shortage after the war; in 1948, there were 54,000 nursing vacancies. Within a decade, the shortages were being entrenched by decisions to cut the number of student places in medical schools in Britain, despite the medical workforce increasing by a third in England and 50 per cent in Scotland over the same period. Instead, the government saw the Commonwealth as a source of the healthcare workers that it urgently needed to keep the NHS going.

The British Nationality Act 1948 gave all British subjects citizenship of the UK and its colonies. A year later, the government began a campaign in the Caribbean to recruit nurses. The theme of many appeals was to 'help rebuild the motherland'. One advert in the *Barbados Beacon* in 1949 called for thirty-one women aged 18–30 to work as nursing auxiliaries in hospitals in Bristol, Cardiff, Dartford, Edinburgh,

Lincolnshire, Loughborough, Manchester and North Staffordshire. It offered a three-year contract. NHS staff interviewed prospective candidates across British colonies and former colonies, to the extent that the Commonwealth became a major source of labour for the health service. By the mid-1960s, there were between 3,000 and 5,000 nurses from Jamaica alone working in hospitals in the UK, and by the late 1970s the student nurse and midwife population was 12 per cent overseas recruits. Similarly, by the time Powell became health minister, over a third of all junior doctors in the NHS were from India, Pakistan, Bangladesh and Sri Lanka.[38]

Some commentators have referred to Powell personally recruiting these overseas workers. There are claims floating around that he travelled to the West Indies to make an appeal for workers himself. There doesn't seem to be any evidence that this trip happened, or indeed that Powell had any active role in recruitment. He didn't seem to think so, either: in 1971, Labour MP Syd Bidwell made this claim in the Commons, saying Powell had 'urged the recruitment of coloured people from overseas into the British hospital services'. Powell was furious, saying Bidwell and other MPs had 'no foundation whatsoever' for saying this.[39] Simon Heffer meticulously combed the Ministry of Health's records and found no suggestion Powell had actively recruited overseas workers. Godber also told Heffer in an interview that this was 'bunk . . . absolute rubbish. There was no such policy.'[40] Instead, it was the responsibility of the regional hospital boards of the time.

Even before his 'Rivers of Blood' speech, Powell wasn't fully on board with so many immigrant workers in the NHS. He did praise their role in the hospital service, but would always qualify it, as he did in a debate about staffing in May 1963. Speaking about increases in the numbers of doctors in hospitals between 1961 and 1962, he broke off, and said: 'And in case anyone should say that this is attributable to the large numbers of doctors from overseas who come to add to their experience in our hospitals, who provide a useful and substantial reinforcement of the staffing of our hospitals and who are an advertisement to the world of British medicine and British hospitals, they constituted only a minority of this substantial increase. The increase in British-born doctors during the period was 455 and of non-British born only 289.'[41]

Anyway, Powell didn't make any efforts to stop the doctors and nurses coming to the UK. What was clear was that he saw them as acceptable immigrants. It was part of a trope that's become known in more recent years as the 'good immigrant': that is, someone who earns their right to be considered acceptable, largely by giving but never receiving from society. That's how Powell could in one speech praise an immigrant doctor who kept alive the health service he felt was being overrun with immigrant mothers.

He wasn't the only person to hold this view of the 'good immigrant' doctor or nurse. In fact, it was widespread in the press at the time. Many newspapers carried pieces remarking with some surprise at the quality of 'coloured' nursing. Here's one from the *Daily Herald* in March 1955, written in the aftermath of a recruitment ban on non-white nursing staff in Swansea: 'Nearly 2,000 coloured nurses work at 300 hospitals in England and Wales, but only once – at Swansea, a few days ago – have white nurses objected to them. The reason is simple. Coloured girls make as good nurses as white, and sympathy and kindness – like sickness – know no colour bar.'[42]

Similarly, in January 1961, the *Birmingham Daily Post* covered a protest from ambulance crews in the city who objected to the employment of non-white staff thus: 'Some people certainly had shown an extraordinary capacity for believing that injured or ill people might suddenly conceive a violent objection to being taken by a coloured ambulance attendant to a hospital where there would be a very good chance of their encountering a coloured nurse or ward maid. The health Service could scarcely function if it were not for the work of immigrants, Irish and coloured. They have come here for work, it is true, but we owe them, as all the hard-pressed workers in this cause, a great debt.'[43]

Powell had assumed that most overseas-born workers would return to their countries of birth and thus enrich their own health services with their experience of NHS medicine. This assumption also seemed implicit in many of the expressions of goodwill towards migrant doctors. In July 1968, just three months after the

Birmingham speech, the BBC celebrated the twentieth anniversary of the National Health Service with a rather downbeat documentary called *Something for Nothing*. It posed many of the same questions we ask about the NHS today, such as: can it really continue to do its job in its present form, or will the government have to cut back on what it can provide? The programme also complained about the continuing decrepitude of many hospital buildings, visiting a 300-bed converted workhouse operating as a hospital. The junior doctors were, the narrator revealed, all from 'India, Pakistan and black Africa', and the majority were intending to return to their own countries at some point. Another interviewee, Dr Jay Sankar, was described as a 'stopgap answer' to the staffing shortages the health service faced.

Some doctors did see their time in the NHS as a 'stopgap' period: practising as a doctor in Britain was a passport to a prestigious job back home. In the early 1990s, the British Geriatrics Society conducted a series of interviews with South Asian-born doctors who had come to the UK in the 1960s and 1970s. Many of them explained that, when they were training, Britain had been held up as the place all ambitious doctors should want to start their career. Dr Bijoy Krishna Mondal came to England from India in 1965 with 50p in his pocket. His father had wanted him to be a doctor and was very clear where he expected him to practice: 'From my childhood, he told me I had to go to England . . . He thought the centre of excellence is UK and I must do my postgraduate and be a good doctor and come back and serve the people in our own community.' He developed an affection for the NHS as 'one of the best things [that] happened', and stayed in the system his whole life.[44]

Medical schools on the subcontinent pointed to Britain: many professors and senior doctors were English. Arup Banerjee came to the UK in September 1960 because he and his fellow trainee doctors in Kolkata were 'primed' to see Britain – rather than the USA – as the place to go. 'In those days after doing your house job, the only thing we used to talk about how to get to the UK, and which line are you going to go, surgery or medicine or gynaecology or what have you.' Banerjee also stayed for his entire medical practice.

One of the reasons the BGS conducted these interviews was so it could probe why there were so many South Asian doctors working in the specialty of geriatrics. Overseas-born doctors held 40.9 per cent of all consultant posts in geriatric medicine and 23.4 per cent in mental illness, as against 8 per cent in general medicine and 8.3 per cent in surgery. Geriatrics, like psychiatry, has long struggled to get the prestige of other disciplines, and the simple answer is that there were more vacancies and therefore less competition for newly arrived doctors applying for jobs.

This subtle discrimination of pushing non-white workers towards the jobs those who had been born in this country didn't want to do was one way the doctors were treated in a dismissive stopgap manner. But there was also outright discrimination. Banerjee observed the difficulty some of his colleagues had in getting people to pronounce their surnames, telling the story of one Sri Lankan doctor who refused an extended contract in one hospital and told the consultant: 'I do not want to work for you. Do you know why? I have been working for you for six months. You still cannot pronounce my name correctly. Which means one of two things: either you are an idiot, which you are not. Or you're not interested in me. In either case I'm not going to work for you.'

Dr Mridul Kumar Datta and Dr Saroj Datta moved to England in 1965 from India and have each served for more than fifty years in the health service. Having intended to stay only for a little while before returning home, they found that they kept getting jobs they liked, and that their children were growing up settled in Blackburn. Like many others, they arrived with only a few pounds in their hands because Indian government policy prevented them from travelling with much cash. They too noticed that 'most of our people were given jobs in the specialty that the locals didn't want to go into: things like psychiatry'. But when I spoke to the very smiley couple, who are still working, having tried and failed to retire as GPs, they dismissed the idea that they'd encountered much outright racism in all their years in the health service, other than a comment from a registrar that doctors' pay was low because there were so many immigrants who were willing to work for less.

For nurses, the reasons for not returning to their countries of birth were rather more complex. There were regular appeals for them to come back and help their health services, often because so many nurses had moved to Britain that there was now a shortage back home. But some were prevented from doing so by what seemed to be a cruel trick: the qualifications they were given weren't the ones they thought they'd be getting. They wanted the internationally recognised State Registered Nurse qualification, but instead found themselves being pushed into the lesser State Enrolled Nurse, which wasn't valid in other countries. Not only did this reflect widely held beliefs at the time about black nurses' limited capacity for training and for reaching senior posts, it also trapped them in the NHS – where, like immigrant doctors, they found themselves working on the wards shunned by white British nurses.

Their experiences of racism were far more overt than what was suggested in the press. Midwives found white mothers refusing to be touched by 'black hands',[45] and their colleagues assigned dirty or manual tasks to them, or expected them to work more night shifts. They also struggled to find accommodation: the signs on properties to let reading 'No Blacks, No Dogs, No Irish' applied to nurses of colour, too, almost as though the British people were happy to have vacancies in their health service filled by immigrants, but only if they disappeared to a cupboard at the end of the day rather than going out into society. In some instances, nurses found themselves sleeping almost literally in cupboards: in 1965, a group of black nurses in Wokingham wrote to their local newspaper to complain that they were being forced to sleep in an old people's ward rather than having official lodgings in the hospital.[46] There were other instances where hospital charities found it hard to get lodgings for non-white nurses.

The mixture of hostility and qualified gratitude towards immigrant healthcare workers was there long before Powell gave his speech. Many British people agreed with what he said, which is one of the reasons he refused to recant. But the effect of sending a rocket up was that Powell made it near impossible for any other politician to talk about immigration. His friend Lord Howard of Rising wrote in a volume to mark 100 years since Powell's birth that the speech 'must rank as Enoch's greatest failure' because 'at a stroke, he made the subject of immigration a no-go area for elected politicians'– including Howard himself.[47] Powell was also wrong in many of his assumptions, including those about healthcare workers. Many of them settled in Britain and spent their entire lives in the NHS rather than go back home as he had expected. More than that, they integrated to the extent that it quickly became impossible to represent the health service in any accurate form without using non-white faces. The history of the NHS is the history of British society. What a strange contradiction that Powell is the man who left such a potent legacy in both – in two very different forms.

4. The fight for rights

Philip Larkin's poem about a tall hospital building is nowhere as famous as 'Annus Mirabilis', which tells the reader that 'Sexual intercourse began / In nineteen sixty-three'. Despite the achievements of this decade, most people do look back on the sixties not for the new hospital buildings or the failed attempts to abolish mental incarceration, but for the sex. The sex that, for the first time, female members of the species could have without worrying about the consequences. The sex that they could enjoy. The sex that they started to talk about in public. Everyone was having sex. Lady Chatterley, Christine Keeler, the career woman, women who just wanted to enjoy themselves. This decade saw the advent of the sexual revolution, and the NHS had a big part to play.

Until this point, sex had been a complicated affair for women. It was intrinsically linked with having children, which was one of the reasons it was taboo outside marriage. There were already forms of birth control and disease prevention around: the British Museum has a charming collection of eighteenth-century 'sheaths' made of animal skin, which were tightened with a nice pink ribbon sewn into the opening. At the time of their operation, though, the principal mode of controlling the size of families was the high infant mortality rate: women might have to go through childbirth after an unplanned pregnancy, but few of their children would make it out of infancy and into adulthood anyway. By the 1960s, children had better chances of surviving, thanks in no small part to the NHS, which was offering vitamins to them and better care to their mothers. Sheaths had come on a bit, so to speak, but were still not particularly comfortable or trustworthy. Other methods such as trying to guess when the woman was fertile were prone to error. It made sex rather tense within a marriage, never mind outside. The *Spectator* carried a piece in 1963, the year Larkin marked as the beginning of sex (albeit not for him), which remarked only half-jokingly: 'It is partly because the British male is left to take all the precautions that so many British women have earned the unenviable reputation of being frigid.'[1] Less abstemious types were still resorting to other methods. In the same year, the *British Journal of General Practice* carried a report claiming 'country girls still jump up and down after sexual intercourse to avoid conception'.[2]

Reports of a birth control pill developed by American scientists started appearing in the British press in the 1950s. Dr Gregory Pincus was the first to create a hormone-based pill which tricked the body into thinking it was already pregnant, and therefore prevented ovulation. The *Times* correspondent in New York reported in July 1957: 'A new drug which, it is claimed, "definitely inhibits ovulation" when taken orally is being manufactured and marketed in the United States by a Chicago pharmaceutical company, GD Searle and Company. Although it has been hailed by newspapers here as an oral contraceptive, its manufacturers make no such claim on its behalf, nor do they seek to promote it for such a purpose.'[3] But its advantages as a means of birth control were clear to all, and in 1960 this new medicine, called Enovid, got its licence as a contraceptive pill in the USA.

Clinical trials of this medicine, which had also been available privately for the treatment of menstrual disorders, began in Britain that year. Those trials were led by local Family Planning Associations in Birmingham, Slough and a number of London boroughs. Volunteers needed to be married, under the age of forty, and willing to have another baby if the tests failed. Some required consent forms signed by both the woman and her husband.[4] The results weren't particularly astonishing, not least because the Birmingham trial, which involved forty-eight women, had tried the very lowest dose possible of the treatment, meaning fourteen still ended up pregnant. But, by October 1961, the Family Planning Association had added Conovid, as it was known in Britain, to its approved list of contraceptives, and in December 1961 Enoch Powell confirmed in the House of Commons that it would be available through the NHS. He was rather curt in his responses to questions about it, telling MPs: 'It is not for me to indicate to doctors when they should decide for medical purposes to prescribe for their patients.'[5] There weren't that many 'medical purposes' for prescribing a contraceptive, though, and Powell's paucity of words was in some contrast to the lengthy and anguished conversations behind the scenes in government about the Pill. These discussions were conducted largely by people who weren't going to be taking it, because though scientists were already talking about an oral contraceptive for men, only women could take Conovid. And there weren't many women walking the corridors of power at this time. But that didn't stop the chaps having plenty of thoughts about how it might affect society.

Their worries were partly moral but also pragmatic. Who should be allowed to take the Pill? If it were prescribed to unmarried women, would the government be encouraging promiscuity? Bruce Fraser, the permanent secretary at the department, mused thus in a confidential briefing note in 1961: 'One thinks of course in terms of married couples but when it comes to avoidance of pregnancy in order to preserve health a woman has, I suppose, precisely the same rights under the NHS whether she is married or living in sin.' Fraser was also concerned about how a prescription to prevent pregnancy for 'health reasons' would really work. In the same note, he warned the minister: ' "Health" includes of course mental as well as physical. Some people may think the arrangement open to what they would call abuse, because what with all this long-haired psychiatry which is getting so fashionable doctors will be ready to describe a case where a mother just does not want her baby for the time being as a case where pregnancy would so damage her psyche that she can be given an oral contraceptive on the taxpayer.'[6] Sin and long-haired psychiatry aside, if any woman could have it, wouldn't the whole thing get a bit expensive? One Ministry of Health note warned, 'If this became really popular as a contraceptive the annual cost at this price could soon match the rest of the drug bill.'[7] It was also a jolt: until now, the NHS had prescribed treatments to people because something was wrong with them. Pregnancy might be something a lot of women, including married ones, might want to prevent. But it wasn't an illness.

The British Medical Association, still predominantly male, wasn't very happy about doctors having to prescribe the Pill to patients. It was a moral matter for the Family Planning Association to deal with, not something doctors, who worked on cures, should concern themselves with. The problem was that the Pill wasn't a sheath, it was a *pill*, and there were quickly concerns about side effects including clots. So doctors would *have* to get involved, if only at an advisory stage. They needed to take a medical history and check if the woman had any other health conditions, including being overweight, which might be aggravated by the Pill. At every stage, the BMA lobbied for GPs to secure extra money for prescribing this pill, whether in the form of an additional charge for the patient, or annual payments from the government to reflect the numbers of women receiving contraceptive advice from their GP.

Strangely enough, many women took a rather different view. Married women wanted the freedom that came with taking something proven to be so effective that they didn't need to rely on their husband fumbling with a sheath at the last minute. It meant they could start to enjoy and even look forward to sex: as Larkin said, sexual intercourse was beginning. By 1962, 50,000 women in Britain were taking the Pill. A *Times* report on the Birmingham trial in 1961 said: 'It is reported that many patients have stated that this method of birth control brings confidence and relaxation to their marital relationship.'[8]

The problem was that in practice only married women were receiving the Pill, in part because of the worries about state-sanctioned promiscuity. Some women would buy brass curtain rings that looked like wedding rings in order to dupe doctors and Family Planning Associations into believing they were married and therefore eligible for contraception.[9]

As the decade wore on, many family doctors started to understand how big a deal this was for their patients. At a meeting in London in 1965, a number of doctors present spoke in glowing terms about the Pill: one described it as 'not so much a contraceptive, more a way of love', with another who was sceptical about its role admitting: 'In the past a tremendous amount of women always had a fear of pregnancy when other methods were used and did not enjoy themselves. Now, the contraceptive pill has done away with all this.' A third, who had a 'large, mixed industrial practice near Doncaster', said, 'We are on the threshold of a social revolution emancipating marriage and I firmly believe that we should be doing everything to encourage the taking of the pill.' He added: 'Can we not persuade the Minister of Health to put the pill on the National Health Service so it can be supplied to all?'[10]

Some doctors couldn't wait for the ministers to be persuaded: Dr Andrew Semple was the Medical Officer for Health in Liverpool in the 1960s and set up a 'mothers' welfare fund', which covered family planning advice for unmarried women, much to the horror of Catholic members of the council when they discovered they'd been funding the Pill 'on the rates'.[11] The health minister by now was Kenneth Robinson. Robinson was a gentle, amenable Labour politician who had a habit of mollifying even the more awkward sectors of the service without having to capitulate to them on everything. He agreed that family planning should be extended to more women, but agreed with the BMA's position that doctors could charge for prescriptions where there was no medical danger to a woman of falling pregnant. He introduced the Family Planning Act of 1967, which allowed unmarried women to receive contraceptive services – and therefore oral contraception. It wasn't until 1974, when the Conservative government embarked on one of its many reorganisations of the health service, that the Pill became free and family planning part of the NHS.

By that point, over a million women were taking an oral contraceptive. The debate had shifted from the morality of letting women decide when they wanted to have children and when they just wanted to enjoy sex, and on to worries about the health risks involved and questions about whether doctors could prescribe the Pill to women without telling their husbands. It is impossible to imagine these kinds of conversations today, but perhaps it is also impossible to imagine a health service that, until the late 1960s, hadn't really been catering to the health of everyone it purported to serve. With the Pill, women's reproductive health, and for the first time millions of healthy patients were brought into regular contact with their doctors.

Cost and morality weren't the only arguments against the Pill. Another was safety, and that case continues today. In 1969, Barbara Seaman published *The Doctors' Case Against the Pill*, which argued women were not being informed of the possible side effects of these contraceptives. She wrote: 'Up to now, pill-users have heard almost exclusively about the pill's effectiveness and convenience. Most of them have yet to hear the full story of its dreadful drawbacks.'[12] Those included the risk of blood clots, strokes, cancer, heart disease and depression. The Pill was a bestseller, but so was Seaman's book. It was published in America but had an impact worldwide, and beyond the drug in question. It meant doctors had to rethink the way they consented patients for medication, even when it was something a patient was asking for. In the same year as Seaman's investigation hit the shelves, British doctors were restricted to prescribing pills containing less than fifty micrograms of oestrogen, as the higher doses were associated with some of the problems listed in the book. The popularity of the Pill fell dramatically: its historian Lara Marks says that 'by the 1970s, within a decade of its availability, the contraceptive had fallen from its pedestal as a wonder drug'.[13]

It wasn't just the Pill that led to tighter regulation of medicines in the UK. The 1960s also saw an historic drugs scandal – one of the worst in the lifetime of the NHS – that affected pregnant women. Thalidomide was a sedative that was prescribed to expectant mothers suffering from morning sickness. It was marketed by manufacturer the Distillers Company under a variety of names, including Distaval, and advertised thus: 'Distaval can be given with complete safety to pregnant women and nursing mothers without adverse effect on mother or child.'

But there had not been any tests on pregnant women. And it took a number of years after thalidomide was licensed in the UK in 1958 before the drug's true adverse effects on babies were spotted. It is estimated that 40 per cent of the 10,000 people affected worldwide died at or shortly after they were born. The babies who lived had multiple physical defects, including shortened limbs, sight problems and heart deformities. It was withdrawn from sale in 1961, but Enoch Powell repeatedly refused calls for a public inquiry into how thalidomide had ever been prescribed to pregnant women.

Harold Evans was then the editor of the *Sunday Times*, which campaigned furiously for justice for the families affected by this disaster. He wrote in his memoirs that 'Powell's intransigence left the families with only one remedy, to sue the manufacturers for negligence.'[14] They eventually won, with Distillers paying out £20 million to 429 children disabled by the drug. The impact on the activities of the NHS went far beyond that: the Conservative government asked Sir Derrick Dunlop to head a Committee on Safety of Drugs in June 1963, which examined the control of new medication. It covered thalidomide, the Pill, and many other new drugs. Then, Harold Wilson's Labour government introduced a Yellow Card Scheme for doctors to report adverse effects of medication, passed the 1968 Medicines Act, which tightened the regulation of drugs, and replaced Dunlop's committee with a Committee on Safety of Medicines. The Yellow Card Scheme continues to operate today, but is now open to anyone to report drug effects.

The Pill had naturally unsettled many Catholic doctors, who found a conflict between the demands of their patients and the teachings of their church. It was in fact as a result of nerves about whether the Pope would condemn the contraceptive that the developers of this medicine introduced a seven-day 'break' in taking it. This induced a period-like bleed, which made the Pill seem more natural, though the Vatican remained unconvinced. Still, the moral turmoil over that drug was nothing compared to the debates around the legalisation of abortion, which followed in the late 1960s.

Abortion didn't begin in the 1960s. It had always been around behind closed doors – a criminal offence, but a last resort for desperate women. Long before the NHS was even being designed, the British government was worried about the number of women having illegal – and in many cases deadly – abortions. It established an interdepartmental committee on abortion, known as the Birkett Committee, in 1937, to 'inquire into the prevalence of abortion, and the present law relating thereto, and to consider what steps can be taken by more effective enforcement of the law or otherwise to secure the reduction of maternal mortality and morbidity arising from this cause'.[15]

Readers who find this sensitive subject particularly painful may wish to skip the next three paragraphs. I have included them because it is important to show that abortion didn't start in the 1960s; it merely became safe. The report listed the methods used to try to terminate a pregnancy, many of which are deeply distressing to read about. They include 'lively Polly', a soap solution injected into the vagina; crochet hooks; a report of the 'broken end of a spatula' being removed from a woman's vagina during labour; 'castor oil in large doses frequently taken in gin'; and ingesting or inserting 'slippery elm', the bark of a North American tree with abortifacient properties. Some of these methods were successful; others landed the woman in hospital or the morgue with sepsis or a physical injury. Around 15 per cent of all maternal deaths at this time were due to abortion.

Feminist campaigners argued to the committee that the primary cause of abortion was economic: the majority of women trying to terminate a pregnancy were unable to afford to look after a child. Here's one account from a woman attending an antenatal clinic in Kensington in 1937: 'My husband got me some pills from the chemist. We were desperate because we hadn't any money and the baby was so small. I wouldn't do it again – I was too frightened. My mother died after an illegal operation. My father was consumptive and she didn't want any more babies. I should never have agreed to anything more than take pills and I won't do that again.' Her abortion attempt failed.[16]

The situation had not improved by the 1960s. One student nurse's diary of her time at St Bartholomew's Hospital in London from 1960 reads thus: 'It's hard to believe that the sordid things one reads about in the papers really happen. We carried out a D. and C. [dilation and curettage: a procedure which removes tissue in cases of miscarriage and abortion] on a girl of 21 who had tried to carry out a criminal abortion on herself by using potassium permanganate. She didn't realise that it made one bleed not abort. There is another sad case at the moment on Harley Ward. A woman has gas gangrene from attempting an abortion under pressure from her husband. She is 31 and dreadfully ill.'[17]

Doctors, meanwhile, could carry out medical abortions that were necessary to save a woman's life. They were advised to obtain the approval of a second physician. They tried to resist pressure from the police to interrogate the patients they treated who were clearly suffering the aftereffects of a termination: in 1914, the Royal College of Physicians passed a resolution saying doctors had a 'moral obligation' to respect patient confidentiality. Some doctors were caught performing illegal abortions themselves.

The Birkett Committee published its report in 1939 and recommended a change to the law, but nothing happened because the Second World War got in the way. By the 1950s, campaigners were growing frustrated and tried to bring legislation to Parliament legalising the practice, which became much safer when carried out in a medical setting. It wasn't just doctors' organisations such as the Royal College of Obstetricians and Gynaecologists who were pushing for a change in the law; even the Archbishop of Canterbury, Dr Michael Ramsey, had said he believed reform was needed.[18] It wasn't until 1966, when a young Liberal MP, David Steel, introduced a piece of backbench legislation known as a private members' bill into the House of Commons that things started to move. Steel was so young – twenty-eight – that one of his party colleagues in the Lords complained that he wouldn't support a piece of legislation from someone of such a tender age. But much of what Steel was proposing in his Medical Termination of Pregnancy Bill had appeared in previous bills, including the requirement for two doctors to sign off an abortion on the grounds that proceeding with the pregnancy would be injurious to a woman's health or the future health of the child.

By this point, it was believed there were around 40,000 women having abortions every year. Only 3,000 of those would have been in National Health Service hospitals, and the research on this in a national opinion poll conducted in July 1966 described 31,000 as being illegal terminations.[19]

In the same month, the House of Commons passed the first proper stage of Steel's bill with an astounding majority: 223 votes in favour and only 29 against. The government had remained formally neutral but indicated it would help with the drafting at later stages of the bill's passage through Parliament. This was effectively ministers giving the green light to a major social change without having to take responsibility for the moral debates about to start in earnest. This was a pattern for many of the big social changes of this era, including the decriminalisation of homosexuality, which also started life as a piece of backbench legislation rather than something introduced by ministers. The exchanges in the Chamber offered a preview of the tenor of the wider public debates to come.

The legislation included clauses which referred to the pregnant woman's capacity as a mother 'being severely overstrained by the care of a child or of another child'. Steel felt this was necessary because otherwise doctors would have far 'too great a responsibility' to interpret the law. But others felt it would introduce what they dubbed 'abortion on demand'. Conservative MP Jill Knight complained: 'This subsection is so wide and so loose that any woman who felt that her coming baby would be an inconvenience would be able to get rid of it. There is something very wrong indeed about this. Babies are not like bad teeth to be keeled out just because they cause suffering. An unborn baby is a baby nevertheless.'[20] Liberal MP William Wells warned that many Irish nurses who were Roman Catholic would be opposed to abortion, and that this legislation would threaten the independence of the medical profession. He tried to get the bill thrown out of the Commons on these grounds.

But it passed. The 1967 Abortion Act, as it was named, legalised terminations up to twenty-eight weeks. It still had the clauses which campaigners felt allowed 'on demand' abortion because a woman might be 'severely overstrained' by caring for a child in it. It also included clauses allowing professionals with a conscientious objection to the practice to refuse to carry one out. Many years later, Steel met a professor of medicine who had been told as a medical student in the late 1960s that the Abortion Act marked 'a historic day because your generation of doctors will never have to confront the consequences of botched abortions'.[21]

Even those doctors who didn't want to refuse were nonetheless surprised by how much demand there was for terminations when the Act became law in 1968. In January 1969, statistics presented to obstetricians and gynaecologists included an estimate that the annual demand for abortions in England and Wales would be at least 35,000. The physician presenting those figures, Dr Thomas L. T. Lewis, remarked that doctors hadn't expected a great shift from the number of abortions performed before the Act. He added: 'How wrong we were. I am afraid that we did not allow for the attitude of, firstly, the general public, and, secondly, the general practitioners.' He also remarked with sardonic surprise that single women were receiving more abortions on medical grounds than married women: 'Since far more married than single women become pregnant it is difficult to understand how medical indications can be so much more frequent in the women without husbands.'[22]

The effect that the legislation had on the workings of the NHS was curious. Professor Rudolf Klein has studied the way the NHS has changed as an organisation, and remarks that the Act 'imposed no responsibility on the Ministry of Health to provide the necessary facilities, nor did it impose on individual consultants a duty to carry out the procedure'. Klein points out that the former would have meant the service finding extra resources, and the latter would have interfered with physicians' clinical autonomy. It meant in some parts of the country abortion was very easy to secure, and less so in others. Often, it was the case that it was easiest to obtain a termination if you lived in a wealthy area: Charles Webster notes that, even by the mid-1970s, NHS family planning as a whole was not even reaching a third of women of childbearing age, and that, 'as with other aspects of the NHS, family-planning services as a whole were least accessible where the need was greatest'.[23] It's almost as though politicians had determined that they would change the law, but not so much as to have to take responsibility for it.

In practice, women seeking a termination were generally referred into the private sector, which picked up the huge demand for these procedures.[24] It continues to be the case today that the NHS funds abortions carried out by external providers such as the British Pregnancy Advisory Service and Marie Stopes International. By 2019, 74 per cent of all NHS terminations in England were carried out by external organisations.[25]

This has to a certain extent taken the NHS out of the continuing fight about abortion, too. There will naturally always be groups who vehemently oppose the termination of a pregnancy on various or even all grounds. In recent decades, the number of attempts to change the legal situation in the UK has petered out somewhat; indeed, the Abortion Act has only been amended once, and that was with the 1990 Human Fertilisation and Embryology Act, which reduced the time limit on terminations to twenty-four weeks. Instead, the fight rages on outside the clinics where the abortions take place, with ongoing debates about whether there should be an 'exclusion zone' for protestors, to protect the privacy of the women attending their appointments. And with the 2022 overturning of the *Roe v. Wade* judgement in the US, which means individual states can now ban abortions once again, UK activists have become anxious that there will be more attempts to change the law here – though our system functions in a very different way.

It is not for a book of this sort to conclude whether or not abortion is right. But it is accurate to reflect that the NHS has, since 1968, become part of an acknowledgement that some women will want to terminate a pregnancy, and that if the health service doesn't provide that safely, many of those women will find another, possibly deadly, way of achieving their aim. In that sense, it has become part of the fight for women's lives.

In another sense, the health service has a shameful record when it comes to unplanned pregnancies. In the years before the Abortion Act, an unmarried woman who decided not to seek an illegal termination and carried the pregnancy to term was shamed and ostracised by her community. Abortions can take place behind closed doors. Pregnancies tend to be rather difficult to hide, and the taboo around any baby born outside marriage was such that women in the 1960s and before came under huge pressure – coercion, even – to give up the baby.

In fact, 'give up' still suggests some agency on the part of the woman, in an appalling chapter in British history in which – as with the advances of the Pill and abortion – the NHS played an integral part.

Forced adoption affected an estimated 250,000 women and 500,000 children in the 1950s, 1960s and 1970s. Women who found they were pregnant outside marriage were immediately treated differently by society, and the health service was no exception. One academic giving evidence to a parliamentary inquiry on forced adoption put it thus: 'Did unmarried mothers experience differences in care? The starting place for a married couple was to ask, "How can we support your pregnancy? How can we help you go through pregnancy with support?" I would suggest that the starting place for unmarried mothers was to say, "We'll withdraw support. You'll be punished across this process." '[26]

Sometimes the punishment was that lack of support, but sometimes it went much further. One of the women affected was Ann Keen, who became an MP but who gave birth to her son when she was seventeen. Her treatment when she went into hospital was brutal. She was denied pain relief: 'I was not expecting the brutality of what happened. When I went into labour, I was told by one of the midwives that was mainly dealing with me that I can't have anything for pain, because "You will remember this so as you won't be wicked again, you bad girl, you won't be wicked again." ' A doctor refused to give her anything other than stitches, and when she moved in the stirrups, she was slapped and told to stay still.

She summoned up the courage to speak to a midwife, who said she would be allowed to see her son in the day nursery for ten days before he was adopted. But on the eighth day, 'I went to collect him from the nursery and he was not there. She said, "Oh, he's gone. Oh, no, no, no, we told you not to get close. And you did. So he's gone." And then she pointed to a building. And she said, "He's over there in that building and his new mummy is coming for him in two days' time. And you can come with me now." And she took me into this cold, horrible NHS bathroom, got me into the bath and said, "Well, let's get rid of this milk," and she grabbed my breasts. She said, "You won't need this." And I knew then I didn't stand a chance.'[27]

Other mothers had similar stories of cruelty in the delivery room.

Diana Defries told a BBC documentary on forced adoption that when she gave birth to her daughter aged sixteen, she was left for hours 'covered with a sheet and a crying baby that I couldn't reach'. Then, her baby was taken away from her, and began howling as she was carried from her mother. Pat Tugwell was seventeen when she had her son, and recalled 'one particular nurse who seemed to enjoy being quite rough when she examined me and I remember her saying to me, "Oh, how did you get like this if you don't like somebody doing this to you?" It was really quite abusive, they were quite abusive. That was horrid, that really sort of hurt me in a way. You know, I was a human being, why could I not have been accepted for that? All I had done was I was having a baby, made a mistake, you know, but that was it. I was still a human being.'[28]

How could people employed to care behave in such a way, let alone be complicit in forced adoptions involving screaming babies taken from equally distressed mothers? The simple explanation is that the NHS reflected society at the time: the behaviour of these midwives and nurses seemed normal, and tells us now quite how roughly young unmarried mothers were treated across the board. There was no formal policy encouraging them to be thus; it was the culture both inside hospitals and in communities, and so no one was pulled up on their behaviour.

But is it really fair to dismiss this as merely culture? The absence of any disciplinary measures for healthcare workers who behaved in this way shows that the NHS had, even if passively, taken a position of acceptance that not everyone who came through its doors was entitled to the best healthcare possible. Maternity services should never have been part of a punishment for a societal taboo. And yet there has still not been an official apology from the British government on behalf of the health service and the many other parts of the public sector that exacted this abuse on women and children.

Women like Ann Keen, Diana Defries and Pat Tugwell might, had they found themselves pregnant in the early days of the NHS, have been able to give birth at home, though of course it isn't clear that they would have been treated with any greater compassion by their families or a visiting midwife. In 1948 it was the norm to give birth away from a hospital: Aneira Thomas was remarkable not just because she was the first baby born under the new system, but also because that labour took place in a hospital. But the maternal mortality rate had also been increasing in the run-up to the creation of the NHS, at more than 40 deaths per 10,000 births by 1937. As the health service became established, two things became clear: one, that maternity services weren't very well organised, and two, that many women wanted the reassurance and convenience of giving birth in a hospital.

A committee on maternity services led by Lord Cranbrook published its report in 1959. It concluded that 70 per cent of all births should take place in hospital, and that specialised obstetricians, rather than GPs, should take charge of deliveries. This dismayed GPs, who complained that they would be denied 'the satisfaction of attending their patients in pregnancy and labour' and that the obstetric knowledge they had obtained at medical school would also be lost.[29] It also turned out to be a rather arbitrary target, chosen partly because it was a nice round number and not far from the then-current rate of 64.2 per cent of births in hospital. Either way, the figure wasn't particularly questioned at the time because women wanted to be in hospital, and by 1968, 80 per cent of all births were indeed taking place in that setting. Indeed, the demand for maternity beds in hospital far outstripped the supply, to the extent that one woman claimed she had booked her place while still trying to conceive.[30]

Cranbrook also disappointed a number of health service campaigners by saying the current provision of maternity services by hospitals, GPs and local authorities – known as the tripartite system – should stay. Obstetricians in particular had hoped the report would lead to a reform which united maternity care under their own control. But they were still increasing their power at the expense of GPs, midwives and others: they were the ones who could decide whether a woman was allowed to give birth in hospital or at home.

Birth was becoming medicalised as a result of the arrival of the NHS, and it wasn't always to the good. Women were spending more time in a medical setting in the run-up to the birth: ultrasound scanning started in Glasgow in 1958, and by 1970 it was possible for doctors to work out the age of the foetus, as well as spotting twins and possible abnormalities. Mothers-to-be believed the official reports and claims in the press that it was safer, and were attracted by the break from domestic chores a hospital stay would offer. But they weren't given much warning of what it would be like to give birth in hospital. The *Sunday Express Baby Book*, a popular 1950s tome on motherhood, rather charmingly told mothers that on arrival in hospital, they would be 'made ready for the delivery, and given an enema and a bath'.[31] Enemas, along with the routine shaving of a woman's body hair, had no clinical necessity: they were merely a formality to make giving birth less messy, presumably for the benefit of the doctor as much as the mother, who was expected to be a bit embarrassed by the whole thing. The book also glossed over the finer details of what labour would involve, reassuring readers: 'In the delivery room, white with bright lights, you will be taken from the hospital trolley to the delivery table. The nurses will be standing by with the doctor and with their gentle help and encouragement, aided by the science they have studied so long, your baby will be born.'[32]

What it didn't mention, though, was that the brightly lit delivery room would see the woman strapped into stirrups for the delivery, despite this not being a position that encouraged the movement of the baby along the birth canal. Doctors would routinely perform episiotomies – a cut enlarging a woman's vagina so that the baby's head might emerge more easily – even when there was little risk of tearing or the baby becoming stuck. Done crudely, they could leave a woman struggling with incontinence, a lack of sexual enjoyment, and in some cases lasting pain from scar tissue. Husbands were rarely present in the delivery room because childbirth remained a taboo, which meant that a woman incoherent with pain had no one to advocate for her.

Here is one account from Jean Louise, who gave birth to three children between 1965 and 1971, and spoke to a project on experiences of maternity called 'Hiding in the Pub to Cutting the Cord'. For the first birth, she said:

My husband was with me throughout (except during the shaving and the soapy water to empty the bowel). It was a very new concept at that time and it helped me deal with the pain and his wonder at our baby was just as great as mine. He was attending a different university from me and as the baby arrived on a Sunday morning he was home with me.

I'd had to have an episiotomy and the pain from the stitches was terrible afterwards. Everyone in the ward had had an episiotomy and there was only one rubber ring [a cushion allowing a woman to sit down with less discomfort]. Whenever I sat up in bed to feed the baby, the pain from the stitches was dreadful. I could feed the baby perfectly well lying down, with him beside me, but the matron wasn't having any of it and being young and new to it all I didn't want to do anything 'wrong' in case it harmed my baby.[33]

Her second child was born at home in 1967, but she was in pain that became so bad she said 'if I'd had the means I would have killed myself'. The midwife sent her husband out of the room, even though he had been rubbing her back to help her through the agony. When Jean Louise found she was pregnant again, she was so terrified of more pain that her mother paid for her to go to a private maternity hospital so she could have a new procedure called an epidural, which wasn't available on the NHS.

Women were fighting for more rights everywhere, including in the delivery room. Sally Willington set up the Society for the Prevention of Cruelty to Pregnant Women in 1960, though she swiftly renamed it to the rather more neutral Association for Improvements in Maternity Services. She complained in a letter to the *Observer* in that year that: 'In hospital, mothers put up with loneliness, lack of sympathy, lack of privacy, lack of consideration, poor food, unlikely visiting hours, callousness, regimentation, lack of instruction, lack of rest, deprivation of the new baby, stupidly rigid routines, rudeness, a complete disregard of mental care in the personality of the mother.'[34]

Another campaigner was Prunella Briance. She gave birth to her second child in 1955. She described it as a 'ghastly birth experience, where I was treated with idiocy and callousness'. She was dropped while being lifted onto a bed, administered castor oil at the insistence of a doctor even though it made her violently sick, and refused a pillow. Her baby was stillborn after getting 'stuck'. Her response to this was to investigate what she saw as the problem of highly medicalised labour in which women were given little agency. She came across the writings of Dr Grantly Dick-Read, a GP in Suffolk who had developed a method of 'childbirth without fear', which would mean not needing pain relief. Briance set up the Natural Childbirth Association in 1956, which soon attracted the attention of women horrified by their experiences on maternity wards – and of the press. Briance wrote a book, *What Every Woman Should Know About Childbirth*, which struck a rather different tone to the *Sunday Express Baby Book*. It claimed that the 'simple antidote' to the need for pain relief was to be found in the Dick-Read system of complete relaxation for the mother, and that this education for the mother 'only involves a few hours of study and practice'. Briance made clear that she didn't like the 'present practice of delivering babies in general hospitals which is quite unsuitably implying that birth is an illness demanding hospitalisation'.[35] She also set up a network of antenatal classes to teach women the relaxation techniques espoused by Dick-Read, as well as campaigning against some of the brutal practices that were routine in hospitals at the time.

Briance's organisation even received a good-luck telegram from the Queen on its foundation, but what was soon to become the National Childbirth Trust upset the medical establishment. The issue swiftly became the subject of a furious battle of letters in the *British Medical Journal*. Doctors warned that 'elaborate training programmes' would lead to a mother considering 'herself an authority on childbirth of any sort whether natural or unnatural' and being 'prepared to enter into long arguments with her doctor about every detail', which would be 'exasperating and unreasonable'.[36] Another letter in April 1957 from an obstetrician thanked Dick-Read for his 'very great service in helping to wean us away from "unnatural childbirth"', but warned that 'the pendulum has always a tendency to swing too far due to excess of enthusiasm, and it is necessary to check it before any actual damage is done either to patients or to the nation's purse'.[37]

It took a long time for the pendulum to swing, in any case. At the time, Briance was swimming against a very strong tide: the general movement was taking the NHS towards *more* hospital births. The Cranbrook conclusions were followed by another committee examining maternity services led by gynaecologist Sir John Peel, which recommended in 1970 that hospitals have the capacity for 100 per cent of all births to take place on a ward rather than at home. The Peel Report stated: 'The greater safety of hospital confinement for mother and child justifies this objective.' But it didn't produce the evidence for this claim of greater safety. Neither did it recommend that women be given the choice between a home and hospital birth. That only came in 1993, when the Conservative government published *Changing Childbirth*, a report giving women more control.

Peel entrenched a change already under way in the balance of power between doctors and midwives. Lorna Muirhead began practising in the 1960s, and rose to become the president of the Royal College of Midwives in later life. She worked on many home deliveries in that time, and was agonised by the half-hour wait for the 'flying squad' of an ambulance, an obstetrician, anaesthetist, midwife and medical student who attended complicated home deliveries. 'Half an hour was a lifetime with a fitting woman, a woman haemorrhaging, or a second twin lying transversely,' she wrote. 'Perhaps this is why I do not share the contemporary views about the merit of home birth, or birth in freestanding maternity units.' She was relieved when the Peel Report recommended all births take place in a hospital, but this advice caused what she felt to be an erosion of her profession – and an overextension in the power of the obstetricians. The doctors 'believed that they bore ultimate responsibility for all pregnancies', and their rightful interventions in complicated labours soon 'spilled over into normal labour'. Muirhead felt her generation of midwives were largely too busy to spot the erosion of their role.[38] But by the late 1970s, a group of them were becoming increasingly upset by what they felt was 'obstetric violence' – part of a wider culture of male violence against women. They set up the Association of Radical Midwives, which held rallies against birth being overly medicalised and against mothers being confined to their beds in hospital against their wishes.

Hospital births are still the dominant mode of delivery in the NHS today, with 2.4 per cent of all live births taking place at home. But Briance, the radical midwives and their fellow travellers did push the pendulum further when it came to the concept of a 'natural birth'. It's still not entirely clear, though, whether those campaigners of the 1960s really succeeded in putting the mother, rather than the system, at the centre.

5. Forwards and backwards

By the end of the 1960s, humans were walking on the moon. They were swapping in human hearts and making them beat in the chests of seriously ill patients. They were working out how to start life outside the womb, and how to examine the body without cutting it open. The moon landings were the culmination of a space race, a global dash to conquer the great beyond. In the medical world, the same era saw similar furious competitions, to pioneer new ways of saving – and starting – lives. The earth almost stopped spinning as everyone stood still to watch the grainy televised images of Neil Armstrong and Buzz Aldrin in their space suits. They were instant celebrities. So were some of the doctors whose pioneering work changed medicine for ever.

Medicine's own moon landing came in the form of the heart transplant. The first such procedure didn't take place on the NHS. By the time a British team managed to get everything in place to perform this operation, which had enthralled the world, they were carrying out the tenth such procedure ever. The first heart transplant took place in 1967, in Cape Town, South Africa. After the operation, the recipient lived just eighteen days, but the doctor, Christiaan Barnard, carried out another operation a month later on a patient named Philip Blaiberg, who survived for nearly two years.

For years, there had been a global race to carry out a human heart transplant. In 1963, British heart surgeon Dr Donald Longmore and his colleague Sir Thomas Sellors applied for a grant from the British Heart Foundation to work on heart transplants. 'We were told that the roars of laughter could be heard two or three blocks away,' Longmore later recalled.[1] But the BHF did give the pair £6,000 – a tidy sum at the time – and they rented a laboratory at the Royal Veterinary College. There, they carried out all manner of surgeries on animals – including heart–lung transplants from dogs to sheep, sheep to pigs and so on – until the college found out what they were up to and panicked. After taking legal advice, the college decided that it would benefit them to have pioneering surgeons working on the premises, but the initial panic was a premonition of the angst to come in the medical world about this surgery. Some surgeons were trying live transplants on pigs, with the animals escaping and running off down the street.[2] Others, including Antony de Bono, a heart surgeon at the Hammersmith Hospital, had to abandon their work because they did not have enough funding to keep experimenting.

When Longmore eventually found a human patient at the National Heart Hospital who was keen to receive a transplant, he found himself surrounded by an angry crowd of colleagues who issued him with an ultimatum. They told him to 'have nothing to do with this disreputable heart transplant business, you'll bring the hospital into disrepute and if you don't promise not to carry on with your research and not to go on in this area, we will materially damage your career'.[3] Longmore ignored them and started trying to recruit donors. In 1968, he found one.

Patrick Ryan was a building worker who was brain-dead after a catastrophic accident at work. He was just twenty-six years old. Longmore raced in his Lagonda to King's College Hospital, and returned driving behind an ambulance carrying Ryan. Together with two other surgeons – Keith Ross and Donald Ross – Longmore kept Ryan's heart going until they were in the operating theatre at the National Heart Hospital. Keith Ross had the job of taking the heart out of Ryan, with colleagues watching in the gallery of the theatre. Not all of them were thrilled by this highly experimental surgery. Dr Jane Somerville was one of the physicians to the transplant team, and was shocked by what she witnessed. 'The absolute horror of seeing a live patient without a heart in their chest . . . I can remember it to this day . . . it was almost a revulsion.' Another doctor, Ann Naylor, a registrar at the time, told a colleague she had been 'very upset after the operation because here she had, as it were, a live human being and then they snatched his heart away'.

In the adjoining theatre, though, was Donald Ross with Frederick West, a 45-year-old patient with heart failure. His new heart was carried through in a bowl of saline, and the surgeons set to work. Keith Ross described the 'intensely dramatic moment' when the heart 'became pink and began to beat when the aortic clamp was released'. He added: 'One was aware, very much I think, while this was going on, that this was a historic moment and slightly unreal in the relative calm of the operating theatre at the National Heart Hospital.'

The world outside the hospital was anything but calm. One of the doctors at the hospital had been so excited that they hadn't been able to contain themselves, and had tipped off the press – meaning journalists were crowding the street waiting for news of the operation, to the extent that it 'looked like a Royal Wedding being watched', with patients hanging out of hospital windows to see what was going on. The transplant team were horrified to discover that their entreaties to leave Ryan's family alone went ignored: Longmore learned that while the dying man's wife was gravely ill, two reporters broke into her parents' home, stole the wedding photograph from the mantelpiece and had a fight over it.[4]

When they emerged from the operation seven hours later, elated by the success of that pink beating heart, the doctors gave a press conference where they – slightly inexplicably – ended up waving Union Jacks in celebration. The national press was delighted: here was the NHS's own moon landing. The operation, the tenth heart transplant in the world, was naturally front-page news, with the beaming faces (and Union Jacks) of the team plastered all over the place.

The reaction of the medical world was rather different. The *BMJ* was flooded with angry letters from physicians who felt the National Heart Hospital had set up a 'circus' of 'somewhat disturbing publicity'. One correspondent wrote, just days after the successful operation had been announced, that 'I and many of my colleagues are disgusted by this type of publicity, which is better saved for film stars, politicians and astronauts', and surmised that the only purpose of a press conference to celebrate the operation was 'to give to a bloodthirsty public lurid details of a surgical undertaking which ought to remain completely confidential'.[5] Over the following weeks, more letters poured in, with J. Kennedy Harper and Helen M. Harper writing that 'it would be difficult to imagine a more undignified, vulgar and tasteless display than that given by the medical personnel concerned with Britain's first heart transplant operation. Rows of smiling faces lined up for full publicity, team ties, Union Jacks and all . . . Words almost fail us to register our shock and dismay at this evidence of abandonment of the traditional code of professional conduct which has so long been part of British medicine. One dreads to think what abuses may result from this approach to what is undoubtedly a great surgical feat.'[6]

It is hard to imagine doctors expecting their colleagues to hide their lights under a bushel today. But the celebrations may have felt rather premature for the family of Frederick West. He was photographed listening to his new heart in his hospital bed, but died forty-five days later. Patrick Ryan's death was marked with an inquest where the coroner had to deal with conspiracy theories that the doctors had in fact murdered him for his heart. *Private Eye* ran a front page the week of West's death featuring the three surgeons (and their flags) with little speech bubbles saying 'one heart' and 'two spades' alongside the headline 'OK, so we goofed, say Heart Men'.[7]

The next few attempts were no more successful and no less controversial. In 1969, the third UK heart transplant operation descended into a bitter debate about whether the doctors removing the organ from 29-year-old student nurse Margaret Sinsbury, who had been in a road traffic accident, had actually been responsible for her death. The case made headlines across the world when it was revealed that doctors in Putney had been keeping her heart beating artificially with a machine until the transplant team could arrive. The medics had decided that she could not recover, but leading figures in the medical establishment and parliamentarians argued that the beating heart meant Sinsbury was still alive. The recipient, Charles Hendrick, died 107 days after his operation at Guy's Hospital. Margaret's parents had consented to her organs being used for transplant, but they were horrified to learn that the heart had not been cremated along with Hendrick's body.

Heart transplants had been world news. But the headlines were now about how they weren't working, and the media storm surrounding the doctors carrying them out was only growing. The surgeons didn't know how to manage a transplanted heart, and they knew even less about how to manage journalists. They ended up hiring someone to do their public relations, John Gorst, who had just finished representing pilots flying for the British Overseas Airways Corporation (BOAC) in one of the many industrial disputes of the time. He started to take control of matters for the individuals concerned, but by this point it was too late for the transplant programme: a clinical moratorium on the experiments was put in place. Sir George Godber, who was in his final years as Chief Medical Officer by this point, spoke to the clinicians working in the field 'to consider whether it would be best to continue work in human patients or to await the outcome of further work in animals'. Those he spoke to 'agreed unanimously' on a letter to the relevant hospitals suggesting that 'further human transplants were delayed until more research had been done'.[8]

It wasn't until August 1979 that a surgeon managed to carry out a successful heart transplant in the UK, when Terence English performed the operation on 52-year-old Keith Castle at Royal Papworth Hospital. Castle was the first UK recipient to even be discharged from hospital after the surgery, and he lived for more than five years post-transplant, having woken up asking whether his football team, Fulham, had won their most recent match. His survival was against the odds, not just because English didn't consider him to be an ideal patient for the procedure, but also because the moratorium on transplantation was still in place.

English was from South Africa, and had started life as an engineer before changing his mind and moving into medicine. He was a confident surgeon, unimpressed by the practices and behaviour of Barnard (and therefore surprised when Barnard ended up being the winner of the heart transplant arms race).[9] He had spent the five years before the successful transplant surgery trying to persuade colleagues at Papworth Hospital – then a pretty small institution in the Cambridgeshire Fens. Not all of those colleagues were receptive to his arguments: indeed, out of the two cardiologists at the hospital, one was 'neutral' in his stance and the other strongly opposed 'on clinical, ethical and religious grounds', to the extent that he repeatedly accused English of removing hearts from patients who were still alive.[10]

That accusation stemmed from an ongoing confusion about whether brain death even existed, and how one might diagnose it. The medical establishment was wrestling with questions that had simply not been conceivable at the start of the health service; now answering them properly was an essential part of maintaining its position of trust in the British psyche. There had, though, been developments – and not just in what constituted 'brain death' but also in the immunology necessary to keep a donor heart working in a new body. By 1978, English had found two patients who might be suitable for transplant. He tried to get approval and funding from the Ministry of Health's Transplant Advisory Panel, but it was rejected: 'I got a letter from the chief medical officer saying no and refusing to let me do one-off operations. I thought, blow you, I'm going to do this anyway.' So he went in secret to the head of the area health authority responsible for his hospital, and she 'tacitly and courageously agreed' to back his two surgeries.[11]

The next problem was that English couldn't find any hearts. And, perhaps more frustratingly, he couldn't find any doctors willing to help him find hearts. He had to try to charm neurosurgeons who might have a suitable brain-dead patient, but the ones he approached were either too busy or opposed to what he was up to. Then, it all changed. On 14 January 1979, a potential donor arrived at Addenbrooke's Hospital in Cambridge. English sprang into action. There is never much time to lose when a transplant is in the offing, but in this instance, things were even more desperate. The intended recipient, Charles McHugh, was by now so seriously ill that his heart actually stopped when the donor organ was on its way to the theatre. The surgeon had to decide whether to go on with the operation at all, as McHugh might have sustained brain damage. He did get on with it, the heart started beating, and a modest press conference was held a couple of days later to try to stop a repeat of the 1968 circus. But McHugh never recovered, remaining on a ventilator and dying seventeen days later.

English's colleagues were horrified: he was hauled into a meeting with Roy Calne, the professor of surgery at Cambridge University whose approval he had sought for a heart transplant programme at Papworth in the first place. Calne told him in no uncertain terms that he had 'set back cardiac transplantation in Britain by five years' and was also worried about the effect on his own kidney transplantation programme.[12] English disagreed, and started waiting patiently again for a donor. On 18 August, he found one whose parents had explicitly said all organs should be used for transplantation. The recipient would be Keith Castle.

Castle was a cheerful cockney. He was also a heavy smoker with a chronic duodenal ulcer and vascular disease. This was very much not ideal, though he obligingly lied to other doctors about whether he'd given up smoking so he wouldn't let English down. The press followed his progress avidly: a reporter for the *Evening Standard* the following year was much taken by the effect of the new heart on Castle's hair, saying: 'Surgeon Terence English has given the once-balding builder a crop of new curls on top of the gift of life.' Blood was 'reaching parts of his body that his old heart had not pumped to for years' and so 'ears that were almost deaf can hear again, and the skin is young-looking'.[13] Castle lived for more than five years after the transplant, having previously been given weeks at the most. English and a number of other heart transplant patients from Papworth attended the funeral at Lambeth Crematorium in July 1985. He spoke to the press after the service, saying: 'Keith was a truly remarkable man who, in his own way, did more for cardiac transplantation than our medical efforts.'[14]

It is the sort of kind comment you might expect at a funeral, but it also raises an interesting question, which is who should really take credit for the establishment of the heart transplant programme in the NHS? The decade-long moratorium meant surgeons were watching advances being made in the US rather than working on the immunosuppressant drugs and other practices essential for getting the recipient up and out of bed. The health service was not a vehicle for innovation in this instance. Perhaps the obstacles thrown up against English and other transplant enthusiasts were entirely justifiable, given the ethical concerns. And perhaps innovation will always need a figure like English who is willing to go around bureaucrats in order to get their way.

The health service did not provide the additional money the programme needed, either. Indeed, in his own book about the health service, Donald Longmore complains that the Department of Health's response to the prospect of heart transplantation was 'nothing to do with "was it a real medical advance?" but "how much did it cost and how could they prevent it becoming commonplace?" '[15] He claims that a 'large team of paperclip counters [were] sent to "investigate" and they came up with prohibitive costs. They took no notice of any facts and leaked to the press a story about the huge resources which would be needed for heart transplantation, which would in turn deny many patients lower cost treatments.'[16]

It was thanks to the British Heart Foundation that Longmore started up his operations, and again to the BHF as well as the National Heart Research Fund that English was able to carry out his successful transplants. That fund was set up by pioneering cardiovascular surgeon David Watson in 1967, after he became frustrated by the number of cardiac patients dying and the lack of research into how to save them. English – who later became president of the BHF – says 'the charities were absolutely essential to getting the work going; they were there before the state and they were the ones who gave us the money that we needed'. He believes that the turning point for the Department of Health came when he and others managed to persuade those paperclip counters whom Longmore complained about to evaluate transplants not just in terms of the raw cost, but also the benefits to patients who, having been at death's door, were able to live good lives after their surgery. Then, he says, the DoH became 'really very good' at running the transplant programme, keeping a tight limit on the number of centres which were permitted to carry out the operations, and withdrawing permission from a couple whose standards dropped.[17]

The involvement of the NHRF and the BHF in the early heart transplant operations shows that the success of the NHS is not just down to the efforts of and money provided by the state. It is also about the charities working in medical research and funding individual hospitals as well. As the English transplant programme expanded, the hospitals involved started asking for more donations. In 1982, hospitals were given more freedom to raise money for their activities through charitable donations. One advert in *The Times* in that year from Harefield Hospital sought to capitalise on a recent BBC Two documentary called *Heart Transplant* that followed its work, pleading: 'Don't let our programme end.' It said the TV series had become 'essential viewing for many people . . . but not as essential as the actual Heart Transplant programme has become for our patients. Long after the TV programme ends our programme must continue but with less than half of the £20,000 needed for each transplant operation provided by the NHS – we must rely on your support. Without your help, lives will be lost, research will stop and the programme will end.'[18]

Today, there is a network of more than 230 charities supporting hospitals and care in certain regions. Much of the funding for medical research comes from charities such as the BHF. The NHS has never been a monolith – more of a web that reaches across society. Perhaps that is one of the reasons the British public feel so strongly about it: they don't just fund it through general (and more recently, hypothecated) taxation, but also through their own donations, inspired in part by the people who, like Keith Castle, walked out of hospital with a new, pink, beating heart.

If the first human heart transplant was a medical moon landing, the first 'test tube baby' was an event bigger than both. Louise Brown was born a decade after the surgeons at the National Heart Hospital completed their first surgery. The years running up to her arrival in the delivery unit at Oldham Hospital had been full of excited, breathless headlines about the possibility of doctors successfully implanting an embryo they had fertilised outside the mother's womb. In this arms race, some doctors even claimed that they'd already succeeded in the first-ever IVF births, with the first – an Italian doctor, Daniele Petrucci – announcing, without any evidence such as, er, babies to back it up, that he'd produced twenty-seven such babies in the early

1960s. Among the British doctors trying to win the race was Douglas Bevis, an obstetrician in Sheffield who claimed in 1974 that he had successfully delivered three 'test tube babies', but refused to offer any further details in case the children spent the rest of their lives being ridiculed about their origins. The difficulties were many: how to fertilise the egg outside the womb – in a petri dish, not a test tube, incidentally – and then implant the embryo in the womb successfully and convince the mother's body that it had conceived, so that a pregnancy could progress successfully. Would there be risks to the foetus of infection or physical damage caused by its insertion?

The eventual winners, Oldham gynaecologist Patrick Steptoe and two Cambridge scientists – the physiologist Robert Edwards and embryologist Jean Purdy – made sure that an NHS hospital was the site of the first-ever baby conceived through in vitro fertilisation. But the NHS can hardly take the credit for their work. They and the other pioneering doctors in this field had to self-fund, and took flak from colleagues who felt that their experiments were getting in the way of their 'proper' work. Steptoe set up in a small disused theatre at the local cottage hospital, Dr Kershaw's Hospital, and relied on local charities for money. John Webster was a junior doctor in Steptoe's team. He later recalled: 'A lot of people felt that this research was done at the expense of Patrick Steptoe's national health practice and this was all done out of hours, we would go along to Kershaw's early in the morning, 6 or 7 o'clock in the morning or late at night, 10 o'clock at night, so all this research was done after doing a busy day in the NHS.'[19]

Edwards read about the work on keyhole surgery that Steptoe was becoming renowned for, and realised that this could help him in the techniques he was developing. Through laparoscopy, they could collect the eggs from a woman's ovaries for fertilisation outside the body. The trio shuttled between Oldham and Cambridge, Steptoe with a rabbit on the passenger seat of his car.[20] The bunny wasn't just to keep him company on the long journeys; it was carrying eggs taken from women who'd been undergoing surgery in Oldham in its womb, to keep them warm. The pair started to try to fertilise and then implant embryos in women desperate to get pregnant. Many of them suffered from blocked fallopian tubes, which made it near impossible to conceive without a complicated and risky surgery. One of them was Lesley Brown.

Lesley, twenty-nine, and her husband, John, had been trying for nine years to conceive, and were growing desperate to the extent that their marriage was struggling.[21] Their GP in Bristol, Dr Ruth Hinton, had read about Steptoe's work, and wrote to him. Unlike other patients who'd come to Oldham, Lesley became pregnant on the first attempt. As her due date in July 1978 approached, the media circus around the hospital grew and grew. A month before her baby was due, Lesley registered high blood pressure and was admitted to hospital, where she was kept in isolation to hide her from the banks of television cameras and journalists assembling outside the hospital. Three weeks later, she was diagnosed with toxaemia, and Steptoe decided to deliver the baby by C-section. First, though, he tricked the press, driving ostentatiously away from the hospital in his white Mercedes and then slipping back in later. Webster recalled that the team even had to prepare the mother 'by torchlight – so no one would see her room light up'. He added:

> Everything was riding on this moment – the whole team was hyped up. If anything had gone wrong, it would have destroyed everything we had worked towards. There was an incredible air of anticipation in the theatre. My job was to hand Patrick the instruments. Gradually he was able to place his hand under the baby's head and I helped push the baby out. The theatre was silent. Louise finally emerged – a perfectly normal, healthy baby girl – and let out a huge cry. Steptoe shouted 'that's what I like to hear, good lung development!' The relief was palpable. It had been a routine Caesarean delivery but we knew history had been made.[22]

There was an authorised camera crew at the hospital. They captured those first cries that Louise made, and the footage was broadcast on ITN and the BBC three weeks later at her mother's request. Lesley lay on the operating table and, after a while, 'the only thing I could think to say to [Steptoe] was thank you'.[23] Meanwhile a team of doctors started the first of a series of checks that went far beyond what was normal for a newborn: they were concerned that this new method of conception might have caused an abnormality in the new baby. Eventually they were able to tell Steptoe, Edwards and Purdy what the three of them had been hoping to hear: this was a normal baby.

The world around the mother and the most extraordinary normal baby exploded. Everyone wanted a piece of this story. But none more so than the many other couples – around one in six – who were infertile and had largely given up the prospect of having a baby. This was a medical breakthrough, an almost inconceivable conception, but it was also a moment of hope. Edwards himself said: 'Steptoe and I were deeply affected by the desperation felt by couples who so wanted to have children. We had a lot of critics but we fought like hell for our patients.'

It was quite a fight. Edwards repeatedly tried to get the NHS and DoH interested in his work. In 1974, he wrote to the ministry arguing that his method 'could avoid many operations now carried out, which could become unnecessary'. The Medical Research Council repeatedly refused to offer funding, with some referees for the grant applications complaining that the publicity the team sought had put them off. Even after the second IVF baby, a boy named Alastair Montgomery, had been born the following year, Edwards and Steptoe found the health service refusing to offer the technique to infertile couples as treatment. In late 1981, Edwards wrote to the Cambridgeshire Health Authority pointing out that 'it is professionally accepted that our approach offers the only hope of conception for some women' and that 'these patients have paid their contribution to the NHS and, now they want treatment, they are not being allowed to receive it'. The local health authority's argument in response was that it couldn't afford what was a very expensive procedure: 'Our current allocation is insufficient to maintain the service that we already provide. There is, therefore, no way in which the Health Authority can meet the expense of NHS patients attending your clinic.'[24]

Edwards, Purdy and Steptoe had realised that if they were going to offer any couples hope of children, they would have to do so privately, and so they set up the Bourn Hall Clinic in Cambridgeshire. Purdy found a derelict country house which she converted into the first-ever IVF clinic, opening in 1980. Some NHS hospitals did start to offer the treatment, but found they were quickly inundated and unable to afford to treat the number of couples seeking their help. By 1984, there were just eight hospitals who ran IVF treatments, and a number of those refused to treat people from outside their area. The problem for the NHS and for couples trying to pay privately for treatment was that IVF was very expensive: each course cost around £3,000. The average annual salary was £6,000, and the health service itself was, by now, under significant financial pressure.

The barriers weren't just financial, of course. This immaculate conception had shaken the world morally, too. Cardinal Albino Luciani, who became Pope shortly after Louise Brown was born, gave an interview in which he appeared to compare the development to weapons of mass destruction, saying:

> I share only in part the enthusiasm of those who are applauding the progress of science and technology after the birth of the English baby girl. Progress is a very fine thing, but not every kind of progress is helpful to mankind. The ABC weapons [atomic, bacteriological and chemical] have been a kind of progress, but at the same time, a disaster for mankind. Even if the possibility of having children in vitro does not bring about disaster, it at least poses some enormous risks. For example: the natural ability to conceive sometimes produces, as a result, malformed children; won't the ability to conceive artificially produce more? If so, won't the scientist faced with new problems be acting like the 'sorcerer's apprentice', who unleashes powerful forces without being able to contain and dominate them?[25]

He went on to worry about whether the process might allow 'baby manufacturing', which would cater 'for those who cannot or will not contract a valid marriage'. The newspapers were full of headlines predicting 'Frankenbabies' and warning of 'rent-a-wombs'; indeed, the very term 'test tube baby' was often used in a rather dismissive tone. It became clear that this medical advance raised huge ethical questions for everyone, not just those with a particular religious world view. The British government set up a committee to examine it, with distinguished philosopher Mary Warnock as its chair.

Warnock's committee, which reported in 1984, had to consider the moral questions around IVF, and other treatments for fertility which had been in use for some time – such as artificial insemination, either by a woman's husband or a donor. Was it acceptable, for instance, to create more embryos than would be transferred, and then allow those superfluous to requirements to 'die'? Then there were the questions that Steptoe, Purdy and Edwards had come up against – of resources. The inquiry considered an argument 'which draws an analogy between IVF and heart transplants, or other forms of "high technology" medical care, and asks whether the country can afford such expensive treatment which benefits only a few, and whether money could not be "better" spent, that is, with beneficial effects for more people, elsewhere'.

Its conclusion was that IVF was 'an acceptable means of treating infertility' and that it should continue under a licensing and inspection regime, which would be applied to artificial insemination by donor. That regime would be administered by a new quango, the Human Fertilisation and Embryology Authority (HFEA). As for whether the NHS should provide IVF, the recommendation was that it should, but that it didn't necessarily need to be made available at every hospital. What was important, the report argued, was that NHS centres were 'distributed throughout the UK'.[26]

Health authorities continued to refuse to fund IVF, though, and by 1985 an investigation by the *Observer* found that NHS infertility clinics were asking couples to donate hundreds of pounds to their research funds as a means of paying for their treatment. The National Association for the Childless complained that 'the government's attitude is that no one dies of infertility' and so it wasn't a priority for funding. At the Jessop Hospital for Women in Sheffield, the *Observer* reported, women were being asked for £350. In other areas, hospitals were closing their waiting lists.[27]

The cost to the NHS didn't just relate to the IVF itself. The method led to many multiple pregnancies because it initially stimulated the ovaries to produce a number of eggs – sometimes as many as twenty – at once, rather than the one which is normally released as part of a woman's monthly cycle. Then, for a better chance at success, doctors would often implant up to three embryos in the mother's womb. A multiple pregnancy carries a far higher risk of infant mortality, as well as the need for intensive care for the infants after birth due to premature delivery. The risks to the mother are also considerable. This all came at no small expense to the health service – as well as being highly traumatic for a couple who may have longed for a child over many years, only to risk losing the babies after birth. Research in 2005 found that the cost to the NHS of a multiple birth was significantly higher than for singleton births – £3,313 for singles, £9,122 for twins and £32,354 for triplets.[28] In 2007, the HFEA launched a campaign, 'One at a Time', to bring down the multiple-birth rate following IVF. At that stage, one in four births were multiples, but the authority wanted to make it 10 per cent. Just over ten years later, it recommended that clinical commissioning groups (the organisations who were at this stage responsible for commissioning care within each area) incentivise single embryo transfer.

Guidelines for the NHS now are that couples diagnosed with a cause of infertility should be referred for three rounds of IVF. But it remains the case that waiting lists are long, and a postcode lottery exists that means women in some areas are offered three cycles on the NHS and in others just one. The treatment today costs the health service around £3,000 per cycle. The HFEA continues to regulate the use of embryos, and has been lauded as a successful and – in the words of one of its former chairs, Ruth Deech – 'very British' institution which has ensured a rational and calm approach to a still-controversial area of medicine. IVF was a British invention. It's a little harder to call it an NHS invention. And it is still hard to say it is an NHS priority today.

The CT scanner isn't just an invention that started within the NHS and is therefore part of the British story thanks to the health service. It is such a British invention that it even has the Beatles as part of its story. The first computerised tomography scan in the world was carried out on a 41-year-old patient at Atkinson Morley Hospital in

Wimbledon, London, on 1 October 1971. It changed medicine for ever, opening up what had previously been a mysterious part of the body. Before the CT scan, there were few ways of detecting problems with the brain: you couldn't carry out exploratory operations on it and X-rays would only show the outlines of the skull in black-and-white, not the grey matter itself.

The CT scan was the invention of an engineer called Godfrey Hounsfield. Hounsfield worked for EMI, the huge electronics and music company, which had made vast sums of money from a band it had signed a decade ago called the Beatles. It employed Hounsfield to work on radar and guided weapons. He was a naturally curious fellow, and became more and more intrigued by the developing world of computing. The idea for a new scanner came to him on a weekend ramble in the countryside (which is, of course, where all good ideas appear). Instead of admiring the flora and fauna around him, Hounsfield found himself gazing at a picnic basket and thinking, 'Wouldn't it be nice if I had many readings taken from all angles through a box?' It's not necessarily a thought many of us have on a walk, and neither is what came next: 'Wouldn't it be nice if I could reconstruct in 3D what was actually in the box from those random direction readings taken through the box, and, of course, turning the three-dimensional object into a series of slices?' Back from his walk and at the EMI offices, Hounsfield's extraordinary mind led him through the practical stages of this experiment using a computer program, and he was surprised by how well it worked. He and his colleagues were 'quite excited' by it, and he then realised that it might be relevant to medicine. So he 'went to the Department of Health . . . waving this piece of paper and saying, look, I can reconstruct a picture, a slice through the body, with great accuracy'.[29]

A number of senior officials at the DoH were quite excited, too. Dr Evan Lennon, the radiological adviser to the department, Cliff Gregory, the Chief Scientific Officer, and Gordon Higson, who ran the Supplies Technology Division at the department and ensured Hounsfield got funding to start developing his discoveries further. EMI matched what the DoH was giving the engineer. Initially, he wanted to build a machine that would scan the entire body, but a group of radiologists from three hospitals – Atkinson Morley, Hammersmith and Northwick Park – and DoH advisers persuaded him to focus solely on the head, because it could be kept still for the twenty minutes it took to produce the scan. Those three radiologists weren't typical of their discipline in the NHS, though. Hounsfield found that the majority of radiologists were 'so steeped in their X-ray pictures that they couldn't really grasp the importance of this at all. They couldn't grasp the sensitivity. They said, so what? They couldn't understand that they would be seeing much more. The result was very discouraging.' EMI's top brass began to wonder if their engineer was working on a vastly expensive white elephant.

Higson took a different view, and placed an order on behalf of the DoH for three machines before Hounsfield had built even one. When that scanner was ready, it was Atkinson Morley that took it. The hospital's neuroradiologist James Ambrose found a patient who was suitable for the first image, and they produced the scan, which was then printed onto film and whisked away to be developed. When they saw it, Hounsfield said: 'There was a beautiful picture of a circular cyst right in the middle of the frontal lobe and, of course, it excited everyone in the hospital who knew about the project.'[30] Previously, Ambrose and his colleagues in neurology and neurosurgery would have had to guess what was going on in the brain based on symptoms. Now, they didn't have to join up the dots to make the picture. It was in front of them: an accurate image of a world previously locked up in bone. Had it not been for the excitement of officials in the DoH, and the clear-sightedness of a number of doctors working in the NHS, this technology might have stayed locked away for much longer.

Much of this chapter has covered advances in healthcare which led to the doctors pioneering them being accused of 'playing God'. The NHS itself has become known as Britain's national religion (more on that later), which is a reference to the high regard Brits hold it in. And institutionally, it does bear more than a passing resemblance to our formal national religion, Anglicanism. Both the NHS and the Church of England were born out of compromise rather than ideological purity: Elizabeth I tried to disentangle the religious conflicts that her father had ignited and her siblings entrenched, with a compromise allowing the Church to be 'both Catholic and Reformed'. Bevan did not set up a perfect service, but the service that it was possible to set up. Where the comparison ends, though, is that the compromises and idiosyncrasies of Anglicanism are well known and often embraced by its adherents. The NHS, by contrast, has always maintained a veneer of precious purity.

The reality is of course quite different, and has been ever since the service's inception. One of the many compromises Bevan *had* to reach when he was setting up the health service was whether hospital doctors could continue to treat private patients. He had feared that not offering the opportunity to continue with so-called pay beds in hospitals would be to lose the consent of specialists altogether, which in turn would make a comprehensive health service impossible. And so it was that, by the 1970s, entire floors of new-build hospitals contained paying patients who could jump the (growing) queues for treatment and enjoyed a better standard of care than their NHS contemporaries. Pay beds had long been a fact of life – Enoch Powell found himself having to fix a situation in the early 1960s where the charging regime for the beds was no longer complying with the legislation enabling them. He wrote in a short memo to civil servants that 'if Charing Cross want a gold bidet in every private room, they can work out the resultant charge and make up their own minds'.[31] It was at that same hospital that, over a decade later, pay beds stopped being a fact of NHS life and became a matter of bitter political controversy.

This was the decade of medical science going whoosh! It was also the decade of British political life sinking into despair. It was a period of discontent and strife, popularly remembered for the strikes, three-day week, power cuts, uncollected bin bags and unburied bodies, and rampant inflation. The health service was not exempt from this turmoil. By 1974, the NHS had undergone a great deal of change, including a vastly controversial Conservative reorganisation led by Sir Keith Joseph. Labour had opposed that, but on winning the 1974 election discovered it would be impossible to reverse the changes, which abolished the original tripartite structure of the service and brought the administrative functions of hospitals, GPs and local authority health services together. For the first time, community services came into the NHS, having existed outside it before, which goes some way to explaining why they remain the poorest part of our health landscape even today. New Area Health Authorities, which followed local authority boundaries, were responsible for the planning and delivery of healthcare. They would be advised by Community Health Councils, which scrutinised the performance of the AHAs, as well as being able to take up patient complaints and advise ministers on policy.

More painfully for Labour on coming into power, the state of the economy meant the party that had founded the health service was unable to maintain its commitment to it through spending: the 1970–74 Tory government increased spending on average by 4.3 per cent a year, while Labour could manage only 1.5 per cent.

The new Health and Social Security Secretary was Barbara Castle. Ironically, given what was to come, she had been a patient in a pay bed herself in the 1960s: a statement from her department, reported by *The Times* in July 1974, admitted that she had 'received treatment for sinus trouble in a private room at University College Hospital in order to be able to continue essential work which, as a Cabinet minister, involved secret papers'.[32] Castle was, by this point, a political icon. The neat, flame-haired, deeply socialist young Barbara Betts had turned up at her first Labour Party conference in 1943 to give a fiery speech attacking her own party's failure to press the government with sufficient vigour and force it to implement the Beveridge Report. 'We want jam today, not jam tomorrow,' she told conference attendees, who were much taken with her. Reporters watching had a similar reaction, to the extent that the *Mirror* put her on its front page as the voice of the party's future. The night editor, Ted Castle, decided to investigate this 'voice of the future' further, and promptly fell in love with her. 'It got me a husband and a constituency,' she joked.[33] She was a minister on and off for a decade as Labour washed in and out of power during the political turmoil of the 1960s and '70s. In 1968, she was the Secretary of State for Employment and

Productivity and personally intervened in a strike at the Ford plant in Dagenham. That industrial action was led by female sewing machinists who had discovered that they would be paid 85 per cent of what equivalent male colleagues were earning. Castle brokered a deal with eight of the strike leaders to end the strike, and this marked the start of equal pay legislation.

Castle had a hot temper, and yet doubted herself constantly, telling her biographer Wilfred De'Ath, of her 'own agonising heart-searchings. You say, "Am I just God's most arrogant bitch?" '[34] Michael Foot mused that she had a 'great capacity for enjoying life, but I believe she gets herself into tight neurotic knots and that these can burst out into great invective against people around her when they occur . . . I've heard her on occasions, at dinner parties where I've been, behave in a way that I think is outrageous; she can turn on people and deride them contemptuously and really let loose.'[35] She was a Bevanite, much concerned not just with preserving the legacy of the man she knew personally and admired deeply, but also with trying to better it. That desire had already led her into trouble: a year after the Dagenham strike, she was responsible for a White Paper called *In Place of Strife*, which was designed to echo Bevan's *In Place of Fear*. The reforms, which she had drafted secretly with Prime Minister Harold Wilson – who was very loyal to Castle – would have restricted the power of the trade unions, including forcing them to hold a ballot before calling a strike. It led to a furious row in Wilson's Cabinet, and Castle was forced to retreat, licking her wounds. So by the time she took on her fourth and final Cabinet position, she was an icon, but one whose power was very much on the wane.

Her solution to this was to embark on what her biographer Anne Perkins describes as 'her boldest, her most political and her least successful' reform yet. It was to take on a 'triumph that had eluded Bevan' and remove the fly in the ointment of his NHS.[36] She wanted to abolish the pay beds.

Castle had long opposed these private beds, writing about them in her own personal manifesto in the 1955 general election. But by 1974, the political landscape was changing enough to make it possible for her to do something about it. By now, there were just 4,500 pay beds in NHS hospitals. As a proportion of the health service's capacity, they were meaningless, making up less than half a per cent of the patients the NHS treated annually. As a political symbol, though, they were irresistible to trade unions (well, some of them) and Labour Party activists at a time of intense industrial strife. Even within the NHS, industrial action was already taking place: a 1973 strike by ancillary workers in the service had made clear that the government couldn't rely on the traditional reluctance to withdraw services that would affect sick patients.

Rumours had been swirling for a few years about the injustice of pay beds in practice. An inquiry by the Parliamentary Expenditure Committee had heard evidence that the beds allowed people to pay to jump the waiting list, and that consultants were deliberately keeping waiting lists long in order to encourage people to move over to their private practice. At the 1973 Labour Party conference, Castle received noisy applause for promising to 'eliminate private practice from our NHS' and that there would be 'no queue jumping'. The party's manifesto at the February 1974 election promised to 'phase out private practice from the hospital service'. Labour returned to power, but without a majority. In the ensuing months, the pay beds issue exploded. In June 1974, the National Union of Public Employees started a strike at Charing Cross Hospital. It had not, as Powell had sarcastically written, installed gold bidets in every private room. But the hospital did have a floor with twenty-two patients in pay beds, which quickly became nicknamed the 'Fulham Hilton'. The NUPE workers refused to look after these patients, a practice known as 'blacking'. The action spread across the country to other hospitals, with NUPE general secretary Alan Fisher predicting that it would lead to the end of private treatment within the NHS.[37] Hospital consultants did not take kindly to this, threatening through the British Medical Association their own work-to-rule action unless Castle took action to ensure Area Health Authorities 'maintain the existing provision of government-approved private beds'. Castle and Wilson were caught in a bind. They still wanted to phase out pay beds. But they also disliked the idea of any patient being refused care as part of an industrial dispute. After a night of talks, in the early hours of 6 July 1974, Castle managed to get a deal to end the strike at Charing Cross and an agreement in principle with the BMA on the phasing out of private beds.[38]

Wilson was forced to call another election in October of that year to try to get a majority. He had spent much of the short session in Parliament since February publishing White Papers to show what a Labour government could do if it had the votes. The party won with a majority of just three. The paucity of the victory lulled the BMA into a false sense of security that Castle wouldn't even try to get her way on private practice in the health service. Castle, meanwhile, was convinced of the need to show her party and the (non-medical) trade unions that 'a Labour government still believed in socialism' and that 'it was possible to be a socialist in Cabinet, to live down for all time the humiliation of "In Place of Strife", to establish her place in the pantheon of Labour heroes'.[39] It wasn't a small ambition, and it led to one of the biggest and bitterest rows since the health service had been created.

Castle didn't initially anticipate how bad things were going to get. She wrote in one memo: 'I do not see that the proposals to control the development of the private sector will necessarily lead to major political difficulties with the medical profession.'[40] She was quickly proved wrong on that front. One of the problems was that Castle was by now also responsible for negotiating a new contract for consultants in the NHS, with the new proposals deeply unattractive to consultants who feared that alongside the abolition of pay beds, it would become financially unattractive for them to accept anything other than a full-time NHS contract.

In August 1975, the government published its consultative document, which proposed phasing out pay beds and licensing any new private-sector beds so that the total never exceeded the combined number of private hospital and NHS beds that existed on March 1974. The medical establishment was furious, sending a lengthy memo to Castle signed by seventeen different organisations – including the BMA, the Hospital Consultants and Specialists Association, the Junior Hospital Doctors Association, the Royal Colleges and the British Dental Association, and the Independent Hospital Group. The memo warned that the proposals would be 'profoundly damaging – to the community, to the NHS, and to the medical and dental professions'. They were, it alleged, 'calculated to lead to a full-scale confrontation between the Government and the medical and dental professions'. It repeated the strongly held suspicion of many doctors that this was just one of the 'first steps towards the elimination of the independent sector of medicine altogether'. The authors of the memo then compared this to the principle of conscription, ending with this warning: 'If the doctrine is allowed to pass unchallenged in the NHS context, there is no assurance that it will not spread further and further on a gradually all-embracing programme. A logical step must be to institute "permits" to control travel – lest it result in migration – and ultimately the justification for the watch-tower, the search-light, and the Berlin Wall.'[41]

Yes, that's right: the proposals to phase out paid-for beds in National Health Service hospitals were allegedly the thin end of the wedge of a totalitarian society in Britain. The BMA was now insisting in communications that it had always supported the NHS, but while it may have forgotten its behaviour in the 1940s, it had not lost the hyperbolic language.

The problem was that each side was as stubborn and intemperate as the other. Throughout the dispute, Castle's own personality – and, she suspected, her sex – made things trickier. Castle, for her part, found the talks a 'misery', and she described the 'petulance' of some of the BMA's representatives in her diaries.[42] She also found her Cabinet colleagues were rather less excited than she was by the row. They ended up having fiery exchanges of letters with Castle, who repeatedly batted down their concerns. Denis Healey, the Chancellor of the Exchequer, was angered that Castle hadn't bothered to clear her policy with him before presenting a paper on it to Cabinet, and demanded she withdraw the paper. Then, in autumn 1975, the Chancellor of the Duchy of Lancaster, Harold Lever, warned her in a series of letters (which he copied to Wilson) that she was about to commit a grave error. He complained that her timetable for restricting private practice was only aggravating doctors' fears about her real agenda, adding, with a line that seemed particularly well-designed to upset the Bevanite Castle personally: 'I am convinced that your time-table needlessly ignores the need for gradual adjustment and the other historic conditions so well understood by Nye Bevan.'[43] Castle privately dismissed Lever as 'the impassioned voice in Cabinet for the constants in private practice who share his bridge tables' and described him as frightened of 'anything socialist'. She was no less forceful with him in her letters back. Wilson, on this, backed her, sneakily talking the Cabinet into what looked like a compromise for Castle by saying the government could be vague about the timetable. His minister spotted his trick, and pretended to accept it 'with a show of reluctance'. 'Harold at work rigging Cabinet is wonderful to behold,' she wrote in her diary.[44]

The prime minister had nevertheless recognised that he did now have a full-scale confrontation on his hands, and tried to quell it by announcing a Royal Commission on the NHS – though he refused to add pay beds to its terms of reference. By November, the consult-ants and juniors were announcing industrial action and Wilson decided he needed someone other than the 'Red Queen', as Castle was nicknamed, to break the stalemate. Lord Goodman, Arnold, was an enormous bear-shaped lawyer known for solving tricky disputes. He secretly acted as a go-between, finding a compromise with the consultants whereby there would be no phasing out of pay beds until there were alternative private facilities available. Castle didn't know until her visibly shocked private secretary told her. The implication was clear: the prime minister and Goodman had been working behind her back and had made it impossible for her to interfere. She was furious and humiliated.

Wilson was in Rome on 2 December, and returned tired and stressed about international matters at 3 a.m. on the morning of the 3rd. He and Castle had a stand-up row in Downing Street half an hour before the talks with the doctors were due to start, the prime minister snapping at Castle that he wasn't going to be told what to do. Castle shot back that her position would be intolerable if he took over the talks, and that the press were already circling her. 'You pay too much attention to the press,' was Wilson's reply, which grimly amused Castle. 'You will be playing into the hand of the Opposition,' she returned. 'Their whole line has been that you should be brought in because it is my "personality" that is preventing a settlement. They said that about Nye, too, when he was fighting to create the NHS. Do you think Clem Attlee would have intervened to take the negotiations out of Nye's hands at a crucial stage?' The shouting match was interrupted by an official who stepped nervously into the room to tell Wilson that Goodman was waiting downstairs. Castle trailed after the pair into the Cabinet room to face the doctors.[45] They did reach the bones of an agreement: within six months of the bill becoming law, 1,000 pay beds would be released to general NHS service. The rest would be phased out only when there were 'reasonably alternative facilities' available nearby.

Castle and Wilson continued to fight in angrily scrawled notes and during sour lunches, not least over a speech she had given about the 'wrecking mood' of the health professions who were taking 'unthinkable' industrial action. The papers duly wrote it up as 'Castle Rocks Peace Talks', which was the front-page splash of the *Daily Mail*. Eventually, the pair hammered out a compromise with the doctors, which they agreed on 15 December.

The agreement was by no means the end of the war, however. The doctors had already been marched up the hill of industrial action by their leaders, who were worried about the impact of marching them back down again. A ballot of the consultants still endorsed strike action, which blighted the health service for the next two months. The juniors were still on their protest against their contract, too, and it was this that caused the greatest strife in the NHS. The doctors described this as a 'heal-to-rule' strike – a play on the usual 'work-to-rule' used in industrial relations. Some moved to emergencies-only cover; others stuck to a forty-hour week. The result was that hospitals across the country were forced to close their emergency departments, and many their maternity services as well. Local newspapers began to list which casualty departments were closing and for how long, and which were only taking cases from certain areas. It didn't take much time for the horror stories to flood in. In Reading, a ten-year-old boy, Derek Giles, was refused admittance to two hospitals after a car hit him and broke his leg. The local paper described him going through a 'four-hour ordeal' in which the ambulance that arrived to collect him could not take him to Battle Hospital in the town because the casualty unit was closed, and he was then turned away from Wexham Park in Slough because the emergency unit there was full. Eventually he was admitted to Heatherwood Hospital in Ascot, where he was 'comfortable', but the distance was too far for his unemployed father – who had four other children to care for on his own – to be able to afford to travel to see him. It being December, the family feared he would have to spend Christmas on his own.[46] At Hayes Hospital, consultant surgeon John Piper and colleagues worked eighteen hours at a time to cover for the eight-hour days the juniors were sticking to. 'The signs of tiredness are beginning to reach the surface,' wrote the *Evening Standard* journalist who interviewed him. Piper was faced with agonising decisions as a result of the staff shortages. 'He had a 66-year-old woman patient on his hands brought to hospital with bleeding stomach ulcers,' the paper reported. 'Normally, he would have had full medical assistance, but none was available because of the dispute. He operated without his normal team.' The operation was a success and the patient recovering well, but Mr Piper pinned the blame squarely on Castle – not his juniors – for the dilemma he'd faced, and the exhausting hours he was working.[47]

By the time the action ended two months later, all parties had sustained serious wounds. Castle only survived in the job a few more months, losing it when Jim Callaghan took over as prime minister. She had sealed her own fate with a number of mistakes, not all of them related to pay beds. She had told Harold Wilson that she was starting to think about leaving government and enjoying life on the backbenches, and though she later changed her mind, she discovered to her horror that Wilson had broken this confidence and passed it on to Callaghan. She also refused to back Callaghan – long a political foe of hers – which meant the new leader had little incentive to keep her in Cabinet in the way Wilson had. And, yes, she was very wounded by the pay beds. True to form, she had a little fight with Callaghan in the meeting where he sacked her, refusing to write a letter saying she was resigning in order to make way for someone younger, and threatening to hold a press conference announcing that she wasn't going voluntarily. She told the new PM that she wanted to stay to finish her pay beds legislation. He exclaimed, 'Heaven help your successor!' On leaving, Callaghan asked to kiss her on the cheek, but Castle simply said 'Cheerio' and walked out.[48]

Castle did get her way on the pay beds themselves: her successor David Ennals carried through significantly amended legislation. But Castle had engaged in an almighty fight to, in effect, move private medicine down the road. NHS consultants could still carry out private practice, often in private wings of the same NHS hospital. They have the freedom to carry out private practice in the non-NHS time built into their contracts today. They can still carry out private practice in rooms provided in an NHS hospital. Indeed, Nicholas Timmins notes with some irony that the dispute 'presaged the real take-off of the private sector', reporting that between 1977 and 1980 the number of private health insurance policies rose 'by a spectacular 60 per cent to 3.5 million, heavily driven by company purchases in order to get around pay policy, but also by a perception that the NHS was no longer coping so well'. This meant that 'by an awful irony, Barbara Castle had become the patron saint of private medicine'.[49] More and more people were seeing the value of private health insurance to give them more control over their care. Among them was a woman called Margaret Thatcher.

6. A Big Bang or a whimper?

Margaret Thatcher's legacy is perhaps the most discussed of any of the British post-war prime ministers. Almost as hotly debated is what she actually wanted to do, her secret motives and whether or not she 'cared' about public services and vulnerable people in society. Her tenure in Downing Street saw sweeping and lasting changes to the NHS, but today the political debate is as much about what she might have wanted to do had she been able to as it is about what she actually did. It taps into the suspicion, which had been there since its inception, that the Conservatives had never supported the NHS and would happily run it down in order to replace it with another model of healthcare. What Thatcher did do to the health service, and perhaps even more importantly what she did to wider British society, is one of the key sources of today's obsession with NHS privatisation. Some of that, as we will see, is a political chimera. How much of what we assume to be Thatcher's own attitude towards the health service will turn out to be the same?

Thatcher wasn't passionate about the health service. Neither in the sense that she had a burning commitment to its design, its underlying principle and its role in the British story, nor in that she was desperate to get rid of it and start again. Her biographer Charles Moore says she never 'ceased to worry that the NHS had the potential to destroy her politically and electorally'. Like most prime ministers, she grew weary of pouring money into the health service without seeing much visible return. But she would repeatedly insist that the 'health service is safe in our hands', and Moore thinks she probably believed that.[1]

The need to demonstrate that it was safe in the Conservatives' hands was the key theme of Thatcher's relationship with the NHS during her premiership. One of her health secretaries, John Moore, reflected to her biographer that Thatcher 'didn't want to talk about [reform]' and that instead 'what she wanted was peace'.[2] Ken Clarke, who was a health minister between 1982 and 1985, and then Health Secretary from 1988 to 1990, remembers her strong attraction to an insurance-based system. 'She wanted to go the whole hog and privatise it completely,' he says.[3] But as attracted as Thatcher was to a different system of financing and providing healthcare, she was also acutely aware that the British public never seemed to agree that the grass might be greener on the other side. Like Enoch Powell, she recognised that the public liked the health service and that her party would get no thanks for trying a different model that may well have worked better. But unlike Powell she was ambivalent about the NHS beyond that pragmatic acceptance: she herself went private for treatment and was happy to discuss that. During the 1987 general election, she revealed that she had private health insurance, telling a press conference: 'I, along with something like five million other people, insure to enable me to go into hospital on the day I want; at the time I want, and with a doctor I want. For me, that is absolutely vital. I do that along with five million others. Like most people, I pay my dues to the National Health Service; I do not add to the queue.'[4]

In fact, she thought it a moral imperative that people who could pay should. Clarke remarked: 'She thought it was disgraceful that people who could afford it relied on the taxpayer to provide their health. She was positively proud of the fact that she looked after her own health and made no claims on it.'[5]

But the wider Conservative movement certainly contained plenty of figures and organisations which wanted this health service gone, and replaced with a better model that worked for patients and cost less. Among them was the Institute of Economic Affairs, a free-market think tank that Thatcher relied on a great deal for her economic policies, and which had always opposed the NHS. The IEA had, incidentally, been deeply disappointed in Powell when he refused to entertain their proposals when he was Health Secretary. They would continue to push for a market-led solution to healthcare in Britain during the Thatcher era, but were again ultimately disappointed – and remain so today.

In opposition, the party had to respond to a Royal Commission on the NHS, set up by Harold Wilson and due to report in 1979. This was in response to the frequent complaints from the BMA and Royal Colleges that the health service was in crisis and underfunded, but Nicholas Timmins explains that it was never given the scope to think the unthinkable in terms of different ways of financing the NHS: 'The committee's membership had been "rigged" to ensure it would not come out with a report opposing the basic principles of the NHS or having any truck with private financing.'[6] The Tory health spokesman Patrick Jenkin studied alternatives including a switch to insurance, but realised he wouldn't have the political space to proceed. Then, as Thatcher began to settle in as prime minister – and as she grew still more frustrated with the health service – she and colleagues including Chancellor Geoffrey Howe encouraged a Whitehall think tank called the Central Policy Review Staff to examine radical options for the size and design of the welfare state, including the NHS. What the CPRS came up with, in September 1982, caused 'the nearest thing to a Cabinet riot in the history of the Thatcher administration', according to Nigel Lawson.[7] It included compulsory private medical insurance and 'the end of the National Health Service'. The paper leaked and caused a political riot, too. When the full confidential documents relating to it were released to the public under the thirty-year rule, it emerged Thatcher and her Cabinet had spent rather more time considering the plans than had been claimed at the time: she had argued it had never been taken seriously, when in fact there had been a half-day discussion of the paper.

In December of that year, she held meetings with the relevant Secretaries of State, including Fowler, with Howe continuing to push for Thatcher and the minister not to 'close off any options at this stage'. But the notes written for Howe in the run-up to these meetings also contained a key line that those searching for the secret plot to scrap the NHS often overlook. 'Given the Prime Minister's concern about the NHS, this may be difficult,' a senior Treasury official, Peter Mountfield, wrote to the Chancellor. It was this concern which meant the CPRS plans never stood a chance. Thatcher herself wrote in her memoirs that she was 'horrified by this paper', but Moore explains the nuance of this: 'Although the report's suggestions were certainly not her own private thoughts, still less a secret plan, they did reflect her direction of travel. Nothing about them upset her, except for the political embarrassment they caused.'[8]

The CPRS recommendations are still held up today as a sign that the Tories had a 'secret plan' to scrap the NHS – one they might yet act on if they get the chance. It is unclear what that chance would be, as the Thatcher years saw all the conditions for a government to dismantle the health service: big parliamentary majorities, a general pushing-back of the frontiers of the state, even the running-down of the NHS in terms of funding and political support that those on the left say is the Conservative tactic to encourage the public to turn against the health service and support a market-led solution instead. Even when the NHS was in such bad nick that Thatcher herself was publicly accepting the premise that it was in 'crisis', to the extent that she pitched up on an episode of the BBC's *Panorama*, the public blamed the government not the principle of the NHS itself. And even at that point in the late 1980s when she ran an internal government review and pushed another favourite think tank, the Centre for Policy Studies, to write its own 'radical' proposals, she vetoed many of the ideas coming from within and outside government as politically unpalatable. The CPS, for instance, wanted changes that would convert the NHS into an insurance-based system from which people could opt out and get a tax rebate.

Her own ministers had their own ideas, too: the Health Secretary at the time, John Moore, had suggested a hypothecated health tax. Moore was an ambitious, unusually (for politics) handsome minister whose star was, at the time, on the rise. He was an avowed Thatcherite, and the prime minister had moved him to Health and Social Security as a mark of how impressed she was with him. But she wasn't impressed with the idea of a hypothecated tax because it would merely lead to higher NHS expenditure, which wasn't what she was after. Secret Treasury documents also make clear that both Lawson and Moore were in favour of 'encouraging growth of the private sector', with Moore keen on tax relief for insurance premiums. Chancellor Nigel Lawson and his advisers wanted a strategy that included 'encouraging the private sector, and introducing more market mechanisms into the public sector, with the aim of eventually blurring the present and very sharp distinction between the two'.[9] That could include, in the long term, compulsory private insurance. In the short term, Lawson wanted to radically extend charging, including removing the exemption for elderly people and children from prescription charges, introducing £5 fees for visits to the GP. That last was particularly politically difficult, and Thatcher wouldn't go near it. She eventually settled on dramatic internal reform of the service, having concluded that the public would never bear anything more fundamental. These reforms allowed the NHS to emulate the commercial sector more, without tackling its funding or design. Thatcher might have had her own ideas and sympathies about what an ideal health service would look like if she were tasked with designing it, but she was also a pragmatist. She went for what was possible – much like the man who set the NHS up in the first place, as it happens. So, if the 1980s wasn't the time to privatise the service, it's not clear when it ever will be.

But the prime minister *was* alarmed not just by how expensive the health service was but also by how many people it employed, and what on earth they were all up to. In 1981, she was 'most disturbed' to discover in the course of a discussion in Cabinet that there had been an increase of 25,000 staff in the NHS since 1979, and urgently asked for a note explaining what was going on. She was particularly unimpressed that there seemed to be a ratio of one administrator to every four or five 'professional staff'. She found herself being harried by Secretaries of State including Michael Heseltine, who wrote to her that he felt 'bitter' given he had been working so hard to cut staffing numbers in his own Department of Environment. The Health Secretary, Patrick Jenkin, tried to argue that this was in line with the party's manifesto commitments. He claimed he and Thatcher had agreed that the pressures on the health service meant 'planned expenditure should be maintained'. This was a commitment he had bounced colleagues into before the election, but Thatcher didn't seem to remember it, scrawling a large '?' next to his words as she read them.

The solution, she decided, was to look into how to control NHS manpower, and to get someone who knew how to run organisations to look at it. Initially, Norman Fowler – now in the Department of Health and Social Security (DHSS) as Secretary of State – approached Basil Collins, the deputy chairman and group chief executive at Cadbury Schweppes. The attraction of Collins was that he had 'achieved outstanding success in drastically slimming down the work-force in the profitable Cadbury Schweppes consortium, with a strike-free industrial relations record'. He was also chairman of the finance committee of the Royal College of Nursing, and seemed keen, initially, to carry out the review. But after a few weeks of thinking about it, he told Fowler he couldn't do it this side of an election, saying he felt 'an inquiry now would cause more disaffection within the NHS and much political trouble'.[10] The attention turned to the minister's second choice. Roy Griffiths was the deputy chairman and managing director of Sainsbury's. He was someone who 'got' the NHS, and wasn't about to recommend the Tories did something drastically different to the model, telling *The Times* that he was of a generation that could remember the days before the health service, and that the Beveridge Report made 'exciting reading'.[11] He had never used the private medical insurance which came with his Sainsbury's remuneration package.[12] Even more relevantly, he had two children who were doctors, which sparked the interest he had in taking on the inquiry.[13]

Bringing in a businessman to look at manpower was a politically fraught move. Sir Derek Rayner, the Marks and Spencer director, was advising the prime minister on efficiency in Whitehall, and warned her that 'there is the risk of an adverse reaction if the inquiry is set up on the explicit assumption that there is over-manning in the NHS'. Thatcher agreed, accepting that while she thought the NHS might be overmanned, it was important to avoid suggesting that when setting up the inquiry. Her private secretary reflected her view that 'to do so would produce a markedly hostile response from the unions and others but more important, it would alienate those medical, nursing and other staff who worked hard to keep the hospital service going during last year's dispute and whose support for, or at least acquiescence in, the review is necessary for its success.'[14]

Griffiths, too, was resistant to the idea that the inquiry should just be about manpower, telling ministers that if staffing was out of control then there were clearly wider management problems with the health service. They agreed, and the effects of this review went much further than one merely on cutting staff would ever have done.

The Sainsbury's boss was joined in the inquiry group by three businessmen: Sir Michael Bett, the board member for personnel at British Telecom; Jim Blyth, the group finance director at United Biscuits; and Sir Brian Bailey, formerly the chairman of the South Western Regional Health Authority. Their task was to: 'examine the ways in which resources are used and controlled inside the health service, so as to secure the best value for money and the best possible services for the patient'; and to 'identify what further management issues need pursuing for these important purposes'.[15]

Up to this point, the health service was managed on the basis of 'consensus' between committees of the key figures in a hospital such as the doctors, nurses and administrators. It was a British way of muddling through, but Bevan himself hadn't been fully convinced by the set-up at the start of the service, predicting that administration would be one of the most intractable problems. Subsequent Health Secretaries hadn't been happy, either: Richard Crossman remarked in his diaries that regional health authorities were like 'semi-autonomous governors in the Persian Empire – they do what they damn well like'.[16] The 1974 reorganisation had introduced a level of bureaucracy into the service that didn't seem to be working particularly well and that never really received the level of commitment necessary to make it work, meaning administrators were already loathed in parts of the service.

There was also the question of who was in charge at the top. Bett and the other group members had a dinner one night with the DHSS permanent secretary Ken Stowe in the course of the inquiry. Bett recounted it thus: 'We asked: "Ken, who is managing the Health Service?" And he said, "What do you mean?" "Is it you?" "Oh no. My job is to advise ministers and to run the Department. I'm not . . ." [. . .] and we went round and round. "No, no, no." "Well, how is the Health Service managed?" It was a question that absolutely flummoxed me and of course Roy.'[17]

When they reported back to Fowler in October 1983, they concluded that it wasn't clear who was running the health service at all, with a phrase that made the inquiry famous: 'At no level is the general management role clearly being performed by an identifiable individual. In short, if Florence Nightingale were carrying her lamp through the corridors of the NHS today she would almost certainly be searching for the people in charge.' Griffiths added that the 'NHS does not have the profit motive, but it is, of course, enormously concerned with control of expenditure'. But, he complained, 'it still lacks any real continuous evaluation of its performance against criteria such as those set out above'. A lack of general management meant it was hard to implement big initiatives. Moving to a managerial system would mean 'the same level of care could be delivered more efficiently at lower cost, or a superior service given at the same cost'. This was not about more appointments, either: 'We should, even in the short term, be talking about a considerable reduction in numbers.'[18]

The letter the group sent to Fowler (it was never intended to be a proper report, though is often now referred to as the Griffiths Report or the Griffiths Inquiry) also criticised the DHSS for getting too closely involved in issues that were for the health service, not politicians – though the experience of any minister before or since will underline that this is a naive complaint given how politically salient any and every aspect of the NHS is and always will be.

The inquiry's biggest change was to end 'consensus management' and introduce general managers, who would be of a quality commensurate with the task ahead of them. Griffiths wrote: 'One of our most immediate observations from a business background is the lack of a clearly-defined general management function throughout the NHS. By general management we mean the responsibility drawn together in one person, at different levels of the organisation, for planning, implementation and control of performance. The NHS is one of the largest undertakings in Western Europe. It requires enormous resources; its role is very politically sensitive; it demands top class management.'

He recommended a 'small, strong general management body' at the centre, 'to ensure that responsibility is pushed as far down the line as possible'. In individual hospitals, general managers would replace the current structure but would work closely with clinicians on their decision-making: 'The time at present spent by doctors in meetings, committees, etc., will be reduced and employed more purposefully.' There was to be a general manager for every regional and district health authority and for every unit. And the government would set up a Health Services Supervisory Board which would decide objectives, budgets and strategies for the health service.

The government chose to accept the recommendations. But it wasn't long before the healthcare professional bodies and unions started to push back against them, fearing a loss of power for their members. The British Medical Association wanted doctors to be the only people eligible to be general managers. BMA council chair Anthony Grabham wrote to Fowler claiming that what Griffiths appeared to want was 'a somewhat autocratic executive manager to take over the running of health authorities'. The Royal College of Nursing predicted that this would be the 'end of nursing', and ran an expensive newspaper campaign with adverts featuring a man in a grey suit and the caption: 'Why is Britain's nursing being run by people who don't know their coccyx from their humerus?' Its members wanted to go further, tabling a resolution at their annual congress in 1984 that general managers must be thrown out of the college because they were no longer nurses. The RCN's national management officer, Ray Rowden, described how angry nurses were: 'I was doing meetings around the country with 300 nurses turning up.' But he later changed his tune, becoming a general manager himself, and telling the *Health Service Journal*: 'With hindsight Griffiths was absolutely right and remains right to this day.'[19]

Griffiths had a huge cultural impact on the health service, and not all of it was positive. Even though the inquiry had recommended developing clinical leadership, very few doctors and even fewer nurses made it into general management positions. One of the reasons was the hostility from their professional bodies as described above. But another was an enthusiasm for hiring people from outside the NHS, partly on the assumption that they would be able to tell the health service what it was doing wrong. When the *HSJ* marked sixty years of the health service in 2009, it named Griffiths as one of the most influential figures but also said: 'The reforms contributed to the "them and us" attitude which still persists between managers and clinical staff and to the demonisation of NHS managers in the media.'[20] Though Griffiths had insisted that the differences between the NHS and business 'can be greatly overstated', many felt he had still missed the nuances of the organisation. Writing in the *BMJ*, Roger Dyson, chairman of the North Staffordshire Health Authority, complained that: 'Like all newcomers to the health service, Griffiths is dismissive of the differences between the NHS and private industry, arguing that they can be greatly overstated. This is a view that all newcomers eventually modify in a greater or lesser period of time, depending on their personal learning curve, and it accounts for the frustrations of many of the new chairmen of district health authorities.' One of the key problems as Dyson saw it was that the new structure would erode clinical freedoms of doctors while also creating managers who were a 'toothless tiger' without real power.[21]

Anthony Dalton, who had joined the NHS in 1955 as a junior clerk, explained the problem to the *HSJ*: 'The big challenge of the health service – and one that does not change – is how to manage doctors. That's what makes NHS management different from education or retail management. At the heart of it is a relationship between a doctor and a patient.'[22] The new outside managers who didn't appreciate this stayed only a few years before leaving for pastures that were rather less populated by angry consultants. There were stand-offs between doctors and managers, who were now tasked with trying to balance the books at a time of serious spending restraint. One manager at Guy's Hospital at the time recalled: 'To save money, managers literally locked – chained and padlocked – some operating theatres to stop some of the cardiac surgeons operating.'[23]

But the old administrators who moved into general management didn't always nail the new role, either. Nigel Edwards, who was an administrator at the time, describes some of the peculiar behaviour of his colleagues: 'A lot of people suddenly had greatness thrust upon them in these new jobs and suddenly forgot that they were administrators and started behaving in rather odd and caricatured ways. Like how they imagined people in business did.'[24] Indeed, the letter to Fowler had recommended a 'more thrusting and committed style of management'. Some managers thrusted rather too much: one senior executive remarks that 'in some ways Griffiths was the start of the culture of bullying and cover-up that we see in the health service today, though that got a lot worse with the Blair government. But because people were now responsible for failings, they were frightened of those failings being spotted at all. It wasn't healthy, isn't healthy.'[25]

For better or worse, the NHS now had a cohort of workers interested in the bottom line, not just clinical decisions. The health service has always had its battles with money, but those were largely staged by politicians. Now, there were managers worrying about the numbers, too.

Meddling with managers was never going to be the only thing Thatcher did with the health service, though. The internal market was the NHS equivalent of the financial Big Bang of the Thatcher years. It came later in her time as prime minister, it shook the health service to its core – and it shook Thatcher herself politically, too. As we saw earlier in the chapter, by the late 1980s the health service really was in crisis, and the public were up in arms. The health service had been under a severe spending squeeze for the whole decade.

In the autumn of 1987 a storm ripped through England. This wasn't metaphorical: the Great Storm is part of the British collective memory, and it hit the NHS. Trees crashed through the roofs of hospitals, leaving hundreds of thousands of pounds' worth of damage. Wards and staff accommodation were evacuated. Southend Hospital was forced to shut. In Redhill, Surrey, the roof of the lift motor room blew off, damaging the air conditioning and meaning that one operating theatre was put out of use for two weeks. Some hospitals were plunged into darkness when the electricity supply cut out and backup generators failed. The storms also caused blood shortages, with the North West Thames region having to turn to other centres to keep up supplies to hospitals. The chaos caused by the weather epitomised the chaos in healthcare, with managers despairing about how to balance their books. A BMA survey of hospital consultants estimated that in 1987, more than 3,000 acute beds closed in England and Wales due to money pressures.

The lengths to which hospitals went to save or bring in money caused storms, too. In Sevenoaks, the health authority decided to close an operating theatre and a female surgical ward for six months to save £420,000. The local MP, Conservative Mark Wolfson, blamed the authority, and said he would be raising the matter with the ministers responsible.[26] At Barts, general manager Dr Ken Grant was keen to open a private ward and sell the hospital's services to others. He explained to the press that 'our NHS allocations have been down by £4,000,000 a year since 1982 although the government recognises that we needed to have 2 per cent more each year to keep pace with demand. It means that we are now working with fewer than 600 beds, although we have the consultant staff for an 850-bed hospital. We should be using this spare capacity to earn money.'[27]

Units were short-staffed, to the extent that operations were repeatedly cancelled for lack of specialist intensive care nurses to look after a patient post-surgery. One of the most prominent cases was that of little David Barber, who at just eight weeks old had surgery to repair a hole in his heart delayed five times due to short-staffing. He was becoming immune to the drugs he was being given to keep him stable, and his parents feared what would happen if he was kept waiting for much longer. His parents took the local health authority to court, arguing that it was failing in its legal duty to provide comprehensive care. But in the High Court, Mr Justice MacPherson ruled that this was not a matter in which the courts could intervene: 'No surgeon should be ordered to perform an operation by the court in circumstances which this case reveals.' His view was that the case was a 'general criticism' of the resources provided to the NHS, and he refused the injunction sought by David's parents, which would force the West Midlands Health Authority to carry out the operation.

Finally, on 25 November 1987, the surgery went ahead. Baby Barber was photographed recovering from the operation in an incubator in the intensive care unit of Birmingham Children's Hospital, his little mouth open as he slept. His mother, Diane, clutched his hand as she told the *Birmingham Daily News*: 'I didn't believe the operation was ever going to happen until a nurse picked him up and carried him into the operating theatre.' She couldn't wait to take him home, but felt terribly for the other children waiting. The paper reported consultant cardiologist Dr Eric Silove saying that 'at least one West Midlands baby suffering a heart defect had died in the last week after being turned away from intensive care' and 'another toddler is believed to have died in transit from Birmingham to a Liverpool hospital'.[28]

The story was front-page news, and inevitably caused a row in the House of Commons, with Labour MPs attacking a defensive Thatcher. Labour MP Joan Ruddock argued that 'the catastrophic nursing shortage arises because of the miserable pay and conditions in the Health Service'. Her colleague Bob Wareing asked: 'As 34 cases are still awaiting operations at the one hospital in which the David Barber case caused such problems, what advice would the Prime Minister give in the light of the fact that David Barber received his operation only as a result of a tremendous amount of publicity being raised by his parents? What advice would she give to the parents of the 34 other cases in that hospital alone? Is it not time that she shook herself out of her arrogance and complacency in dealing with the matter?'[29] When Thatcher replied, she was interrupted by jeering from the opposition benches as she argued that the operation had gone well and the number of paediatric nurses had increased along with the money. Internally, though, her policy advisers were warning her that there was a serious shortage of nurses, particularly in London. Her press secretary Bernard Ingham, meanwhile, began to worry that Labour was becoming more effective with Robin Cook as its shadow Health Secretary, and warned: 'It is clear that the Opposition, in concert with the *Daily Mirror*, intend to exploit every sob story that emerges from the NHS. This subject is a useful – and emotive – means of diverting attention away from their lack of policy.'[30]

Ten days after his operation, David Barber passed away. The doctors insisted that there was no evidence the delays in his surgery had contributed to his death, but his parents were, of course, grief-stricken and horrified, not least because they had been preparing to bring him home.

Two days later, the presidents of the three foremost Royal Colleges – of Surgeons, of Physicians, and of Obstetricians and Gynaecologists – signed a joint statement entitled 'Crisis in the NHS' in which they warned that the NHS had 'almost reached breaking point'. It read: 'Each day we learn of new problems in the NHS – beds are shut, operating rooms are not available, emergency wards are closed, essential services are shut down in order to make financial savings. In spite of the efforts of doctors, nurses and other hospital staff, patient care is deteriorating. Acute hospital services have almost reached breaking point, morale is depressingly low.'[31] David's own surgeon, Mr Babulal Sethia, became part of a campaign to 'rescue' the NHS. He told the *Daily Telegraph* the following year: 'This is a major teaching hospital and the standard of care should be no less than what would be normally expected in other developed countries. I am afraid to say that we are just failing to live up to that.'[32]

On the same day that David Barber finally had his operation, the government had unveiled a set of reforms. A White Paper called *Promoting Better Health* changed the way GPs were paid so that they had more incentive to encourage patients to join their lists. It also set targets for family doctors to do more vaccinations, more cervical screenings and more health promotion sessions. If that was controversial with the profession, other measures such as charges for eye tests and dental examinations would anger the public. The paper came alongside cuts to funding and plans – first trialled by John Moore in a party conference speech the previous month – to allow hospitals to rent out space in their buildings to businesses such as florists and gift shops. Moore's party-pleasing address was interpreted by reporters as 'hanging a "For Sale" sign over the National Health Service' because he argued he wanted to break down the barriers between public and private healthcare and allow hospitals to spend money in order to make a profit.[33] His shops idea was striking, not just because of what it would entail for the character of hospitals, but also because it seemed to require him to amend the original 1948 National Health

Service Act. Despite the fuss it caused, though, it was not going to raise the money the NHS needed. Something big needed to change.

Thatcher was always anxious about the potential of the health service to undermine her popularity. The opinion polls were now increasing that anxiety: a Gallup Poll in January 1988 for the *Telegraph* found that more than two-thirds of voters disagreed with the statement 'the National Health Service is safe in the hands of the Conservatives'. This was a hike from the previous May, when 55 per cent disagreed with the statement. Her former chief of staff David Wolfson became anxious that it was going to enable a leadership challenge from Geoffrey Howe, who was loitering with intent at the Foreign Office. He had given a speech where he appeared to back the idea – now circulating and occasionally backed by the prime minister herself – of a radical review of the health service. Wolfson wrote to Thatcher warning her of this: 'I believe you are now more at risk than with the Falklands or Westland. In both those crises you are able to look at the facts and formulate a strategy to deal with the facts. You are now unable to formulate a strategy to deal with the facts. You are now unable to formulate a strategy to deal with a crisis which you maintain does not exist.' Thatcher had an interview with David Dimbleby on the BBC's *Panorama* looming in the next few days, and so Wolfson offered her what he claimed was the 'most critical and best' advice he had given her. He thought the intervention of the Royal Colleges back in the autumn was a way to open up 'the debate about the future of health provision and funding'.[34]

And so it was that Thatcher pitched up to the *Panorama* interview with something new to say. She told Dimbleby: 'We are already looking at the demands that will come in future, but we know there has to be a limit and therefore we shall continue as we did in education: make our own inquiries, our own consultations. Believe me, people flood in to see us and of course, John [Moore] sees them. And then, when we are ready, we shall come out with our own proposals, just exactly as we have done for other things.'

This did allow the prime minister to seem as though she was gripping the situation, but what would these proposals be? The ideas from the Centre for Policy Studies and her own ministers were, one way or another, unworkable, and yet something needed to be done.

That something was already in circulation in the health policy world. Back in 1984, the Nuffield Provincial Hospitals Trust had asked a Stanford University figure, healthcare economist Professor Alain Enthoven, to write up his own thoughts on the health service. He duly published a paper, 'Reflections on the management of the National Health Service: An American looks at incentives to efficiency in health services management in the UK'.[35] The premise on which he did the review was that the NHS was beloved by the public, but was going to be under increasing pressure to meet all the demands on it. He made clear that 'I do not sense any serious demand for radical change in the NHS', which meant his preferred model of healthcare maintenance organisations, which were a growing source of healthcare provision in the US, wasn't an option. Beyond that sort of dramatic overhaul, Enthoven approved of the Griffiths Inquiry's recommendations as 'very sensible ideas', but added: 'If the structure and incentives in the NHS are not changed more fundamentally, these changes are likely to be little more than cosmetic.'

The NHS, he wrote, 'relies on dedication and idealism'. 'It is propelled by the clash of the interests of the different provider groups. But it offers few positive incentives to do a better job for the patients, and it has some perverse ones.' Some of those perverse incentives included that 'a district that develops an excellent service in some specialty that attracts more referrals is likely to get more work without getting more resources to do it'. On an individual level, consultants had little incentive to clear their NHS waiting lists because that would reduce the demand for their private paid services. Key in Enthoven's paper was the criticism that 'somehow, the interests of the patients get lost'. This was exactly what Thatcher was interested in. Her fascination with reform was not just about making the state smaller; it was also about stopping public services from being loaded in favour of the people and organisations providing those services, with little thought for the consumers.

Enthoven's solution was an 'internal market model' for the NHS under which 'each district would resemble a nationalised company' and would 'buy and sell services from and to other districts and trade with the private sector'. The beauty of the internal market was that it would force the NHS to come up with costs for different treatments and procedures – something it wasn't doing at present. When he published the paper, he discussed it with David Willetts, who was in the policy unit. It was also read with care by officials in the Department of Health, who knocked it back on the grounds it would mean the government spending more money.

As Thatcher's policy advisers thrashed through the various ideas in circulation in 1988, the internal market started to look like the most workable one. Willetts, now at the CPS, wrote a note a couple of days after her *Panorama* interview, which reported that 'a consensus is emerging, both within the Health Service and among commentators, about sensible ways to reform the NHS'. One of those was 'to develop an internal market, with the best hospitals winning more "customers" and more funding'. Willetts reminded Thatcher of something that had been niggling away at her for a while: that the health service took little notice of the cost of operations, to the extent that 'Guy's can do 600 heart operations for roughly the same cost as 200 heart operations in St Thomas's' (these two hospitals were a couple of miles from one another in Central London, and eventually became part of the same NHS trust). Similarly, there was a gap of £800 in the cost of cataract surgery between hospitals in the Trent region because 'patients stay in one hospital for ten days and for two days in another'. The internal market would 'make doctors servants of the patient because they need to win his custom'.

Willetts went further than Moore's policy of allowing hospitals to rent space to shops. 'There are enormous possibilities here which go way beyond simply putting a florist by the hospital entrance.' What about allowing local companies to sponsor wards, for instance. 'Why not the Glaxo wing and the Marks and Spencer kidney unit?' It would involve local people and 'moreover, no private company wants its name associated with a badly-run or slovenly authority'.[36]

This note formed part of the considerations of the working group on the NHS, which consisted of the prime minister, Nigel Lawson,

Chief Secretary to the Treasury John Major, Tony Newton and John Moore. It was publicly announced, but then met in secret.

The Department of Health, reported a Treasury official to Lawson, was 'very lukewarm about the internal market, which they see as adding a lot of administrative overheads to no purpose'.[37] But it was the favoured model within Downing Street, and it soon emerged that it was the favoured model among NHS professionals who got on with the government. Timmins describes a series of meetings in March and April of 1988 with doctors and managers whom Number 10 trusted, and reports one figure who was there saying: 'These were just awful. Margaret at her worst. We would have two- or three-hour meetings and she would end up screaming like a fishwife and complaining about the bloody consultants and the hospitals, and her doctor friends had told her this, or told her that, or we would end up with unbelievably rambling conversations in which we failed to get to grips with anything.' Slowly but surely, though, it became clear that the internal market was the only game in town.

In the middle of this, Thatcher moved the beleaguered Moore, who felt his time overseeing Health had 'destroyed' him.[38] She split the leviathan DHSS in two, sent the incumbent to deal with Social Security and brought in Ken Clarke as Secretary of State for Health. Clarke is known today as one of the more lefty Conservatives: pro-European and concerned about the direction of his party more widely. In Thatcher's era, he was what was known as a 'wet': a moderate who didn't fully embrace the red in tooth and claw free-market views of his leader. But he was not a mollifying character and was still very pro-market. Moreover, he didn't like the way the producer held all the power in public services. Like Thatcher, he wanted to tip the balance in favour of the consumer. He shared her analysis that the left hand of the NHS had no idea what the right hand was doing. He had been a health minister already, which was perhaps why he had a stronger belief in the health service than his boss: there are very few politicians of any stripe who leave the Department of Health feeling less in favour of the principles of the NHS, and they are often more cognisant of its real need for more money than the government of the day will allow. That's not to say he didn't think it had some very silly elements to it, describing it as being run in a 'comically bad fashion' prior to Griffiths.[39]

Clarke set about designing this new internal market. Alongside the Enthoven plans, he also drew on a paper written in 1985 by health economist Alan Maynard, which proposed GPs becoming 'fundholders': they would be the ones in charge of the budget for the different levels of care, whether day-to-day primary care or hospital-based secondary care, for their patients. Each patient, Maynard suggested, should have a value which would then help form the GP's budget for primary care and all other services. Alongside this was a move to 'self-governing hospitals', which would allow hospitals to opt out from the control of local health authorities and turn them into separate legal entities with their own boards of governors. This was the start of the NHS 'trusts' that we know today.

These ideas then went through a great deal of to and fro between Clarke, Thatcher, the Treasury, and Clarke's own department. He later recalled returning from one meeting with Thatcher to tell civil servants about the internal market plans, only for the permanent secretary to reply: 'Oh, that's very interesting, Secretary of State, congratulations! I'm afraid at the moment the department is up to its ears, we are very committed and we don't have any civil servants we can put on this. I'll see if we can find a team.' Clarke ignored them and put together his own team.

Clarke was as idiosyncratic a figure back then as he is today: he delighted in smoking cigars in meetings and wrote up many of his policy ideas for the reform of the health service while on holiday in Galicia. He wasn't just prepared to fight vested interests; both he and the prime minister enjoyed developing policy through having blazing rows, and there were plenty of those as they tried to work out what they wanted. He also had to work with the Treasury on something Thatcher had become personally quite obsessed with, which was the tax relief for private health insurance. Eventually, he and Lawson managed to persuade her to keep the tax breaks for pensioners only, though Clarke joked he was happy with this compromise because 'in my view nobody would ever sell private health insurance to elderly people anyway'.[40]

What those rows and compromises led to was a 1989 paper called 'Working for Patients', which detailed the new internal market for the NHS. Alongside Enthoven and Maynard's ideas was the 'purchaser-provider split', something Clarke felt was the 'the most significant change after 1948'.[41] The purchasers would be health authorities and GPs. The providers would be hospitals, which would have greater freedom, and other services. This would force the NHS to buy the care it wanted from the best provider – whether NHS hospitals or the independent sector. That last covered both private and charitable organisations, ranging from private hospitals to addiction charities. All providers had to compete for business, thus driving up standards and down costs. And because purchasers were commissioning and choosing providers, they would, for the first time, have a real view of how much a service should cost.

The impact this would have on the structure of the NHS was profound. It was also an awkward cultural fit for many working in the service. Enthoven himself reflected in 1999 that 'the "market" idea proved to be counter to the culture of most people in the NHS, a culture of dedication to public service, not one of competitive buying and selling'.[42] He also accepted that it was nigh-on impossible to split the NHS from the political world: there would always be pressure on local MPs to save an ailing constituency hospital, and even moving the NHS Executive to Leeds, as Clarke did, would not stop the Department of Health from feeling forced to get involved when bedpans were dropped.

'Working for Patients' was launched with more than a little fanfare, and the reforms proceeded through more than a little opposition and turmoil. The government spent a cool £1 million on the launch, which included Ken Clarke taking a boat trip down the Thames to Limehouse, where he spoke to an audience of NHS managers and clinicians. The press conference itself was broadcast around the country. A fifteen-minute film about the reforms was played to managers at the launch, closing with a statement from Thatcher herself. It was full of the sort of praise that she and all other politicians always felt bound to include in public discussions of the NHS. 'The National Health Service at its best is without equal. Time and again the nation has seen just how much we owe to those who work in it.' She claimed the reforms would 'put the needs of patients first' and would 'provide even better health care for the millions and millions of people who rely on the National Health Service'. It was a pretty anodyne address given the nature of the reforms. It was almost as though Thatcher was more concerned with reassuring people that she wasn't doing anything serious to alter the health service other than making it work better for them. Indeed, she was still nervous about the reforms and continued to swing between confidence and anxiety about them for the rest of her tenure.

But the launch initially got, in Clarke's words, 'an extremely good reception'. He told a witness seminar on the internal market in 2018: 'Astonishingly, we got really good write-ups. I remember Margaret thought it was marvellous and embarrassed me by commending it at the beginning of a Cabinet meeting on how to present policy. Of course, with the greatest dismay, I expressed my opinion that I did not think it would last more than five minutes and I hoped she was braced for having the political battle to end all battles before we got any of this implemented, which she thought was a curious reaction on my part. I think she thought we had solved the whole thing by this presentation.'[43]

Naturally, that was not how things panned out. Having reached this point in the book, you will probably be able to predict the stance of the BMA, which is that it was against the reforms. Clarke joked that the union found itself fighting in favour of the 1974 reorganisation, which it had at the time bitterly opposed. Like every other Health Secretary, he found the BMA 'impossible': 'In the 1970s and '80s I dealt with just about all the trade unions. The BMA was the most difficult, most extreme, most militant and most accustomed to getting its way. They couldn't understand why a minister wouldn't give way.'[44] The union spent more than £3 million on an advertising campaign opposing the reforms. Some of the campaign was about the reforms; much of it was, as is the case throughout the history of health service battles, more personal. One poster asked: 'What do you call a man who ignores medical advice? Mr Clarke.' Clarke refused to do the pilots of the new freedoms for hospitals, partly because to do so would be to capitulate to the BMA, which would have annoyed him. Instead, hospitals could become trusts in waves, which he felt was sufficiently piloting the self-governing policy anyway. 'Of course, if any of those had quickly gone belly-up, we would have to have gone back to the drawing board rapidly, so we were piloting, in effect,' he said.[45] Within the Royal College of General Practitioners, there was a row over whether to oppose fundholding on the grounds it would hurt patients, with those GPs who wanted the institution to be in favour of it being labelled 'quislings' by their internal critics.[46]

'Working for Patients' led to the National Health Service and Community Care Act 1990, which came into effect on 1 April 1991. William Waldegrave took over from Clarke as Health Secretary in November 1990. It quickly became obvious to him that Thatcher 'was extremely nervous about anything to do with reform of the health service . . . She told me: "Ken stirred them up, I want you to calm them all down". Ken had stirred them all up not just by being Ken but also by initiating a programme of reform. She clearly signalled to me that if I thought it wasn't well founded, I could ditch the whole thing.' Waldegrave sat down and did a 'crash course in the underlying theory of the purchaser–provider split' and became convinced it was right. He was also aware that, with just five months before it went live, the 'leadership of the health service would have been completely discombobulated if we had changed direction suddenly'.[47]

Thatcher continued to be worried about the changes even after she had been ousted in November 1990 as prime minister and moved to observing (or, many suspected, nagging) from the backbenches. Just weeks after she had left office, in January 1991, she had a meeting with her successor, John Major, where she checked that the government was still pressing ahead with the reforms. Major assured her that 'there was no question of backtracking on this'. But Major was well aware of the delicacies around these reforms: briefings warned him 'Mrs Thatcher was very concerned about the plans to reform the NHS'.[48]

Waldegrave's approach was to try to introduce the reforms in a way that didn't rock the boat too much. What helped him was that, despite the way the national debate had indeed been thoroughly stirred up, the implementation of the reforms was already well under way. In December 1990, there were fifty-seven new NHS trusts. At the big launch of that April, there were 306 fundholding practices – of which a number were run by members of the BMA Council who had spoken against the policies. By 1994, most hospitals, ambulance organisations and other health service providers had become trusts, with all of them eventually doing so. The internal market and fundholding were much more popular in practice than they had been in theory. Indeed, as Timmins argues, the person who had come closest to derailing the changes was Margaret Thatcher herself.

Beyond whether people liked the reforms is the more important question of whether they actually worked (these are very different points in an ideological system such as the NHS, where it has always been possible to dislike something that works very well and vice versa). It depends on what the measure of success is, of course: for Thatcher, that was whether the health service was becoming more efficient and whether it was paying due attention to the patient rather than being generally minded towards the interests of those working in the system.

An analysis by the King's Fund in 1998 found that there was an increase in efficiency in the NHS that could be attributed to the reforms, that GP fundholders were able to keep down prescription costs better than non-fundholders, and that it seemed to improve the responsiveness of providers. But it added that there was 'only limited evidence that trust status made hospitals more efficient than they would otherwise have been'. In fact, rather than breaking up a monopoly of healthcare provision, the market had in many ways just created new ones. The report explained: 'Although the conditions for competition between individual trusts existed in most parts of the country, there is no evidence of widespread competition between trusts. The incentives faced by purchasers and providers seem to have led to a series of bilateral monopolies.' It was similarly dismissive of the possibility that the reforms may have improved care, saying that 'there are some concerns that different trusts had conflicting incentives which threatened the continuity of care'.[49] Virginia Bottomley, who became Health Secretary in April 1992, felt fundholding forced general practice to modernise: 'The joy to me of both fundholding and the GP contract is that they incentivised laggards to immunise, to cancer screen, to do all the things they should have done.'[50]

Naturally, different GPs had different views of how well fundholding worked for them and for the system as a whole. Michael Dixon, a GP in Devon, wrote in the *BMJ* in 2016 that while its full potential hadn't been realised, 'the provider-purchaser split has had successes'. He felt that 'as clinicians we have matured from regarding ourselves solely as individual patient advocates (which is not sustainable in a health system that is free at the point of delivery) to balancing this role with the duty to the greatest good for the greatest number'. In the same article, Maynard – who came up with fundholding – was far less impressed. He argued that: 'The history of the evolution of the internal market since 1989 is characterised by politicians' promises of an elusive utopia. All reforms are experiments. NHS reorganisations since 1989 have been characterised by unevidenced structural change and high and escalating regulatory costs that might better have been spent on patient care. They have shown that competition in healthcare is "mission impossible". The internal market is neither effective nor cost effective.'[51]

The boards of the new self-governing hospital trusts also contributed to the macho management style that had been developing since Griffiths. Their members tended to be Conservative-supporting business figures who wanted the internal market to be seen to be working. Nicholas Timmins argues that this led to 'something of a reign of terror as the new activist chairmen (and they mainly were men) along with the hospital general managers – who had all, unilaterally and overnight, restyled themselves "chief executives" – alighted on poorer performers with the instruction to "clear your desk by tomorrow"'.[52] Waldegrave agrees with this: 'One of the unintended side effects was that those leaders who wanted to take their hospitals into trusts were powerful types who wanted to run their own show. This probably played to a certain kind of character who read the wrong books about management and thought macho management was necessary. We moved to a system where people were in charge but were they really accountable enough?'[53]

Duncan Nichol, the chief executive of the service at the time, protested against the culture of 'macho management' in 1992.[54] But the NHS was becoming a breeding ground for bullying. That culture has festered right up to the present day, to the extent that it is now very hard to find anyone who doesn't think there is widespread bullying – whether of staff in underperforming hospitals and units or of whistle-blowers to safety threats – in the service. It cannot solely be blamed on the habits brought into the NHS by businessmen, though. As we shall see in Chapter 8, on New Labour, the culture was also exported from the dysfunctional and macho world of politics, too.

Labour had never supported the internal market, and promised to abolish it in the 1997 election campaign. But Neil Kinnock, the party's leader until July 1992, told Nicholas Timmins that he wouldn't have scrapped the split, either, because it would have wasted time, and would instead have focused on keeping both purchasers and providers in the public sector. What actually happened when Labour finally made it back into government was that it kept many of the foundations in place, with the purchaser–provider split remaining. The Scottish and the Welsh NHS both abolished the internal market in 2004 and 2009 respectively: from 1999, devolution meant health went from being the preserve of the relevant Whitehall departments – Department of Health, Scotland Office, Wales Office and Northern Ireland Office – to being something controlled by the devolved governments of these countries within the UK.

But New Labour in England extended many of the market principles of 'Working for Patients': foundation hospitals and the use of the independent sector to clear waiting lists were just two prominent examples. Thatcher once joked that her greatest legacy was Tony Blair because of the profound effect she had on the left of politics. That was very clearly true in healthcare.

For England, it was only in 2017 – with integrated care systems, which brought together the purchasers and providers of healthcare at a local level – that the split came to an end. Two years later, the two management bodies for the health service, NHS England and NHS Improvement merged, which meant there was no national split between commissioning and providing either. In the same year, the health service started to move away from payment by results for healthcare. The Johnson government then pushed ahead with a Health and Care Bill, which gave integrated care systems a statutory footing. The internal market had finally died, having never really lived a full life anyway.

What the Thatcher decade unquestionably led to was an era of permanent upheaval for the NHS, as its structures were reorganised and the purchasers in particular rearticulated in slightly different ways by different governments and successive Health Secretaries. The 1974 reorganisation under Sir Keith Joseph had arguably been the start of that, but the 1980s reforms cemented it. This is somewhat ironic, given how nervous Thatcher herself was about shaking up the service.

Perhaps its most enduring legacy in the eyes of the public, though, was the NHS blue lozenge. Despite it being one of the most recognisable logos in the world today, it has not been with us since the inception of the service.

The story – untold until now – of how that logo came about involves a fight, naturally. Richard Moon was a successful designer who in March 1990 was invited, along with others, to come up with a design for the NHS Management Executive. The brief initially called for a 'logotype', which meant it had to be made from letters only, but Moon was later told it must include a high-profile illustration along the lines of the Labour Party's red rose, or the Conservative party torch – but using navy blue and cream. He dismissed this brief as 'political suicide' because the government was 'closing hospitals left and right. If they introduced a flashy trademark that looked like they'd spent any more than £100 on it, politicians, press and public opinion would shut the project down before it had begun. This would have been a disaster, as it would have also shut the door on tackling some serious issues we'd discovered during our research.'[55] In his pitch, he revealed his company had uncovered confusion and mistrust throughout the NHS, so a new logo on everything would solve nothing. Conservative ministers, he feared, were keen to exploit the fragmentation of NHS services. His plan was to bring them back together under a single brand. His company settled on a colour which he had seen in nurses' uniforms in West Africa and had found very compelling: a mid-blue, known in the design world as Pantone 300.

Moon won the bid, and when a few months later the logo appeared in the wild for the first time, its launch was deemed a success. The reason officials were happy with the way the logo had landed was that no one had noticed it. Moon says: 'The Department of Health tested it out surreptitiously by placing it above the head of Ken Clarke when he introduced the successful reforms in July 1990. A photo of Clarke with the reform document under the logo appeared in the *Financial Times* the following day. Its appearance was regarded by both the Department and my company as a huge success – *because nobody had commented on it.*' But the logo was then little used outside three hospitals Moon went on to work for. He recalls that 'the Major government did all it could to smother' the logo, and 'hundreds of hospital trusts were effectively bullied into creating their own brand and marketing programmes'.[56] But the Major government didn't kill off the logo entirely. It was still there when the Conservatives left office in 1997. In the years that followed, Moon achieved his aim of creating a logo that would reassure the public in times of pandemic, when they sought advice, and when they received letters. It was commissioned at a time when the NHS was becoming more and more disparate. In the end, it was instrumental in solidifying the service in the public consciousness.

It took years for some of the consequences of the internal market to become obvious: that's always the case in healthcare reform, or at least the case with reforms that are given the luxury of a bit of time to bed in before politicians shake things up again. But it was never going to be very long before the wishful thinking that said politicians wouldn't get involved in dropped bedpans was exposed for what it was. It was inevitable that before long a Secretary of State was going to get embroiled in the sort of row about hospital closures that the reforms of the 1980s were supposed to make impossible. It was obvious to most working in the healthcare world that the location of that row would be London.

In fact, it had been obvious that there would be a row about the NHS in London since the 1950s. The trouble was that it was the kind of row that few politicians wanted to have: they knew that the basic problem was that there were too many big, world-famous hospitals in too small an area taking up too much money. But no Health Secretary wants to be the one to close hospitals. Especially not august institutions like Barts.

St Bartholomew's Hospital was founded in the twelfth century; it survived the dissolution of the monasteries, the Great Fire of London and the Blitz, and still has a grand entrance built in the time of Henry VIII. It has murals by Hogarth and featured in Arthur Conan Doyle's Sherlock Holmes novels. Pre-dating the NHS by some 800 years, it was much loved as part of the fabric of London and the medical world, and was now – for the first time since Henry VIII – facing questions about its future.

Those questions came in the form of the Tomlinson Report. This had been commissioned by William Waldegrave, who could see that the internal market was having a particularly tricky impact in London. The reason for this was the concentration of hospitals in the city, all now competing for a limited amount of money and having to justify their existence like never before. More than that, the hospitals were in the centre, and patient demand seemed to be moving to the edges. It was finally becoming impossible to ignore that London hospitals, while world-famous, were not working well. At the same time, many of these hospitals were busily commissioning new buildings, as though they were definitely the ones to expand even as the debate moved inexorably towards a programme of closures. The minister had been shown two big building schemes, at St Mary's, Paddington, and at UCH, the latter of which was due to cost about £300 million. His response was 'I have no rational basis for making this choice', because both schemes should not go ahead. But there was an election in the offing, and so someone else needed to look into this in a way that meant it wouldn't become an issue until a while after polling day. So Waldegrave commissioned Sir Bernard Tomlinson, who had been the chair of the North East Health Authority, to lead an inquiry into how to change all this, promising that this would finally bring an end to the failure to take unpopular but necessary decisions.

In the event, it did force unpopular decisions, but Tomlinson also highlighted why it is that the political system will always try to avoid taking them, even when there is a clear case for doing so. Virginia Beardshaw had chaired an investigation by the King's Fund a year before Waldegrave commissioned Tomlinson, and described the atmosphere in London: 'I went round and everybody without exception said there were too many hospitals in London and the one next door should shut.'[57] Perhaps this insular attitude is not a surprise given the NHS was just the latest, relatively short, episode in the long and distinguished history of these institutions – the health service's seventy-fifth anniversary coincided with the 900th year of Barts. Perhaps, though, it also shows how resistant the service as a whole can be to change.

The day before Tomlinson's report was due to be published, all hell broke loose early after pressure group London Health Emergency leaked the report to the Press Association. It contained proposals to close Barts, Charing Cross, Queen Charlotte's, the Royal National Throat, Nose and Ear Hospital and the Hospital for Tropical Diseases. And it would call for St Thomas's and St Guy's to merge and operate from a single site. It concluded that there were more acute (meaning where patients receive short-term, active care, including elective surgery, for a severe condition) beds per head in London than in other parts of the country – 3.9 per 1,000 people to 2.5 per 1,000 respectively. The capital contained 15 per cent of the population but 20 per cent of NHS resources went to it, and acute spending amounted to £260 per head, compared to £173 in other cities. 'The problems of the inner London hospitals,' Tomlinson wrote, 'are plainly not due to overall lack of resources.' He predicted that the demand for inpatient beds in the inner London hospitals was going to fall, and that by the end of the decade, between 2,000 and 7,000 beds could be surplus to requirement. It wouldn't be enough for individual hospitals to slim down: the report pointed out that this would leave 'fixed costs, overheads and under-used buildings'. Instead, there needed to be a 'managed run-down of the most vulnerable hospitals', and then their entire sites taken out of use, their services relocated and staff redeployed.[58]

Health union the Confederation of Health Service Employees estimated 20,000 jobs would be lost under the changes outlined by the report. Hector MacKenzie, general secretary of COHSE, said the report 'threatens to do what the Government has tried to do with the mining industry', adding 'the rest of the world will think we are mad to close down world-famous centres of excellence because a rigged market has diverted funds out of the capital'.[59]

When he was giving the press conference launching the reforms, Sir Bernard was interrupted by a staff nurse from UCH who shouted: 'It is utterly insane, outrageous and revolting. How can they say there are empty beds when we have cancer patients on our waiting lists?'[60] That interjection set the tone for much of the row. Tomlinson himself complained he had been harangued in the street by members of the public who recognised him. Ainna Fawcett-Henesy, one of the members of the London Implementation Group set up following the inquiry, found herself being called a 'traitor' by members of her own nursing profession for taking that side. The Royal College of Nursing was at the time taking the stand that not one single nursing job should be cut. Tomlinson did not heed that. So the row wasn't just about historic institutions and their buildings; it also became about nurses losing their jobs. A toxic combination if ever there was one, and especially under a government run by the Conservative Party, which rarely had the permission of the public to do as it pleased with the NHS in the way Labour did.

By the time Tomlinson reported, Virginia Bottomley had taken over as Health Secretary. Bottomley had, in her own words, 'come from a medical mafia', with many family members working as doctors. She was on the left of her party, and liked and understood the health service. She described herself as someone who could calm things down in the health world, a 'glazier' while other Health Secretaries needed to break windows. Bottomley was characteristically stoical in the face of furious opposition and decided 'to make sure we tackle the problems that weren't going to go away', including getting on with the London problem. She would need all the stoicism she could muster just for this fight, let alone any others.[61]

Insisting that the report was merely 'advice to the government' rather than official policy, Bottomley told MPs: 'What we are considering – and it is a sensitive and complex matter – is how we can ensure that London services are matched more effectively to the needs of Londoners. The great institutions – the teaching, postgraduate and acute hospitals, which go back many years – are no longer appropriate to a health service where hospitals all over the Home Counties are able to offer advanced and sophisticated treatment.' As she sat down on the green benches in the House of Commons, she knew she would face fury from the MPs all around her. It came in two forms. The first was connected to the wider Conservative NHS reforms: Labour's David Blunkett called on Bottomley to 'accept that the reversal of the internal market and the commercialisation of the health service are a prerequisite for the ability to put London's health care back on its feet'. The second was more local: MPs don't tend to applaud the closure of their local hospitals for the local, let alone the greater, good. And they didn't in this session. Backbenchers told her that 'Londoners will not let her close Bart's' and made clear they weren't convinced by the claim other closures would improve healthcare in their part of London. Bottomley politely acknowledged 'the great loyalty that every individual constituency Member of Parliament has to his or her own particular institutions', but insisted that there needed to be change.[62]

One of the factors in the noisy opposition to the plans from the trade unions at least was that it represented a wedge for opposing the principle of the internal market more widely. Take this letter in the *Pinner Observer* in March 1993, from Jack Gilbert, who was secretary of the Harrow Trades Union Council: 'The application of market principles in London is inappropriate. It is recommended that the operation of the purchaser-provider system be stopped throughout the Greater London area and that funding the NHS as it was before the implementation of the 1990 NHS and Community

Care Act be reinstated. All trust applications should be turned down and existing trusts returned to direct management.'[63]

But the upset went far, far wider than trade unions. Even former Conservative health minister David Mellor joined the campaign against the changes when the Queen Mary's Hospital in Roehampton, part of his constituency, was threatened with losing its burns and plastic surgery unit and its A&E and becoming a largely outpatient hospital. Queen Mary's was another historic hospital in London, though rather younger than Barts. It was a stately home designed by Thomas Archer and converted to a military hospital in the First World War, and had started to take on NHS patients when the health service was founded. One of the babies born there, a few years before the NHS started, was now the prime minister. In 1961, Queen Mary's joined the NHS. By the 1990s, it was running acute services, many of them in the long, high-ceilinged Nightingale wards that Enoch Powell had hoped to see the back of when he was building the modern health service. It had an emergency department run by Dr John Thurston. He was exasperated that the A&E he had spent fifteen years building up was coming to an end, telling the *Guardian* 'the review is completely illogical. They claim that closure will lead to shorter waits. How can it do that?'[64]

The A&E threat came from a review carried out by the regional health authority; the burns unit closure from Tomlinson. Both sparked local fury. Mellor opened a new ward in the A&E in November 1993 and told his local newspaper: 'Any minister who accepts this report should seek immediate admission to Broadmoor. This whole process is about cuts and I cannot imagine the public will put up with it. I wouldn't be surprised if they didn't wreak a terrible revenge. It is absurd that this whole process is going to be concluded at the same time as the local elections.'[65] He launched the petition alongside the Conservative MP for Richmond and Barnes Jeremy Hanley and actors including June Whitfield. That's the thing about a London hospital closure in particular: there are always plenty of big names living nearby to help out with the campaign.

Backbenchers like Mellor weren't the only Tory forces against Bottomley. Michael Portillo, the Chief Secretary to the Treasury, complained in December 1993 that she was being 'unwise' in announcing some of the reforms with 'only a matter of a few days for consideration by my officials, and only a matter of hours for me'.[66] Bottomley went ahead anyway. But the way in which she made the announcement had also caused some consternation in Number 10: a memo from Jonathan Hill expressed concern about the plan to put it in a written answer. Written answers to questions are quite low-profile as things go in Parliament, with hundreds of questions coming from backbenchers to government departments every day. They are published without fanfare and are often used by ministers who want to sneak out unpalatable information. That was the argument Hill made when he wrote to Major:

> My strong view remains that we should seek to make one announcement, rather than two. If we do Bart's separately, we should not delude ourselves that the announcement of some extra money for the London Ambulance Service or for Homerton or UCH/Middlesex will be enough to offset the hammering we will receive from the [*Evening*] *Standard*.
>
> I am also not certain that announcing the closure of Bart's A&E by Written Answer is very clever in the present climate where we are being accused of stifling debate.
>
> I gather that Virginia is very keen to get the announcement out of the way before Christmas and will no doubt say that the news is starting to leak, but the last time that argument was used by Michael Heseltine, we can remember where that led us!

That last was a reference to a row that nearly ended Heseltine's political career in which he had claimed in a written answer that the government was considering more money for a high-speed floating train called Hovertrain – when in fact ministers had already pulled the plug. Major agreed with Hill, writing in the margin 'very true!'[67]

In some instances, there were even more surprising groups who were interested in how the review panned out. Some of the members of the Implementation Group were visited by a succession of figures from the political establishment, including Black Rod (responsible for security on the parliamentary estate), the head of MI5 and the

Metropolitan Police Commissioner. All of them argued that it was impossible to close the casualty department at St Thomas's because of its key strategic position for the safety of Parliament. It is where sick politicians are treated (Boris Johnson was admitted to St Thomas's when he was seriously ill with Covid in 2020), where the victims of any terror attack on Westminster are sent, and the ideal place for a sick MP to stay when there are crucial votes (the party whips will sometimes insist on an MP being brought across Westminster Bridge in an ambulance, and wheeled out in a chair or even a stretcher into the voting lobbies when the government is worried it is going to lose a vote).

Bottomley still insists that 'the medical leaders knew you needed fewer, better hospitals', and that the success of the reorganisation hinged in part on her getting on with the recommendations to close Barts. She describes Admiral Sir William Staveley, chairman of the Royal London Hospital NHS Trust at the time, and Sir Derek Boorman, chair of the Barts trust, coming to her and saying: 'Secretary of State, if you back down on Barts, we will both resign.' She adds: 'You know, so we just had to take it forward because you couldn't continue to have more and more hospitals. There had been reports repeating the message that we needed fewer better hospitals with critical mass for global excellence in research, teaching and healthcare. It was the time for acting, not options.'[68] The Royal Colleges, too, were reasonably supportive. But not all medics were in favour, especially not the ones who worked in departments and hospitals earmarked for closure. If the reaction of Dr John Thurston at Queen Mary's seemed emotional, it was nothing in comparison to the response of doctors at Barts.

Barts was world-famous, and now the campaign to save it quickly gained the same status. A couple named Rob and Barbara Bonner-Morgan were instrumental in setting up the Save Barts Campaign, which involved doctors protesting outside the hospital wearing their white coats, the City of London attempting a rescue bid which would have made Barts a private hospital, and the Arthur Conan Doyle Society of Tokyo donating money purely because of the Sherlock Holmes link. At one point the Queen even appeared to wade into the row: she was reported as telling the dean of Barts' medical college in a private conversation that she was 'very anxious' about the threatened closure. NHS campaigns are rarely without a bizarre element, after all. Barbara Bonner-Morgan wrote a book about the campaign, with a poem which had as its payoff: 'Never invoke the wrath of the ordinary people or you release a tiger!'[69]

Tomlinson and Bottomley had released a tiger, and ultimately that tiger won. Barts became a major feature of the 1997 general election campaign, with Labour's aspiring Health Secretary Frank Dobson promising to halt the closure. Dobson's motivation was this: 'I am not having a blue plaque on the wall of Bart's saying "founded by Henry I in 1123, closed by Frank Dobson in 1999".'[70] When his party duly won a landslide, he did as he promised. Cancelling the Barts closure was a Labour decision. But it was hardly a great step away from the theme of the eighteen years of Tory reforms of the NHS that preceded it. Yes, there was much that was radical. But the real earthquakes that many feared never happened for the simple reason that they were not politically possible. Thatcher wasn't the ideologue she was caricatured as – and she understood that, just as Bevan had in 1948. And that's why for the rest of the NHS's lifetime, there will never be a proposed hospital closure – no matter how well-argued or sensible – that doesn't have a band of local politicians lining up to block it.

7. Infected

John Eaddie's friends didn't know he was dying until it was too late to say goodbye to him. By the time they found out that the rare pneumonia he was suffering from was going to kill him, he was unconscious. One of them recalled: 'I remember the doctor saying he's not going to survive, him lying there unconscious, sort of strapped up to stuff, and that was it. We never spoke to him again.'[1] It was 1981, and they were crowded around his bedside in the Royal Brompton Hospital. It was only then that they found out he wouldn't survive. And it wasn't until forty years later that they found out from an investigative journalist that John was the first British victim of an illness that shook the world and the NHS. He had died of AIDS.

At this point, though, AIDS didn't have a name, and medics were still working out how this mysterious illness afflicting mostly gay men was spreading. In 1981, doctors in Los Angeles described a cluster of pneumocystis pneumonia in five young gay men. This was a rare lung infection, and even more unusual in patients who, as the authors of the report to the US Centers for Disease Control and Prevention noted, had previously been healthy. Two of them had already died. Then there was a strange outbreak of Kaposi's sarcoma, a rare cancer which normally affected people with weakened immune systems, among gay men in New York and California. It became clear that something that attacked the immune system was spreading – and to begin with, it seemed to be spreading only among gay men. 'Gay-related immune deficiency', or GRID, quickly became nicknamed 'gay cancer' and even 'gay plague', which suggested it was an illness sent to punish people for their sexuality.

How was this plague spreading? Was it a sexually transmitted disease? Could it travel through the air? Where had it come from? Researchers theorised that it may have spread from central Africa, where a similar syndrome seemed to be present in heterosexual couples. Other doctors suggested they had diagnosed the illness in infants born to women involved in sex work or who were using intravenous drugs. One patient, Gaëtan Dugas, a Canadian flight attendant, was smeared as the spreader of the virus in the States because doctors studying the virus in March 1984 wrote him up as 'Patient O', with the 'O' standing for 'Out of California'. That 'O' was misread as a zero, and Dugas, who died in March 1984, was vilified for his promiscuous lifestyle.

By the end of 1981, the illness had reached Britain. A letter in the *Lancet* on 12 December 1981 described a 49-year-old male who had been referred to the Brompton Hospital, 'having presented elsewhere with a 3 month history of weight loss, 3 weeks' general malaise, and progressive breathlessness on exertion. He had been fit before this illness and did not abuse drugs or smoke. He was a practising homosexual who travelled to Miami, Florida, annually to visit homosexual friends.' He died ten days after being admitted, the doctors reported, suggesting that 'we believe this to be the first report of this relationship of disease in the UK, and suggest that the diagnosis be considered in 187 male homosexuals who present with an unexplained respiratory illness'.[2] That man, who was known only as 'the Brompton patient' for forty years, until ITV journalists Paul Brand and Nathan Lee tracked down his identity, was John Eaddie.

The team treating Eaddie had no idea what they were dealing with, or how big his illness was going to become. It was – until recently – the worst epidemic the NHS has dealt with. In many ways, it was a vindication of the national health system. It was certainly a vindication of the individual doctors and nurses who, despite rampant societal prejudice against the patients they treated, did their best to make their drawn-out, desperate deaths a little less awful.

From John Eaddie's death in 1981, the disease spread. By the end of 1984, there had been 108 cases and 46 deaths in the UK. In 1982, doctors started to diagnose the syndrome in heterosexual women, leading to a new name: 'acquired immune deficiency syndrome', AIDS for short. In the same year, a 37-year-old man called Terry Higgins collapsed while DJing at Heaven nightclub in London. He was rushed to St Thomas's Hospital with what was initially believed to be pneumonia. He had been suffering from headaches for a while, but had dismissed them as nothing to worry about. One of his friends, Martyn Butler, said: 'To some extent, I'm pleased he had no idea what was coming, that he was so ill he was never going to get out of the bed.' Terry died on 4 July 1982. His partner, Rupert Whitaker, later told the BBC about that day:

> The last time I went, I was going to take some Lucozade and some ice lollies for him. I went up to the ward and there were curtains around Terry's bed at the time. And I was standing just a few feet away and I could see there was quite some activity inside and I just stood there. Then one of the nurses and one of the physicians came round and said: 'Sorry to tell you, but Terry's just died.' And they had been trying to resuscitate him as I had been standing at the end of the bed, well, just a few feet away from the end of the bed. And it was – yeah – that was very hard. It was a very hard thing to see and hear.[3]

Terry's cause of death was toxoplasmosis: by this stage HIV had not been described, and GRID or AIDS was still something most people in Britain thought was a disease afflicting only American gay men. As tests for this new disease advanced, Rupert and Martyn decided to set up a charity to raise awareness of AIDS and fund research into what was causing it – and how to treat it. That charity was named after Terry – the Terrence Higgins Trust – in an attempt to humanise an illness that was already heavily stigmatised.

Brian Gazzard saw the impact that the trust and other charities had on the way the government responded to what was turning into a new epidemic, and a frightening one at that. He was another doctor who treated early AIDS patients before it was known what this new disease was. He was working as a consultant at St Stephen's, now part of the Chelsea and Westminster Hospital in London, 'and along came a man who turned out to be one of the first HIV cases in this country, and we didn't know what was the matter with him. I'd sent my senior registrar to San Francisco on a different project, and he wrote to me saying "there's a new disease sweeping the States" and of course, bizarrely, the very following week the patient appeared in our department with a condition called pneumocystis carinii pneumonia. It was the only time everybody thought I was very clever, because I looked at the X-ray and said, this is PCP, because I'd been forewarned the week before.'

That patient initially told Dr Gazzard that he was monogamous, which turned out to be slightly inaccurate. 'About 150 of his partners came to see me and they all had the same syndrome.' The doctors at St Stephen's started to organise themselves. They took over much of the private wing of the hospital, as it had single rooms so the patients could be isolated from one another. At the height of the epidemic, Gazzard was running two wards of forty patients each, with about five or six dying a week. With each diagnosis, he would have to explain to the patient that 'I'm very sorry, you know we can't cure you, but we can at least make sure you die with dignity'.

Many of their medical colleagues were fascinated by the clinical practice and research they were doing: 'There was a waiting list of several months to try to join our department. Doctors were queuing up to come and try and work for us. Because although for the patient it was absolutely devastating, medically it was absolutely fascinating: you had a new disease, with all sorts of psychosexual issues involved, and then you have a range of 30 to 40 previously unbelievably rare diseases connected with the central problem. And nobody really knew how to manage any of them. So it was a very interesting time.' Others were less positive: the medical director at the hospital came to Gazzard and complained: 'You are ruining the hospital's reputation. People won't come here because they are worried about being infected, and you're taking over the private wing of the hospital.' Looking back, Gazzard remarks that the opposite was true: Chelsea and Westminster is now renowned worldwide for the work it did with AIDS patients in the 1980s, and still does today. He also feels that the way the health service responded to the illness represented 'the NHS at its best':

> Ken Clarke, who was health minister first of all, came to see me nearly every week to ask me if he could do any more to help with what was going on. And then Norman Fowler did the same thing. And it was one of those occasions where really everybody rose

magnificently to the test. We clearly needed more money. So they gave us money. We clearly needed more staff, so they gave us more staff. It wasn't just me who was impressed: people from the States used to come over and they'd say: 'But you've not asked him about his insurance yet.' And I'd say, 'No, that's not actually relevant.' 'But you've ordered an MRI scan, and that's very expensive: how's he going to cover it?' They found it very difficult to believe that everything was free at the point of contact.[4]

The Terrence Higgins Trust and other campaigners made sure ministers and the medical establishment paid attention. In 1985, Chief Medical Officer Donald Acheson set up the Expert Advisory Group on AIDS. One of the medics at the first meeting recalled that the officials offered a 'flattering, patronising, inappropriate response' in which they encouraged the doctors themselves to take the initiative and talk to the media about the disease, rather than getting the government involved. At the second meeting, Acheson was chairing, and 'very quickly recognised the importance' of what was going on. It was at this point that he started to warn the then health minister, Norman Fowler, about what was going on.[5]

Of course, not all healthcare professionals responded well or made the right judgements, particularly in the early days of the epidemic. Many AIDS patients were too ill to leave their beds. But one, a young man admitted to Monsall Hospital in Manchester in 1985, found that he didn't have any choice. After asking to go home to die, Roger Youd was detained under public health legislation introduced that year, which made it illegal for anyone to knowingly spread an infectious disease. Monsall was a Victorian isolation hospital. The 29-year-old patient was ordered to stay there for three weeks after local medical officer Dr Anna Jones and the Chief Medical Officer, Donald Acheson, argued that because he was bleeding profusely, he posed a risk to the wider community in a way that most AIDS victims didn't.

His detention was lifted on appeal because the city council said Youd's condition had improved and therefore couldn't justify his continued detention. In any case, Youd was 'now said to be willing to remain in hospital'. The Terrence Higgins Trust brought the appeal, and its spokesman Les Latner told the press after the hearing: 'Now he knows that he can leave he is quite happy to stay. Once people had explained to him that he was in no condition to leave he agreed that hospital was the best place for him.' Latner was critical of the way the doctors had, as he saw it, rushed to take legal action against Youd: 'The man said that he wanted to go home to die. He was haemorrhaging, he was so weak he could hardly have walked out of the door. The doctors should have persuaded him to stay instead of rushing off to the courts. His parents didn't even know he had AIDS until they read the court report.'[6] But the judge hearing the appeal said the original order was legal – something often missed by those citing this case. What the case did do was to galvanise the gay community in Manchester and beyond to start campaigning actively for the rights of AIDS patients and for more support. The Terrence Higgins Trust began to receive calls from other people who were anxious that they might be detained if they came forward for testing. In the event, Youd was the only patient detained under the Public Health Act. He died a few months later, in January 1986.

Gazzard's team used single rooms on wards for their AIDS patients. This was a sensible infection control measure, not just because it wasn't clear how the virus spread but also because each patient was suffering from a variety of different AIDS-related illnesses, some of which were infectious for other immunocompromised people, such as fellow AIDS sufferers. But the single rooms also made the life of someone dying of a highly stigmatised illness even lonelier, as it meant wary staff could easily avoid them.

As the virus became better known but remained poorly understood, fear about it spread through the healthcare community. Within this was a terror of catching it, along with judgement of the gay men suffering from it.

Sue Reeve worked as a nurse in London from 1980 onwards, and recalls the anxiety of some colleagues charged with looking after AIDS patients. 'One of my friends was doing agency work at the Hammersmith Hospital and I can very clearly remember them telling me that they were on the ward with AIDS patients who were in side rooms, and the regular staff were not happy to be going in and providing care. My friend would go in and would find a week's worth of detritus and food trays that hadn't been cleared out. They told me that some staff were only giving patients toast because that was something they could slide under the doors without entering the room. It became known as the "toast diet".'

When Reeve trained to be a district nurse in 1985, a doctor gave her group of trainees a talk in which he told them 'AIDS . . . would be more appropriately called "acquired-immoral deficiency syndrome"'. One of her patients was a man living in South London with his partner. He was dying. Reeve was referred to him to offer him emotional support. 'I was quite nervous,' she admits. 'There was a lot of anxiety. But I was absolutely determined that I was going to do my utmost with him. He was going to get better care than the rest of my patients as far as I was concerned. He then became very sick and moved back to his family in the north of England where he died. I remember going to his funeral which was all young gay male couples who were obviously just thinking "when is it going to be me?"'[7]

Understanding of the illness advanced and a disparity grew between the professionals who were regularly in contact with AIDS patients and those who were only occasionally. In 1985, porters at the Hammersmith Hospital refused to go into the room of a man who had just been admitted with AIDS. One district nurse in the late 1980s, when the ways of transmission were well known, asked a colleague to visit one of her AIDS patients for her, and later discovered that this colleague arrived at the patient's home in a hazmat suit. The hazmat suit and other extensive but inappropriate applications of personal protective equipment were a common theme among workers who didn't fully understand what the real risks of AIDS were. Ambulance workers were anxious about performing resuscitation, and again some donned what one doctor described as 'space suits' to try to protect themselves.

Sue Carrington was a nurse working in haematology in Bristol at the start of the epidemic. In an interview she said: 'There was a huge amount of publicity about it. There was a lot of finger-pointing at people who were gay or drug takers, which was sad. But because I worked on the haematology unit, they were fairly well informed about AIDS. But when I worked on a general ward and in theatres there was more fear around it because people didn't understand it as much.' She described an operating department assistant turning up to surgery later in the epidemic with 'all this gear on. Full PPE, mask and everything. And this patient was like a child. He was a teenager and it was so inappropriate to have this like, zombie spaceman walking towards you. This operating assistant wasn't even going to be in theatre. It really pissed me off, it angered me. And I was in charge so I told him off.'[8]

Some doctors tried to reassure colleagues. In 1985, Dr Stuart Glover of Ham Green Hospital appeared on a *TV Eye* documentary on AIDS where he very pointedly examined his patients with his ungloved hands. Another doctor, Dr Anthony Pinching, a clinical immunologist at St Mary's, Paddington, told the documentary that 'AIDS is not a very infectious disease. In fact one of my colleagues has called it one of the least infectious diseases I have ever seen. I think it's important to understand what that means. We are talking about a disease which can only be transmitted by very intimate contact, that is to say sexual contact or direct blood-to-blood inoculation. It is not a disease that is spread by any other means.'[9] In the event, the risk of transmission from patient to doctor or nurse turned out to be very low. By 1987, there were just nine reported cases of such transmission worldwide. Some risks were easier to avoid than others: for example, needles were redesigned to make it harder for healthcare workers to accidentally prick themselves with an unsheathed needle.

There were also fears that healthcare professionals who were themselves HIV-positive could unwittingly spread the virus to their patients if they were performing certain procedures. The *News of the World* tried to 'out' two doctors working as GPs in London and who were undergoing treatment for the virus. The London health authority managed to get an injunction preventing the newspaper from printing their identities, which had been obtained from medical records passed to the reporter by a hospital employee. But on 15 March 1987, the paper ran a piece headlined 'Scandal of Docs with AIDS', complaining that the DHSS had refused to answer questions about whether any GPs infected with AIDS were currently working in

NHS surgeries, whether Sir Donald Acheson thought it appropriate for a doctor with AIDS to carry on treating patients in gynaecology, and whether there were any doctors suffering from AIDS as a result of homosexual relationships. That article was found to be in contempt of court, and the paper was issued with a £10,000 fine.

Then, the *Mail on Sunday* published a piece in November of the same year that revealed a consultant working in the renal unit at the London Hospital had died of AIDS. Public fear was mounting.

Internal government briefings at the time remarked that even though there were no known cases of such transmission in the world, it might be difficult to detect given the time lag between infection and the development of AIDS. There were also worries that dementia – which many AIDS patients seemed to develop along with other illnesses – might impair the judgement of a positive healthcare worker, and so lead to accidents in care. The General Medical Council issued guidance that anyone who thought they had been infected must get tested and have regular medical supervision if they turned out to be positive. Those who didn't take the necessary actions would be disciplined.

This didn't fully satisfy Thatcher, who was worried that the medical community was being too complacent about the risks of transmission from doctors or nurses who were still asymptomatic. Her special adviser John O'Sullivan wrote her a note which complained that the Department of Health and Social Security was trying to block testing all doctors for HIV on spurious grounds. He wrote that officials were employing the 'familiar technique of greatly inflating minor practical difficulties', including claiming that doctors might refuse en masse to be tested even if it were made a contractual requirement. 'I doubt that even the medical profession is so arrogant as to risk the public hostility that such an attitude would provoke,' he wrote. In another briefing to the PM, he added: 'I would not like to be the Minister for Health, nor indeed the President of the General Medical Council, when the first patient died of Aids contracted from a doctor who had concealed his infection.'[10]

There were more deaths that kept this fear alive. Dr David Collings was working as a surgeon at the Royal Devon and Exeter

Hospital when he went down with what he thought was flu in March 1988. A day later, he was diagnosed with pneumonia and admitted to a general ward at the hospital. He went downhill rapidly, moving to intensive care. Just five days after being admitted, he started to wonder whether he had contracted something far worse than his current diagnosis and asked for an AIDS test. He was positive. He died twelve days after his first symptoms, leaving his family – a wife and a young baby – stunned. Dr Collings had been working in his native Zimbabwe for five years before returning to Britain in 1987. It was in the African country that he was suspected to have caught the virus while performing surgery, but the case naturally sparked concern among the 300-odd people he had operated on since starting back in the NHS. The hospital set up a helpline. Some medical colleagues said the case underlined the need for AIDS to become what was known as a 'notifiable' illness, which meant it must by law be reported to the government. But AIDS never became a notifiable illness, and one of the reasons for this is the fear that it would further stigmatise the disease and make potential carriers even less likely to check their own status. Because Dr Collings had caught AIDS while treating people, he was described in the press as a hero. The same veneration was absent for those who were gay.

The public were terrified of AIDS. But they also had no idea how it spread or whether they were at risk. The assumption on the part of heterosexual people was that because the illness had, in its early stages, seemed to pass between gay men, they didn't need to worry unless they went near an infected person. Even health service workers were still terrified of catching the illness through touching a patient without adequate protection.

The solution came in the form of two touches. One was light; the other heavy-handed. Both became iconic.

In April 1987, Princess Diana agreed to open a ward at the Middlesex Hospital. It wasn't her first hospital ward opening, and it wasn't her first medical venture; by this point she was patron of the British Heart and Lung Foundation. But the striking difference here was that this ward treated AIDS patients.

Diana was used to having images of what she wore beamed around the world. But on this day, the focus was on what she *didn't* wear. Shane Snape was a nurse on the ward treating nine AIDS patients and was himself HIV-positive. 'The lead-up to Princess Diana coming was will she or won't she wear gloves,' he said afterwards. 'I'm pleased to say she didn't wear gloves.'[11] She shook his hands and made a point of touching the patients with her bare hands, sitting on their beds, talking to them, and then asking if they might pose for photographs for the press. Most of them didn't want to be identified at all, or hid because they were deeply unhappy with the sensational way the newspapers had covered the epidemic. One, though, agreed to be photographed shaking the princess's hand, albeit without his face in view. 'He was dying,' one of the nurses explained later. 'And he thought, well, so what, I'll do it.'[12]

Everything Diana had done was entirely deliberate. She told the media: 'HIV does not make people dangerous to know. You can shake their hands and give them a hug. Heaven knows they need it.' Buckingham Palace sources further briefed journalists that 'she did this to explode the myth that Aids, spread through promiscuous sex and tainted blood products, could be caught from ordinary activities, such as shaking hands.'[13]

Diana's visit lasted just forty minutes, but it wasn't the only one she made to AIDS patients in the UK, or abroad, in her life. The gentle touch of her hands on the bodies of dying men changed attitudes to AIDS, not just in Britain but around the world. Snape described it as giving AIDS a 'Royal Approval', which would 'break down this stigma to what's attached to it'. Martyn Butler, co-founder of the Terrence Higgins Trust, described 'a pre-Diana and a post-Diana AIDS', with it becoming 'fashionable' and 'acceptable' to care about people with the illness.[14]

Around the same time, government ministers were coming up with far less gentle ways of educating the public about AIDS. Norman Fowler was the Conservative Health Secretary between 1981 and 1987, and by 1985 was aware that AIDS was becoming a serious problem in Britain. By 1986, it was occupying so much of his time as a minister that an adviser noted in a memo to Margaret Thatcher that 'AIDS has been absorbing most of the energies of both Tony Newton [a health minister] and Norman Fowler for the past few weeks' and that she should ask him whether 'more of the "normal" NHS management work' was being taken on by others in the department.[15] Fowler was horrified by the attacks on gay people, and concerned by rising diagnoses in heterosexual individuals, and he realised something needed to be done to educate the public. But he found that his prime minister was rather anxious about what this might entail. 'My first battle was to get everyone including the government to take it seriously. I didn't have a great deal of support from the prime minister, who had a rather curious attitude to HIV and AIDS. She didn't quite regard it as purely a moral issue as some did, but she didn't really want to talk about it at all. And she never really changed from that. I know that when she appointed my successor John Moore it was made clear to him that "Fowler has gone, he's made too much of this AIDS issue, now get back to cutting waiting lists".' Along with Acheson and the Cabinet Secretary, Robert Armstrong, Fowler came up with a way of dealing with Thatcher's squeamishness about both the illness and the necessary advice for avoiding it. They set up a Cabinet committee which was chaired not by Thatcher but by her deputy, Willie Whitelaw. 'There was no way the prime minister could interfere with it, and because half the Cabinet were there already they were signed up to what we did. It was the internal bureaucracy allowing us to get things done.'

Thatcher continued to demur on public awareness campaigns, though. Fowler says her initial preference was for 'having advertisements in public lavatories rather like VD', but this didn't seem to him to encapsulate the scale of the threat. Venereal disease wasn't killing people in large numbers like AIDS was.[16]

Initially the government placed adverts about AIDS in the newspapers. One of those advertisements said, in large type: 'WHAT KIND OF PEOPLE GET AIDS? THE KIND THAT DON'T KNOW THE FACTS.' It included pictures of a woman with a baby in a buggy, a man in a suit and a young man in a T-shirt, to illustrate that everyone was at risk. In smaller type, it said:

The AIDS virus is not just caught by drug addicts and gay men. Many more men than women are infected so far. But all men and women can catch it and pass it on. It depends on how you behave.

The only ways you are likely to catch the AIDS virus is through sex with an infected person – and by sharing needles if you inject drugs.

You can't tell if someone is infected. They can look and feel completely well – and not know they have the AIDS virus. Probably 30,000 people are already infected in the UK. Don't join them.

The text moved to the 'explicit' section. It instructed men to wear a condom and to 'beware of casual sex', adding: 'Sex which might damage the anus, vagina, penis or mouth is particularly dangerous if one of the partners is infected. Anal sex involves the greatest risk and should be avoided.' Then, it told drug users not to share needles or other equipment, warning: 'Just one fix with an infected needle can give you the AIDS virus.'

This level of detail about sex upset Thatcher and her advisers to the extent that the prime minister asked to ensure that they did not breach the Obscene Publications Act. A memo from David Willetts in the policy unit told her: 'Norman Fowler is proposing to place explicit and distasteful advertisements about AIDS in all the Sunday papers. The AIDS problem is now so serious that we must do as he proposes, though the advert could open with more facts about the spread of AIDS.' Thatcher wrote back: 'Do we have to do the section on Risky Sex? I should have thought it could do immense harm if young teenagers were to read it.' It seemed to have escaped the prime minister's notice that the campaign was warning about the dangers that risky sex held for passing on a disease that people were so frightened of they were refusing to have social contact with anyone gay, let alone someone known to have the infection. Moreover, it was an insight into the way Thatcher had been brought up and the company she kept that she was so worried that people would learn about risky sex for the first time from a government campaign. Fowler's argument, however, was that 'there will still be criticism but I think we must accept that is a necessary price to be paid'.[17]

In the event, no complaints were made about the adverts, and Willetts concluded in a later note to Thatcher that 'public education measures which only a year ago might have been attacked for bad taste will be more acceptable now'.

Fowler, still worried by the small scale of the government response to the epidemic, then developed an idea for a nationwide leaflet drop at the same time as TV advertisements. Both would be a first for the UK. He also wanted a ministerial broadcast to 'explain to the public why we are undertaking a public education campaign on this scale'. Thatcher blocked this request on the grounds that it 'would not be appropriate to have the first Ministerial broadcast for eight years on this subject'. The government was paying more attention by this point, in part because – as a memo in November 1986 noted – 'the spread of the disease is going to affect the community generally, and not just sub-groups such as drug addicts and gays'. Concern was also rising about the costs of the disease. They would be, private briefings to Thatcher indicated in the same year, 'enormous – about £20,000 per person with the disease'. There were anxieties that the prime minister's sensitivities about the matter were 'acting as a brake' on efforts to combat AIDS. Her press secretary, Bernard Ingham, was dismayed that a dinner between twenty-four editors of provincial newspapers and the prime minister in October left the journalists with the impression that she was 'cautious' about a house-to-house leaflet drop, despite their own enthusiasm for the government to 'counteract the damaging effects of the sensational treatment of the issue by such papers as the *Sun*'.

Thatcher wasn't the only one concerned about Fowler's plans. Lord Hailsham wrote to Willie Whitelaw worrying that an unsolicited leaflet would not be popular: 'The appearance on every doormat of the document in question is liable to cause controversy or even offence, and might well spread panic instead of creating a cautious approach to sexual practices and drug injections.' It was, he complained, 'expressed in language dangerously vague and sometimes almost ludicrous'. In another letter, he worried that 'there must be some limit to vulgarity'.[18]

Fowler also wanted a television advert that would stop the leaflet going straight into the bin. He turned to the advertising agency TBWA, which had been working on government health campaigns for a number of years. Malcolm Gaskin, who ran the agency, agreed with Fowler and others that the best approach was 'to attack the disease itself rather than the people who had it, which is how other agencies might have gone about it'. The way of attacking the disease was to scare the living daylights out of television viewers in just forty seconds. 'Scaring people was deliberate,' Gaskin reflected in an interview with the *Guardian* in 2017. His colleague David O'Connor-Thompson came up with a memorable phrase: 'Don't Die of Ignorance'. The agency chose director Nicolas Roeg because he was good at a 'doom and gloom sci-fi aesthetic', and he pulled out all the stops on that front.[19]

The advert opened with a volcano erupting, followed by workers chiselling letters on an enormous tombstone. Actor John Hurt provided a rasping, serious voice, which warned: 'There is now a danger that has become a threat to us all. It is a deadly disease and there is no cure. The virus can be spread through sexual intercourse with an infected person. Anyone can get it, man or woman. So far it has been confined to small groups, but it is spreading. So protect yourself and read this leaflet. If you ignore AIDS, it could be the death of you. So don't die of ignorance.' His closing words were accompanied by the tombstone crashing to the ground, and the 'Don't Die of Ignorance' leaflet landing on top of it, followed by a bouquet of funereal white lilies.

The advert was designed to shock, and it naturally divided opinion. If it wasn't blocked by Thatcher and her colleagues, it wasn't encouraged either – Fowler says the Treasury refused to give his department any more money to cover the campaign, so there was a scrabble within Health to fund it. But Fowler felt it was a price worth paying.[20] Research by his department found an 82 per cent recognition rate, with people surveyed saying they had changed their behaviour because of it.

The epidemic continued, as did the attempts to work out how to stop it. Thatcher was regularly horrified by some of those measures. The Minister of Health David Mellor wrote to her in April 1989 with a plan for a national sex survey of around 20,000 people, which would help inform forecasts of the future spread of HIV, funded in part by the department. He was backed up by Ken Clarke, whose private secretary wrote a note for Thatcher arguing that 'a survey of people's sexual behaviour is needed for these forecasts' and that 'the pilot service shows that it is possible to get truthful answers'. Next to that last, Thatcher scrawled, 'How do you know?' She was, her private secretary Caroline Slocock replied, 'absolutely opposed to such a study of sexual attitudes and behaviour and does not think that it is necessary in order to forecast future AIDS cases. She believes that people would rightly be deeply offended by questions of the kind proposed and she feels strongly that the government is not entitled to intrude into their privacy.' Neither the government nor government money should be involved in any way if the survey still went ahead.[21]

Later that year, Thatcher was sent a 'National AIDS Manual' written by the National AIDS Trust, which was funded in part by the Home Office. An aide warned her that 'far from being neutral, this material legitimises all kinds of deviant behaviour'. Indeed, the manual went into great detail about safe sex, offering suggestions for how people might satisfy their sexual urges without having penetrative intercourse, including through fantasies and a long list of sex toys. It also used vernacular language to appeal to people, with headers such as 'If you're going to fuck despite the risks'. A terse letter from her private secretary to the Home Office complained that: 'The Prime Minister recognises that sexually explicit material may be necessary for communication in this area. But she considers that, in this case, the borderline between the permissible and the pornographic would seem to have been crossed. She feels very strongly that a publication of this sort should not be financed from government funding'.[22] She did, however, accept that it was necessary not just to talk about sex but to talk about sex outside monogamous relationships, gently disagreeing with the Chief Rabbi who suggested it would be more effective to teach abstinence.

Fowler is, by and large, one of the heroes of the government response to the AIDS epidemic, in the same way as Brian Gazzard, Stuart Glover and Anthony Pinching are among the NHS heroes who pioneered the treatment of and encouraged compassion towards the people who caught and died of it in the early years. But it is worth taking a step back and remembering that this expenditure and these scary adverts came from a Conservative government, not a Labour one: the Tories are often concerned about government getting too involved in the way people live their lives, in the form of the 'nanny state'. Not only did AIDS itself necessitate a major programme of health education, it also appears, Rudolf Klein argues, to have converted the Thatcher government to spending money on preventive health measures.[23]

In September 1985, Thatcher was invited to open a £30 million blood products laboratory at Elstree. The purpose of this lab was to ensure a British supply of special blood plasma to avoid any need for blood products from abroad. It sounded like a good way of showing that the government was protecting people with haemophilia. But her private secretary Mark Addison wasn't so sure. In a memo to her diary secretary, he wrote: 'My own feeling on this is that the Prime Minister should stay clear of AIDS (!), even when it is a question of opening laboratories to help innocent victims.'[24] The implication was that the disease was too controversial even when 'innocent' people were involved, and that gay men or drug addicts somehow deserved the suffering and death that was coming to them.

The Elstree laboratory was necessary because of one of the biggest scandals in patient treatment in NHS history: that of contaminated blood. In 1983, twenty-year-old Kevin Slater was diagnosed with AIDS. He died two years later. He hadn't caught it from a sexual partner or from injecting drugs. He had caught it from the products used to treat his haemophilia. His brother Paul also had the clotting disorder, and also died of AIDS more than a decade later, aged thirty. In the intervening years, the scandal ballooned.

People with haemophilia were managing their illness with blood products called factor VIII and factor IX. They contained the proteins which encouraged the blood to clot and were missing for haemophiliacs. The NHS supplied these factors, but sourced them from around the world, including the United States. There were many problems with this supply chain, some of which were already obvious. For one thing, in the US, blood donors were paid, which created an incentive for certain disadvantaged and high-risk groups – including prisoners and drug addicts – to come forward. It would take just one infected donor to contaminate an entire pool of blood. The appeal of the factor products was that haemophiliacs could use them at home, rather than having to trundle to and from hospital endlessly for treatments including transfusions.

The press started to pay attention when a second haemophiliac, Terry McStay, died. In November 1984, the *Daily Mirror* reported that 'a man in Britain has died from the homosexual disease AIDS after being given a blood transfusion'. He was, the newspaper pointed out, not homosexual. The report added that both McStay and the first victim (Slater) 'had received transfusions of Factor 8, a blood clotting product imported from America – where the disease is known as the "gay plague".'[25] The response from the government was to order gay men not to give blood, and blood donation workers to quiz potential donors on their sexual orientation.

Other haemophiliacs were starting to worry. Haydn and Gareth Lewis were brothers with the illness, and had started to hear stories in the early 1980s about fellow sufferers dying. They had experienced the liberation of being able to treat themselves at home thanks to the factors and cryoprecipitate, a part of plasma rich in clotting factors. Gareth described his early days of being a haemophiliac thus: 'My first memories of it were, like milk bottles, pints of milk bottles hanging from drop stands . . . and there was whole blood in one and pure plasma in the other and they were just pumping it through your body to stop any internal bleeding . . . Just weeks and weeks of lying on the bed, having sort of pure plasma and whole blood pumped into you to stop the bleeding.' From his mid-teens, Gareth was treating himself with cryoprecipitate and then recombinant factor. It gave him 'something I've always wanted': control over his illness. But then they grew anxious. A friend of Gareth's who was a biochemist got in touch in 1982 and told him to stop taking factor VIII because he was aware something was wrong.

Haydn, the older of the two, described going to see the

haematologist in Cardiff who was responsible for his care, Professor Arthur Bloom, 'and he seemed to reassure that the risk was so small that it wasn't worth not having treatment'. In 1984, though, Bloom got back in touch to say he might need the brothers to come in and get tested. 'I thought then, well, that's a bit strange, about a year ago he was saying that there wasn't particularly anything to worry about and everything would be okay.'[26]

Both Haydn and Gareth tested positive for HIV, and found out on the same day – Gareth in a corridor of the University Hospital of Wales. Haydn described the fallout:

> Even then when we were told it seemed – and maybe as the doctors the logic is that to tell any patient something you always try and put it across in a way where you're not going to alarm them unnecessarily. Well, he must have been very good at it because I didn't particularly think there was any problems when I came home, but then when I, as soon as I told Gaynor [his wife] of the result then there was a lot of tears and emotions going around as to what was going to happen. And by then, '85, I suppose the reality is that I had read a little bit about how it progresses and what it affects and what the prognosis is if it progressed . . . and it was pretty alarming, frightening.[27]

For Gareth, the diagnosis led to the swift end of his marriage: 'I was told I would be dead in two years and wanted to become a loony lunatic, travelling the world, and my partner at that time just wasn't interested. And her parents reacted rather strangely, wouldn't come in the house any more.'

This meant some people assumed that Gareth was gay, because he was known to have AIDS and his marriage had broken down. He found some members of his local rugby club where he used to go drinking wanted him to stay away. After he gave a TV interview, his car was covered in red paint. 'It was AIDS scum, gay plague and all this, you know, that's what we were dealing with.'

Another victim, who spoke to the campaigning Labour MP Diana Johnson about her plight, was infected with HIV and hepatitis C from a blood transfusion while she was in childbirth. When she went to the doctor, his initial reaction was: 'What have you been doing: injecting, or sleeping around?' The implication was that her lifestyle was why she was in this position, and she was, understandably, mortified.[28]

Even though the media narrative was largely that haemophiliacs were 'innocent' victims of the disease, that didn't filter through to communities where even infected children were shunned. Lee Turton was diagnosed with haemophilia soon after his birth in 1981. Four years later, his parents, Colin and Denise, were told he was HIV-positive as a result of the blood products he was given to manage the condition. When the press and his local school found this out, the little boy was ostracised, with other parents saying he should be barred from classes and one teacher saying they would refuse to teach him. Denise said, 'He wasn't invited to friends', he wasn't invited to parties, which was very hard not only for him but for his sister.' They moved to Cornwall so they could start a new life without anyone knowing their son's diagnosis. Lee started to get sicker in 1988, going from a 'happy little boy' to a child in immeasurable pain. Denise described him as being unable to 'walk far, he couldn't breathe, he couldn't eat, he was eventually fed through a tube'. The family were in and out of hospital with him as he continually contracted infections. He died in January 1992 at home, having repeatedly pleaded with his parents to take him back from the hospital. After his death, the Turtons discovered Lee had been also infected with hepatitis C, in common with many other patients.

Denise's description of the decline and death of her son comes from her evidence at the Infected Blood Inquiry, which was finally set up in 2019 to examine when it became clear that blood products were contaminated and haemophiliacs and people receiving blood transfusions were in grave danger, and how much was really known. The estimates of the number of people infected in the UK range from 5,000 to 30,000, and 3,000 are believed to have died.

It took a long time for the victims to be taken seriously. The inquiry itself was set up after years of campaigning by victims and MPs whose constituents had been infected. Diana Johnson was one of the key forces behind this campaign, taking it on after meeting Glenn Wilkinson, who had been diagnosed with hepatitis C after an operation to remove two teeth at the Hull Royal Infirmary.

Wilkinson was angry that he had never received answers to his questions about what had happened to him and how it had been allowed to happen. Johnson then 'realised it wasn't just Glenn or a few dozen people, it was hundreds, no, thousands, of people'. What she then discovered was that health ministers of all stripes had ended up stonewalling those affected. 'The Department of Health always had the line of "there's nothing to see here, no, move on". And every minister that I've ever spoken to, was always being told, no, there was nothing that they needed to worry about.'[29]

Johnson, along with MPs from across the House of Commons, pushed for a public inquiry into what had happened, but only succeeded when it was politically expedient for a government to do it. The Theresa May government, wounded after losing the Conservative majority in the 2017 snap election, was still trying to set up an agreement with the Democratic Unionist Party when the Northern Irish party – to everyone's surprise – signed a letter saying it would vote in favour of the inquiry in Parliament. At this point, the Tory whips panicked and warned May she could lose a vote in the Commons, which would highlight her weakness, and the government quickly capitulated to the demands for an inquiry.

Johnson is a Labour MP – from the 'party of the NHS'. She was shocked by the difference between the health service that had been there for her when she needed it most, and the behaviour of that service when it got things wrong. She points to a phrase from Bishop James Jones, who worked with the victims of this scandal – having previously chaired the Hillsborough Independent Panel and the inquiry into the deaths at Gosport War Memorial Hospital. In his report on the Hillsborough disaster, he wrote about the 'patronising disposition of unaccountable power'. The victims of the contaminated blood scandal were treated badly for years because those in power could – and that includes the NHS.

Hepatitis C and AIDS weren't the only frightening illnesses in the 1980s. This decade saw the resurgence of antibiotic-resistant 'superbugs' in NHS hospitals. Penicillin-resistant *Staphylococcus aureus* was well known even when the NHS was being set up, and by the 1950s some medics were raising serious concerns. The problem was that penicillin and other antibiotics – first developed for use at the start of the Second World War – were wonder drugs, and the medical establishment more widely didn't want to have to back away from them. Accompanying what now appears to be their vast overuse was an increasingly relaxed attitude to hospital hygiene, because it was assumed that antibiotics would stop a patient from catching anything anyway. The obsessive polishing that Enoch Powell had ridiculed in his time was becoming a thing of the past. Now, it was obsessive prescribing. Antibiotics were prescribed pre-emptively to stop infection – and for viruses, which they could not treat.

By the 1950s, antibiotic use was routine. And by this time, staphylococcal infections were starting to become part of the backdrop of life in NHS hospitals. In 1956, St Bartholomew's Hospital suffered a serious outbreak on one of its surgical units, with thirty-one infections in two months. Researchers studying the spread spotted that one of the surgical staff themselves was a carrier (this is very common, with around a third of the general population carrying the bacteria on their skin, in nasal cavities and elsewhere on their bodies) and spreading it to the patients. *S. aureus* was found on bedclothes, bed curtains and other soft furnishings on the wards.[30]

By the end of the decade, it was becoming clear that the NHS needed to deal with infections that were spreading and couldn't be held in check by wonder drugs. In 1959, Exeter microbiologist Brendan Moore was responsible for the creation and appointment of the first-ever infection control nurse, at Torbay Hospital. Two years later, a new bug was spotted: this one became known as 'methicillin-resistant *Staphylococcus aureus*' – or MRSA. An article appeared in the *British Medical Journal* from Professor Patricia Jevons, who described resistance to the antibiotic methicillin, which had only recently been introduced (marketed as Celbenin) and was widely seen as the end of antibiotic-resistant *S. aureus*. The man who discovered that penicillin could be used as an antibiotic, Ernst Chain, had declared: 'No more resistance problems, methicillin is the answer.' Not everyone was all that worried by Jevons's discovery, arguing that doctors could move to different types of antibiotic and that all would be well. One of those who went on to be a leading figure in the study of what he himself described as a 'terrifying organism', Professor Gordon Stewart, said that 'when the first strains [of MRSA] were isolated, they didn't seem to matter very much' and that they seemed to 'spread without doing much harm'.[31] That started to change quite quickly, though, not least because the infection itself could spread at quite some speed. An outbreak at Queen Mary's Children's Hospital in Carshalton saw around forty patients infected, with one child dying. As the 1960s advanced, there was increased scepticism about using antibiotics in an indiscriminate fashion.

Tackling the bugs took a lot of work and time. Dr Joe Selkon, for instance, was a microbiologist who started work in the 1950s. He described working at Newcastle General Hospital and being 'amazed at the number of staphylococcal infections occurring in our surgical patients and the complete absence of adequate extract-ventilated rooms for the isolation of patients who had multi-drug resistant staphylococcal infections'. He then spent the next few years building isolation rooms with the ventilation he thought was necessary. But by the end of the decade, the doctors at Newcastle General were 'in serious trouble': in 1968 they discovered methicillin-resistant staph in thirty-seven different patients. 'Quite clearly, our hospital did not meet the requirements of a place that does no harm,' he recalled. The local health authority allowed them to build a separate isolation unit with twelve beds, which enabled them to cut MRSA infections: by 1994 they were getting no more than three patients with MRSA in any one year.

The health authority then demanded the hospital change the use of this ward to the treatment of AIDS patients, because MRSA was 'no longer a problem'. The rates shot back up. Selkon was infuriated, too, by the Department of Health, describing it as 'the most dangerous organism we have' because of the policy in the 1990s that forced hospitals into accepting excessive surgical admissions in order to cut waiting lists – or face having their finances cut. He recalled one conversation at the John Radcliffe Hospital in Oxford when he tried to close a ward to new patients. 'The Chief Executive said: "Certainly we will do that, but you realise that it will cost us £500,000 if we don't meet our expected patient put-through rate: think of the hospital, please." And I foolishly conceded.'[32]

Another problem was the way more basic infection control measures were squeezed because of costs. Dinah Gould was a nurse working in the 1970s and reported that, on the orthopaedic wards, 'we weren't allowed to put gloves on because gloves were expensive and they might hurt the patient's feelings'. Even when changing the bed of a patient with severe diarrhoea, 'all we had was handwashing soap to remove this stuff'.[33]

Gould became an infection control nurse in the 1980s, and struggled to get colleagues to take simple measures such as hand hygiene seriously. She described the NHS as paying 'lip service to infection control' until the late 1990s, when clinical governance forced a change. By this stage, 'the premises in which healthcare was being delivered were very far from being clean and they were certainly not free of dirt'. In 1998, the National Audit Office estimated that there were at least 100,000 cases of healthcare-acquired infections and around 5,000 annual deaths at a cost of £1 billion.[34] Gould struggled with her job description: 'I think that people just hoped that I would make a general improvement and somehow wave a magic wand, so I'd learned that there were wards where I was very welcome and the wards where I was very welcome were always the pristine clean ones where I didn't need to go. The wards where people didn't want me to go were the wards that needed the attention.'[35] It was a strange irony that at the same time as AIDS patients found themselves eating only toast shoved under their doors and some staff were turning up in hazmat suits, other workers were forgetting basic hygiene.

It was in the 1980s that things got much more serious. An epidemic strain of MRSA turned up in London, with the Royal Free being one of the first hospitals where this much more contagious variant emerged. Cases started to rise throughout the decade and into the 1990s. By the late 1990s, 'superbugs', as they were now popularly known, weren't just something Gould and other infection control nurses worried about. They were part of the popular imagination about the NHS. The BBC broadcast an episode of *Panorama* titled 'Superbugs' in 1996. The medical press were hardly less restrained, with the *Lancet* heading one piece on vancomycin-resistant *S. aureus* 'Apocalypse Now!' Politicians started fighting over whom to blame for superbugs, though strangely it never seemed to be themselves or their own party when in government. MRSA even became a major battleground in the 2005 general election campaign, with Conservative leader Michael Howard describing MRSA as the new 'British disease' – an old term from the 1970s and '80s when the 'trade unions were out of control'. This disease was 'in our hospitals', which 'are supposed to cure you, not kill you'.[36] This was personal for Howard: his own mother-in-law had died from a hospital-acquired infection. But it was also personal for a lot of voters, who were now frightened of going to hospital in case it made them sicker than before they'd walked through the front doors.

By the mid-2000s, MRSA wasn't the only scary superbug rampaging through hospitals. *Clostridium difficile* was another antibiotic-resistant infection, which was easily carried and transmitted. Between October 2003 and June 2005, there were two serious outbreaks of *C. diff*, as it was popularly known in the health service, at Stoke Mandeville Hospital in Buckinghamshire. At least 33 patients died after developing the infection, with 334 people infected overall. The Healthcare Commission found the hospital was not isolating patients properly, and was also dysfunctional. It also reported that there was a lack of handwashing facilities and a lack of training in infection control, as well as staff shortages.

Maidstone and Tunbridge Wells NHS Trust suffered two outbreaks in 2005–6. The first wave affected 150 patients, and a number died where the infection was definitely or probably the main cause of death. Then, between April and September of the following year, another outbreak affected 258 patients. In total, the trust had more than 500 patients who developed the infection, with 60 dying. When the Healthcare Commission investigated, it again found filthy conditions despite a recent attempt to improve hygiene at the hospital. Issues included 'bedpans that had been washed but were still visibly contaminated with faeces'; patients who were desperate for the toilet being told to 'go in the bed' because there weren't enough staff to take them; and staff being 'too rushed to undertake hand hygiene, empty and clean commodes, clean mattresses and equipment properly, and wear aprons and gloves appropriately and consistently'.[37]

By 2005, hospital workers had a new dress code including 'bare below the elbows', which meant rolled-up sleeves, no watches or jewellery, and a crackdown on ties. White coats were not allowed either. Hospitals also became adept at closing off wards and isolating individual patients. Less eye-catching but more important was the programme set up at the same time by the health service to reduce healthcare-acquired infections, which involved experts visiting hospitals and improvement teams set up in trusts. The programme did lead to a change in attitudes and practices. Hospitals became cleaner, safer, and the debate in the political world moved on to whether outsourcing cleaning contracts had led to this state of filthiness. One study of 126 NHS trusts in England between 2005 and 2009 found that the incidence of MRSA infection was 2.28 for every 100,000 bed days for trusts which outsourced their cleaning, and 1.46 for trusts with in-house cleaners.[38] The reason this was political was that it was the Thatcher government that had allowed hospitals to save money by contracting out their cleaning. This enabled some politicians to tell a story about what happened when a public service lost control of some of its functions to the commercial sector, and about the effect of the profit motive on standards. For some matrons, the contracts represented a loss of power over their wards – something Andy Burnham, a health minister in the later years of the New Labour government, highlighted in a report he wrote after spending weeks shadowing NHS staff.

That's the NHS for you: where even the question of who cleans the bedpans can become a major political issue. As for who was in charge of them well, that led to an even bigger battle.

8. Control freaks

'You put your faith and your lives in the hands of the NHS and you feel no need to question it. She fell back on the NHS and still believed in it . . . She never imagined it would come to this.' This, for Mavis Skeet, was the end of the line. She was dying of oesophageal cancer. The 74-year-old's faith in the health service turned out to be ill-founded when, after being diagnosed with the tumour in December 1999, the operation to examine it further was repeatedly cancelled. The first time, the anaesthetist at Leeds General Infirmary had gone down with influenza, which was particularly bad that winter. Indeed, there were so many flu cases in the ensuing weeks that Skeet's operation was cancelled another three times in the space of five weeks, each time at the last minute and each time because the hospital had simply run out of intensive care beds. By January 2000, the tumour was inoperable. Skeet died in June that year.

Her daughter Jane was incensed, giving the press the above words as she explained that the medical team had said 'the five-week delay caused it to spread', adding: 'She always felt it was understaffed, underfunded and the doctors overworked but she never imagined it would come to this. The government say they are dealing with the situation, but they obviously are not.'[1]

Skeet's death quickly came to represent something bigger: a fear that the NHS itself was coming to the end of the line. This had been years in the making, but time was now running short. Some of the battles that shaped the NHS have been about how it runs, some about who is in charge. This one was going to be about whether it would survive at all.

The NHS had become used to what Nigel Crisp, then chief executive of the Oxford Radcliffe Hospital Trust but later the chief executive of the service, describes as 'managing decline', with crumbling hospital buildings and huge drops in staffing and training. 'The

NHS was really in quite a lot of trouble. A&E at the end of the '90s was really bad. I mean it really was, in a lot of places, and even in the John Radcliffe, which is a first-class hospital,' he says. 'Even the big, classic, NHS giants, the Guys and the Tommys, their A&E departments were pretty poor and the little hospitals were really rather poor. So there was a very, very obvious sense of decay. I remember the A&E at West Middlesex, where it was sort of detached from the rest of the hospital, so if you were admitted, you were stuck on a trolley and taken out in the rain across to somewhere else. This was a period when people were talking about the "third world NHS", which is an insult both to the NHS and to the third world, of course.'[2]

The quality of the healthcare that remained open was poor, and the public were noticing it, too. Malcolm Alexander was the director of the Association of Community Health Councils for England and Wales and was responsible for the 'Casualty Watch' survey that these statutory bodies ran, providing data on A&E trolley waits. He describes the situation in King's College Hospital's A&E department in the late 1990s: 'There was trolley after trolley after trolley, just nine inches apart in A&E, and others placed in the corridors. The conditions were appalling, with people lying there for many, many hours. When you walked into the A&E entrance, a symbol of how bad things had become was the pigeon nesting on the ledge above the entrance. There were just so many seriously ill patients.' That was what prompted the regular Casualty Watch survey where the health councils would collect data at 4 p.m. on a Monday: how long each patient had been waiting, what was wrong with them and how long they would be there. Alexander felt there was a divide between the way the public tended to view the NHS through their local A&E, and the way the non-emergency doctors saw it: 'It seems strange to us but A&E for many doctors was just the place where the "mob" came in. I thought it was the front line of critical care.'[3]

The Conservatives' spending plans had squeezed the health service to the extent that, by 1997, patients languishing on trolleys in hospitals had become regular news items. Some of the waits were harrowing; others deadly. In 1995, Michael Curtin discovered his wife, Maggie, lying dead on the hospital trolley she had been on for nine hours while waiting for treatment. She had been rushed to Northwick Park Hospital with severe shortage of breath as a result of her cancer. Maggie was well known to staff there because of her illness, but it was a busy time, and her husband claimed that she was left unattended for long periods and that it took thirty-one hours for her to get a scan confirming a pulmonary embolism – a blood clot on the lung. Michael wrote to Virginia Bottomley:

> Is this good health care? Perhaps my wife's life could have been saved had she been attended by the team of doctors and nurses who were familiar with her case. There was a lack of continuity.
>
> Instead, I was left to discover Maggie dead. The report [into what happened] edges around this. Can you imagine anything more unbearable as finding your wife dead in a hospital bed? What if my children had rushed up to give their mum a big get-well-soon kiss?[4]

These kinds of stories were difficult for the public to forget. Tony Blair's rebranded New Labour scented an opportunity, and seized it as it built up its campaign for the 1997 general election. Aware that no one actually reads manifestos, Blair launched a short 'pledge card' with the five priorities for his party in government. Number three was: 'Cut NHS waiting lists by treating an extra 100,000 patients – as a first step by releasing £100 million saved from NHS red tape.' He made similar promises in party political broadcasts, telling voters: 'Ask yourself this question: these Tories get back in for another five years, will we even have a National Health Service in the way that we've known it and grown up with it?'[5] The manifesto itself went into more detail, saying: 'Labour will cut costs by removing the bureaucratic processes of the internal market. The savings achieved will go on direct care for patients. As a start, the first £100 million saved will treat an extra 100,000 patients. We will end waiting for cancer surgery, thereby helping thousands of women waiting for breast cancer treatment.'[6]

These pledges were typical of New Labour in its early days: attention-seeking but without much behind them. The truth was that the *number* of patients waiting was far less important than the amount of *time* it took for them to get treatment. There wasn't a

New Labour health policy as such. Blair himself is very clear that 'I hadn't thought deeply about the NHS in a systemic way'. He says that 'in 1997, it was a very simple deal: the NHS was creaking really under the Conservatives; there had been substantial under-investment in the public realm and our job was to repair that investment'.[7] This lack of systemic thinking didn't stop him making one of his most memorable claims on the eve of the poll: that the country had '24 hours to save the NHS'.

It turned out, though, that the NHS had a lot longer to wait than just twenty-four hours. On winning his landslide majority, Blair appointed Frank Dobson as Health Secretary. Dobson was a joyfully sweary socialist, an Old Labour type – not part of the new establishment in the party. He loved the NHS, but not in the way that Blair believes was ultimately healthy. Reflecting on appointing Dobson, Blair wrote in his autobiography: 'At the helm of the NHS, I had put Frank Dobson. This, in itself, indicated how little I understood when first in office. The truth is Frank was genuinely and, to be fair, avowedly Old Labour. He was one of the many who considered New Labour a clever wheeze to win. He didn't understand it much, and to the extent that he did, he disagreed with it.'[8]

Dobson himself complained about the tendency of Downing Street under Blair wanting 'an initiative every 20 minutes'.[9] The pair met on 6 May 1997 to discuss what they wanted to do with the health service, and Dobson duly produced a rather lengthy note for Blair. He was, unsurprisingly, enthusiastic about ending the internal market and wanted to secure 'contingency plans for coping with winter pressures'. He had also, elsewhere, set in motion plans to deal with some of the more controversial aspects of Virginia Bottomley's London hospital reorganisation, including stopping the closure of Barts. He examined the six options for reforming the way the NHS was resourced: no change; social insurance; a core service with 'top-up' charges for amenities; a 'more rational system of co-payments to replace the current ad-hoc charges'; hypothecated taxes; and greater use of public–private partnership funding. But while he insisted that 'we must be prepared to consider change, given the pressures on the service and our commitments on general taxation', he then dismissed most of them as either being too expensive or against the core principles of the service.[10]

New Labour was a rebrand of an old, tired party. Perhaps it wasn't surprising, then, that the party had similar designs on the NHS. Until this point, the now world-famous blue lozenge logo hadn't been plastered all over the health service. Dobson argued:

> The concept of a *National* Health Service treating and caring for people close to their homes in every part of the country has been undermined by the substitution of competition for cooperation in relations between different parts of the NHS.
>
> This sense of fragmentation has been reinforced by the plethora of new names, slogans, logos and liveries deployed by the Trusts. Besides ending the fragmentation caused by internal competition, I believe we must consider the symbolic advantages of just one logo and livery for all the NHS.[11]

That one logo and livery was the blue lozenge that Richard Moon had designed back in the early 1990s. Deliberately sidelined by the Conservatives for many years, now it was going to be *the* NHS logo. Dobson's department came down like a ton of heavy blue lozenges on anyone using the wrong logo. It might seem a small, operational moment in the history of the NHS, but it was arguably highly significant as a means of firming up the British attachment to its health service. The NHS blue lozenge has become one of the most recognisable brands in the world. The service today is protective and prescriptive about the brand, and the public expects it to be so. Research carried out for NHS England in 2016 described it as 'the most well-known and trusted brand in the UK'. This level of brand awareness is something most commercial organisations spend millions trying to achieve: the survey found that more than half of people could describe the lozenge and letters design, and 87 per cent knew it was blue or white. It also revealed the level of attachment people had to this identity: the public were 'worried' about NHS organisations failing to use the lozenge, and 'for many, this would imply privatisation, or a loosening of the high standards of quality they expected – and felt they received – from the NHS'. They were even 'negative about the use of other colours' in the logo, which was strictly Pantone 300.[12]

But at this time, the branding wasn't going to help with the wider public dissatisfaction with the health service. It didn't matter if the NHS became more recognisable and coherent as an organisation if it wasn't treating patients in a timely or dignified fashion. The British Social Attitudes Survey put public dissatisfaction with the service at 50 per cent in 1996, but it was still high – at 39 per cent – three years after Labour came to power. Dobson very quickly realised from his meetings with health officials that the waiting list pledge made in the election was not only the wrong one in terms of numbers versus length of time, but also impossible to meet for a good few years because of the financial constraints upon the service.

Those financial constraints meant the NHS became part of one of the things this Labour government went down in history for: bitter infighting. The cracks between Blair and his Chancellor, Gordon Brown, were opening up by the day. These were the years of frenzied media briefings by advisers, and the Treasury already had its own operation in place within a few months of Labour taking power. Early on, Dobson's attempts to get more money heading into the winter months led to a furious spat between the two camps: the Treasury had reluctantly signed off on an extra £250 million, but would announce it only as part of a wider story that showed it being tough on spending. In October 1997, Blair's spin doctor Alastair Campbell remarked with some disgust in his diaries that 'GB [Gordon Brown] was adamant that a straight "more money for health" story was a bad story', and described the scramble between him and Treasury spinner Charlie Whelan to brief political journalists in their own chosen way.[13] It didn't land well. A private memo from Blair's right-hand man and 'Prince of Darkness' Peter Mandelson to the prime minister a couple of days later complained of the 'autonomous and unhelpful operation of the Treasury's media relations', which had led to the 'ridiculous situation of being put on the *defensive* yesterday on NHS funding because of the cack-handed way it was briefed'.[14]

The row over that £250 million was symptomatic of the poison that was already seeping through the government – and which would cause bigger issues for the NHS in years to come. But it was also an illustration of the approach the administration was taking to health: a lump of money here, a reversal of Tory policy there. Even the big restructures of Conservative reforms weren't quite as dramatic as billed; the internal market went but the split between the organisations providing the services and those commissioning – known as the 'purchaser–provider split' – remained. There was no big systemic change: a confidential memo from a policy unit awayday in July 1997 had concluded that 'radical change would probably wait until second term'.[15]

The problem was that the public continued struggling with the waits for treatment. The Casualty Watch carried out by the Community Health Councils in January 1999 found waits were considerably shorter than the previous year, but that patients 'still had to wait for unacceptable times (28 hours 43 minutes for one patient by the time of the survey)', and that services were 'tightly stretched' and vulnerable to events. It reported the miserable case of one patient thus: 'Trying to imagine what 26 January must have been like for just one patient at Manchester Royal Infirmary – the 10th longest wait in the list – brings home how distressing such waits must be. A 74-year-old woman attended A&E with chest pains at 8.11pm on Sunday evening. At 4.45am the following morning – i.e. after an 8 1/2 hour wait through the night – a decision was taken that she should be admitted. By the time of Casualty Watch some 11 hours 45 minutes after this decision, she was still waiting on a trolley in A&E.'[16]

The tightly stretched services the survey had warned about ended up in crisis again the following winter, as the flu set in. Mavis Skeet was by no means the only patient who missed out on treatment that was needed. The Casualty Watch for January 2000 had more terrible stories, including a 71-year-old woman with a fracture who had been waiting forty hours and forty minutes on a trolley at Northwick Park Hospital. In Redbridge, a 57-year-old man with abdominal pain had been waiting twenty-two hours and forty-three minutes on a trolley. The Norfolk and Norwich Hospital ran out of space in its mortuary and ended up having to hire a refrigerated lorry to store thirty-six bodies. The ambulance services were struggling to cope, receiving twice the number of calls they were used to. One doctor at Whiston Hospital, Greater Manchester, said he had seen 100 cases of viral pneumonia in just one week – triple the number he'd seen in any week of his 28-year career.

This crisis was serious not just because of the numbers or the individual stories, but because of the long-term consequences. By this point it had become clear that the problems with the NHS weren't about a bad spell or a difficult winter, but something more existential. The service wasn't the envy of the world: it compared poorly to its European neighbours on funding, cancer survival, heart attacks and patient satisfaction. Everyone working in the service and in Downing Street at the time agrees: the fear was not merely that Labour would lose voters' trust on the health service but that the health service itself was in danger of losing public support.

Alan Milburn became Secretary of State for Health in October 1999 after Dobson left to campaign (unsuccessfully) to became London mayor. Milburn was one of Blair's neighbours, both geographically and politically. He was, in his own words, 'an angular young man in his 40s from the North East'.[17] Others described him as blunt – controlling, even. Nicholas Timmins says he had a 'touch of the bully'.[18] He had been the Minister of State for Health in the early days of the government, had then moved to the Treasury, and by this point was seriously worried about whether the NHS would survive. He had personally seen the cost of the waiting lists: a friend of his, Ian Weir – who worked for the *Northern Echo* newspaper in his Darlington constituency – had been waiting over a year for treatment for his heart disease. He died waiting. It shook Milburn, who felt that 'the NHS was on a slippery slope: public confidence was falling, waiting lists were rising. And of course, what was worrying was that the politics had changed as well, in that the Conservative Party was moving towards a position of greater antipathy to the NHS and a greater sense that a different model would be might be required, like state subsidies for private health insurance. And once you had that, you had effectively the middle classes opting out, or, you know, being given a state-sponsored route to opt out: at that point, the universality of the NHS, as an instrument for fairness within British society was under real threat.'[19] Nigel Crisp agreed, writing in his memoirs that 'there was a real question at the time about whether the British National Health Service could survive'.[20]

Milburn wasted no time in communicating his concerns about how serious matters were: just two days after taking the job, he told a dinner of the great and the good in the health service and Royal Colleges: 'Listen, guys, the NHS is drinking in the last chance saloon.' He warned them that the service simply couldn't carry on doing more of the same – that the government was happy to put in resources but there had to be reform alongside it.

His message was soon underlined in an unlikely and – at the time – seemingly rather unhelpful manner. Just days after Mavis Skeet found out her tumour was inoperable, Labour peer and world-renowned fertility doctor Robert Winston gave an interview to the *New Statesman*. He was palpably furious with his own party, professionally and personally. He accused the government of being 'quite deceitful' about the state of the service, arguing: 'We gave categorical promises that we would abolish the internal market. We have not done that. Our reorganisation of the health service was . . . very bad. We have made medical care deeply unsatisfactory for a lot of people. We have always had this right but monolithic view that there should be equality throughout the nation at the point of delivery. All very good stuff, but it isn't working.' Most potently, he recounted the case of his 87-year-old mother, admitted to hospital a few weeks before. 'She waited 13 hours in casualty before getting a bed in a mixed-sex ward – a place we said we would abolish. None of her drugs were given on time, she missed meals and she was found lying on the floor when the morning staff came on. She caught an infection and she now has an ulcer on her leg.' He added: 'It is normal. The terrifying thing is that we accept it.'[21]

The article was incendiary, and tipped the politics in favour of doing something big – and fast. The Blairite spin machine went full throttle. Campbell reacted furiously to a line in the interview where Winston casually remarked that Cherie Blair was having a Caesarean section for the Blairs' fourth child at Chelsea and Westminster Hospital. This was in part because Cherie herself was upset, threatening at one stage to make a complaint to the GMC about Winston. Campbell stopped Winston from doing more interviews and forced him to issue a statement where he 'supported the general direction of our policy, attacked the Tories, and denied the remarks about Cherie'. The prime minister, though, was more anxious about the professor's remarks on the NHS. The story about Campbell trying to 'nobble' Winston dominated Westminster, but the papers were also going to town on the comments about the 'deceitful' health policy.[22]

Blair decided it was time to say something big on the health service. The Gordon Brown problem hadn't gone away, but the prime minister decided that rather than having private meetings with his Chancellor to get the money before announcing it, he'd do things the other way round. He turned up on the *Breakfast with Frost* programme on BBC One that Sunday and told interviewer David Frost that he planned to dramatically increase health spending. He wanted, he said, to be 'in a position where our health service spending comes up to the average of the European Union, it's too low at the moment so we'll bring it up to there'.[23] This was a huge increase. It would mean rises starting at £2.5 billion every year – and going up even more later. Brown was furious, telling Blair 'You've stolen my fucking Budget!'[24] and complaining that the prime minister's solution to every problem was more money.

Blair and his health ministers and advisers were adamant that Health did need more money, though. 'He did have a point. The announcement was a bit of a bounce, to be honest,' admits Blair sheepishly. 'But the money wasn't a big problem. Our disagreements were really about policy: I always had, and still have, an enormous admiration for his intellect and, you know, he's a big heavyweight in anyone's language, but I was absolutely convinced you had to go down this investment and reform path, and the reform was very important but you weren't going to get the reform unless you made good on your pledge to the health service.'[25]

Brown was cornered, and duly announced the extra money in his 'fucking Budget' a few weeks later. Health spending would rise by 6 per cent in real terms every year. Milburn, meanwhile, was beavering away on a plan for the NHS that would cover the improvement and reforms that came alongside the cash. He was joined in this endeavour by an adviser called Simon Stevens, who had worked for Dobson and then stayed in the department for its new boss. Stevens was an unusual hybrid: he was intensely political and was a Labour councillor in Brixton – though prior to that he had run the leadership campaign for a young Boris Johnson at the Oxford Union debating society. But he was also a creature of the health service, having joined its management training scheme in 1988 at Shotley Bridge General Hospital. There, like all trainees, he rotated around the different aspects of the service, including working as a porter. He went on to manage mental health services, hospitals and primary care in various regions of England. One friend told the *British Medical Journal* that Stevens's career had shown him 'the rough end of the NHS': his predecessor in one post had died by suicide. He was a sharp, intellectual sort who knew how to run organisations – and run politicians, too.

Stevens and Milburn didn't have long to write the plan, but by July they managed to produce a document of 150-odd pages containing 300 targets and almost as many uses of the word 'change', just to drive home what was going on. Even more strikingly, its preface wasn't the usual slightly meaningless self-congratulatory waffle that you find at the start of most government documents. It was signed by the presidents of the Royal Colleges, the unions, the Local Government Association, key charities and think tanks. Together, they declared that they supported ten 'core principles' of the health service, which were as follows:

1. The NHS will provide a universal service for all based on clinical need, not ability to pay.
2. The NHS will provide a comprehensive range of services.
3. The NHS will shape its services around the needs and preferences of individual patients, their families and their carers.
4. The NHS will respond to different needs of different populations.
5. The NHS will work continuously to improve quality services and to minimise errors.

6. The NHS will support and value its staff.
7. Public funds for healthcare will be devoted solely to NHS patients.
8. The NHS will work together with others to ensure a seamless service for patients.
9. The NHS will keep people healthy and work to reduce health inequalities.
10. The NHS will respect the confidentiality of individual patients and provide open access to information about services, treatment and performance.[26]

None of this was exactly a crusade against motherhood and apple pie. But the reason Milburn had bothered to get all these organisations on one page was to show that 'what we've managed to do is win an argument that the one thing that was not an option was the status quo'.[27] They were signed up to what was going to happen: they all recognised the 'last chance saloon' risk and were delighted that something was happening that would save the service. When Milburn unveiled his plan in the House of Commons, many of the figures who had signed the preface were watching in his Whitehall office. They started banging the table in celebration at what was happening.[28]

It meant the plan was 'sticky within the NHS': this wasn't a set of ideas but something that was definitely going to happen. Milburn's own wife, a doctor, went to a regional briefing about the plan where the message had – mostly – got through. The civil servant leading the session told the audience, 'You've got to understand that what the Secretary of State is really after here is to really change the NHS because he keeps saying that the NHS is engaged in a gunfight at the OK Corral.'[29]

The full document did emphasise Milburn's 'last chance saloon' warning. It was brutally blunt about the sickness afflicting the service. 'The NHS is a 1940s system operating in a 21st century world,' it read. There was some swagger: 'These are the most fundamental and far-reaching reforms the NHS has seen since 1948.' But this *was* an enormous shake-up. It ended what Stevens later called a health policy that was 'simply the sum of the individual decisions made by clinicians and local health authorities', a 'hands-off approach' that no longer worked.[30] Now, there were national standards, and national pressure to meet them.

The key changes were to what patients could expect: the long waits in accident and emergency departments would stop, with a limit of four hours from arrival to admission, transfer or discharge for any patient. By the end of 2005, the maximum waiting time for an out-patient appointment would be three months, and for inpatients, six months. By 2004, patients could expect a GP appointment within forty-eight hours, and there would be up to 1,000 specialist GPs taking referrals from their fellow GPs. Patients could expect their tests and diagnosis on the same day in hospital so they weren't going back and forth to different appointments. There was a set of seven 'must do' targets, which included the waiting times; improvements to patient satisfaction; reducing mortality rates from heart disease, cancer, suicide and undetermined injury; narrowing health inequalities; and trusts reaching benchmark costs of care.

The targets were there to focus the mind. But they were not at all easy for the health service, even with the extra money. That was very clear at the time. The solution of the Blair government was one that came quite naturally to its key figures: control freakery.

One senior figure in government at the time explains that Blair 'fundamentally saw success in the health service as being absolutely central to New Labour's project. They had to demonstrate that they could run and modernise the major public service in the UK.'[31] The pressure was huge, and the system responded to that pressure. In Number 10, that meant a powerful new NHS Delivery Unit led by Michael Barber. Meanwhile, in the Department of Health, Crisp – now the NHS chief executive – set up his own team to focus on making sure trusts were hitting their targets, and finding out why they weren't. It was, he later wrote, a 'real command and control approach', and involved obsessive attention on the figures. Chief operating officer Neil McKay, director of finance and performance John Bacon and director of performance Duncan Selbie were all figures who worked on this, and were able, at the end of each year, to tell Crisp 'which patients had not been treated in time, which hospitals were not meeting targets and what was being done about it'. There was a 'sheer grind' and 'attention to detail' in order to achieve the big improvements in the plan.[32]

Others around at the time describe this activity in more colourful terms.[33] 'Nigel was definitely on the receiving end of a lot of Alan [Milburn]'s impatience,' says one figure. 'We were all relentlessly focused on meeting these targets and finding out what was wrong. I wouldn't say it was a shouty culture, but yes, quite rigorous.' One manager disagrees: 'It was a shouty culture, and a sweary one too.' A former senior civil servant is even less complimentary:

> Quite quickly the health service adjusted itself so the figures that it produced satisfied the people who wanted that particular outcome, even though the clinical judgements about whether it was right to focus resources here rather than there were many and diffuse. It became a sort of mania, it became a thing unto itself.
>
> Neil McKay's job was to go around bullying people. They'd ring up health service chief executives and would get a million reasons why it was that in this huge Sheffield hospital trust, for example, performance had fallen short on this particular target this month, and be berated uphill and down the dale, and careers threatened and all sorts – it was horrible. It very quickly became a horrible environment, and it's one of those things where pressure from the top starts to get multiplied, because people want to have the right answer to give to Blair.

Trust chief executives from the time don't look back on it fondly. 'You'd have this conversation with Neil McKay,' recalls one. 'And you'd explain to him in five different ways why it wasn't possible to deliver what he was asking for. And he'd say, right, I'm stopping this conversation, you will deliver this and I expect it to happen. And he'd just put the phone down.' McKay accepts that the drive for delivery was rigorous. He points out that ministers had a right to demand good progress: 'I don't recognise the comments about me personally, but I do accept we sometimes needed challenging, robust discussions. All of us felt more accountable for ensuring the government's plans for the NHS were implemented and targets achieved. Some (a minority) struggled to bring about the changes that were needed and sometimes we felt changes in local leadership were necessary. When this did happen, we bent over backwards to help and support people who needed to move on. It's sometimes a tricky balance knowing where to draw the line when managing performance.' Another regional director didn't bother phoning chief executives. Instead, he would turn up at their homes – in one case at ten o'clock on a Sunday night.

It wasn't just the officials. Milburn describes himself as 'angular', others prefer the word 'angry'. 'You didn't want to be invited to sit on the sofa in his office,' says one senior chief executive. 'Because it was heading for him shouting at you and using really foul language.'

This culture had a long-lasting effect on the NHS. Patricia Hewitt, who became Health Secretary in 2005, reflected that 'I've no doubt at all that the targets, particularly on waiting time, compounded that command and control – the pre-existing command and control culture – and exacerbated the risk of bullying and harassment, and not listening to what was really going on'.[34]

The pressure was greatest in A&E, not least because this part of the hospital service was having to recover from being, as Crisp put it, 'really bad'. On top of that, there were the usual Blairite presentational concerns: the prime minister saw emergency as being the 'shop window of the NHS'[35] and therefore was particularly keen for it to improve. Now, no patient could spend more than four hours in the department, otherwise they would 'breach' the target. The consequences of a breach – which quickly became a commonplace in A&Es across England – were that trusts lost power and people lost jobs. Trusts that failed to meet the targets were threatened with being put into special measures, including getting a new senior management team. In the run-up to that, the enforcing team in the Department of Health would put calls in to the chief executives of the trusts to warn them that if they didn't shape up, they'd be out on their ear. Timmins reports chief executives dubbing the waiting times 'P45 targets'.[36]

This fear among senior hospital figures then filtered down through the levels of management and into clinical practice. One junior doctor working in the south-west of England in the 2000s recalls: 'You'd literally be in the middle of a discussion with a patient and you'd get a nurse in the cubicle all of a sudden saying, "He's going to breach, he's going to breach!" And they'd get carted out and taken off to the medical admissions unit or somewhere like that where it would start all over again, no improvement for the patient but at least we hadn't breached.'[37]

Emergency physicians therefore developed what Dr Adrian Boyle, president of the Royal College of Emergency Medicine, calls a 'complicated relationship' with the four-hour target. Boyle has practised in emergency departments in the south of England, Yorkshire and East Anglia. Prior to the introduction of the target, he explains, emergency care was often 'deprioritised' by hospitals. Now, the very clear four-hour waiting time meant the management were paying attention, as meeting the target was seen as a measure of how well a hospital was functioning: if people were getting stuck in A&E, it was because there weren't beds elsewhere in the building for them. 'It suddenly got lots of attention on the fates of people in emergency departments. And certainly, prior to this, the low acuity patients would wait for ever and ever and would become very aggressive. But the four hours meant that people were waiting less time and getting less frustrated and less aggressive.'

But the fear of the breach also caused all manner of gaming, which Boyle and his colleagues became used to. In some hospitals, he says, 'There were an awful lot of people painting a line on the floor to say, this is an off-the-clock area, if you move patients into this bit of the department, they are no longer in the ED.' Hospitals ended up 'cooking the books . . . So they would go, are you absolutely sure the time was collected appropriately? Could we bring it back five minutes?'[38]

Michael Barber was pleased, though, that the A&E target was 'met on time in December 2004 and rarely missed for almost a decade until the NHS was, absurdly, allowed to stop paying attention'.[39] Note the use of 'allowed' there: this was a command and control approach, which saw the NHS as something that must be harnessed and constantly kept in check rather than left to its own devices.

Blair is unapologetic about the depth charge he sent through the service to make it meet its targets. 'My position on targets was you should try and make sure they are reasonably flexible and you should try and make sure that you're constantly revisiting and renewing, but in what other walk of life would you spend literally billions of pounds and not say we want some outcomes! I agree of course that targets can be crude. But they focus the mind, so again I would say whatever downside was massively outweighed by the upside and we would never have got those waiting lists down.' This attitude continues today, particularly among politicians responsible for allocating money to the health service: when the NHS wins some more funding, the accompanying message from the Treasury, briefed out through political journalists, is that it still can't really be trusted with it.

All the New Labour and health service grandees from the time are adamant that the relentless and sometimes ruthless focus on meeting targets was the only way to get things done. But they also agree that things would not have improved without another much more controversial policy. The NHS was going to make use of the private sector to drive down waiting lists. The NHS Plan had made clear that 'ideological boundaries or institutional barriers should not stand in the way of better care for NHS patients'. This led to independent-sector treatment centres. ISTCs were privately owned but only served NHS patients. They were often newly built and carried the NHS branding, sometimes alongside the logo of a private company like BUPA, BMI or Capio. They didn't feel like traditional hospitals: there was no accident and emergency department or ambulances parked out the front, which gave them a calmer atmosphere. The first one opened in 2003, and the first wave of centres saw twenty-five open, with another ten in the second. By 2007–8, their work represented 1.79 per cent of all NHS elective activity.

ISTCs were designed to alleviate exactly the pressures that had led to Mavis Skeet being put off so many times: hospitals were struggling to carry out their diagnostic procedures and elective surgeries because emergency care often got in the way. ISTCs were not a politically easy proposition: they involved the private sector and so immediately the age-old cry of 'privatisation through stealth' went up. They were the source of a row that actually delayed the launch of Labour's 2001 general election manifesto because Brown and Blair were shouting at one another backstage about the role of the private sector in the health service. The tensions weren't helped by Milburn then telling a think tank in 2002 that the new relationship between the NHS and the private sector was 'a relationship that is for the long term. It is not a one night stand.'[40] There were concerns that the private sector might still try to treat the relationship like a casual encounter, though, focusing on getting what it wanted – not what was good for both participants. Detractors warned that the focus of the commercial provider would be on profit rather than quality, and that the centres would leach from the NHS by cherry-picking the easier cases without having to bother with the donkey work of training staff and so on.[41]

Some of these concerns were well founded, though one purpose of the ISTCs was to help plough through the backlog of operations and thereby free up the NHS to focus on the more complex patients. They were also initially designed to encourage innovation, and even ruffle a few feathers among consultants who would see a threat from other providers to their services and so buck up their own ideas about their NHS work – rather than their private practice. The innovation aspect never really took off, in part because the DoH ended up writing very risk-averse contracts. Instead the ISTCs served another purpose, which also irritated the left of the Labour Party and many in the health world: competition. The mere suggestion that an ISTC might be set up in an area often gave the existing services a jolt. Simon Stevens called it 'constructive discomfort', arguing that 'health care improvement requires a source of tension to overcome the inertia inherent in all human systems'.[42] By the time Alan Johnson became Health Secretary in 2007, he was convinced that even stopping proposals for an ISTC meant the system was working:

> We were getting that constant 'You're privatising the NHS' all the time from the left. And that was really because we were going to places where they had these long waiting lists for elective surgery and saying, 'Can you tackle that? Have you got the capacity to tackle that?' 'No, no, we haven't got—' 'Oh right, we'll introduce an independent treatment centre . . .'

I cancelled more than I authorised because once you went to a place and said, 'Okay, if you can't cope, we're going to introduce some extra capacity,' you suddenly found that these surgeons were coming in on a Saturday morning instead of going to the golf course, to get the waiting lists down. So the galvanising effect is just brilliant.[43]

Blair argues: 'It was definitely the combination of more money and choice and competition that changed things.'

ISTCs did have a more profound effect than just making existing services shape up in some areas: one NHS orthopaedic ward in Southampton closed in 2006 in order to meet targets set for ISTC treatment at the nearby centre in Salisbury run by Capio. Angus Wallace, a professor of orthopaedic and accident surgery, complained in 2006 that while many patients were 'living pain-free lives as a result of the surgery carried out much earlier than would have been possible in the early 1990s', this had 'occurred at a price' – both in terms of the quality of the procedures and the effect the ISTCs had on training doctors. He wrote in the *BMJ* that 'the number of patients we are seeing with problems resulting from poor surgery – incorrectly inserted prostheses, technical errors, and infected joint replacements – is too great'. 'Inadequate training' had led to 'several serious errors', and 'training the country's up and coming surgeons' was in jeopardy because the simple cases that they learned their craft on were no longer available in the teaching hospitals where they worked, having all been farmed out to the ISTCs.[44]

But it is true that the use of the private sector changed the way the NHS functioned, and indeed represented an end to a Berlin Wall (erected by Labour, as we saw in earlier chapters) between the two sectors, to the extent that Stevens argued in a 2004 paper – written once he had left government and moved to the US to work in the truly private system – that 'the era of English "exceptionalism" in health care is over'.[45]

This wasn't the only instance in which Blair and his comrades were accused of wanting to privatise or in some way run down the NHS. The NHS Plan didn't just contain targets; it proposed a new way of organising the hospital service. It promised that trusts that performed

well against targets would receive greater freedom. Like the ten principles in its preface, this sounded quite uncontroversial, but what it
actually meant wasn't a small detail. It sparked an almighty row both
in Parliament and in the health service. But the reform – the creation
of foundation hospital trusts – has endured.

About six months after the NHS Plan was published, Milburn and
his colleagues spotted a problem. The money was in the system, the
targets were out there and the scary calls were going into hospitals
that weren't catching up. But waiting lists still weren't falling. On top
of that, consultant productivity was dropping. 'We had this moment
of reflection,' says Milburn. 'Where we said, well, hold on a minute,
what are we missing here? Because we can tell these guys what to do
but they're not doing it. And then you quickly work out actually
telling people what to do, particularly when it's over a million people,
doesn't really work. Running the NHS like a nationalised industry
was never going to work.'[46] In short, you couldn't be a control freak.

He called in chief executives of trusts that had earned three-star
ratings from the Healthcare Commission and asked them what would
help. He was expecting to hear the words 'more money'. Instead,
they said: 'More freedom. We just need to be trusted to get on with
the job. We're good enough to do it.' Milburn was at the same time
shaken that he had been forced to intervene in a local scandal in Bed-
ford, forcing the resignation of the chief executive Ken Williams
after the hospital was exposed for storing bodies on the floor of its
chapel rather than in the mortuary. The minister found it distasteful
he should have been involved at all.

Not long after that, Milburn found himself in Spain trying to
recruit more doctors from the health service there. He was surprised
when he arrived at the Ministry of Health in Madrid to find that a
group of unemployed doctors were outside the building protesting
about the lack of vacancies for them – something that has been
unimaginable in the entire history of our NHS. As he worked with
his Spanish counterparts to entice some of those surplus doctors over
to England, Milburn got to know a little more about the Sistema
Nacional de Salud (SNS). He found many similarities with the NHS,

but was particularly struck by how much more independence the organisations within the SNS had. In particular, he liked the look of a general hospital in Madrid, the Hospital Universitario Fundación Alcorcón, which was run by a private company and had a governance structure that included local government, staff, trade unions and community representatives. He wanted to do the same thing in England.

Milburn had already crossed the Rubicon to using the private sector in the NHS. Now he wanted to emulate parts of it by using competition, patient choice and a concept known as 'earned autonomy' – that is, if a hospital performed well, it would receive greater freedom over how it ran its affairs and, crucially, its money. The plan was for acute hospital trusts to become 'public benefit organisations' that were independent of the Secretary of State for Health and the strategic health authorities. Instead, they were accountable to their boards of governors and a new regulator: Monitor. They could run up surpluses, operate with deficits – and keep the surpluses rather than see their hard work absorbed into the system without a trace. They wouldn't need to ask permission from the government every time they wanted to do something. In short, they were in charge, rather than those at the centre of government. The three-star organisations who told Milburn they wanted more freedom would be the first to be invited to become foundation trusts, while others would be helped to reach the necessary standards to apply in the future.

To get the waiting lists moving, the money a trust received would be dependent on the amount of work it was actually carrying out. This sounds very logical, but was not the case up to this point in the NHS. Trusts were, at the time, receiving what Milburn's adviser Paul Corrigan describes as a 'bung' of cash: 'They'd all get a bung, some because they were complete basket cases and some would get a bung because they were doing very well and could do more work.' The new idea was that the trusts would get paid for the work they actually did. This was 'completely revolutionary', explains Corrigan. 'People said, "No, that's not going to happen. Honestly, honestly, don't be daft."'

It was also a completely revolutionary concept for the Labour

Party, which still had a hugely emotional commitment to the concept of a monolithic NHS. 'I underestimated the power in people's minds of the NHS being the last really powerful nationalised industry,' admits Corrigan. The changes he and Milburn developed were so big that the immediate assumption within the Labour movement was that this had to be privatisation.[47]

The row in the party was enormous, and went all the way to the top of the government. Milburn was constantly being accused in the House of Commons of wanting to privatise the NHS by the back door – firstly by weathered old socialists who'd spent their lives on the Labour backbenches, and then by his own predecessor Frank Dobson, who warned that party members were also against the policy: 'We believe that it will be damaging and divisive, not just for the NHS, but for the Labour Party as well.'[48] Labourites didn't like the idea of more competition between hospitals – not least because they'd been so happy about the abolition of the internal market. They disliked the new payment system, which focused on how much work a trust was doing, though it was quickly and inaccurately badged 'payment by results' when there was in fact no payment for quality. They felt the very structure of the new trusts would in effect be doing away with public ownership.

The Conservatives also opposed the new policy, but in the opening debates on the legislation, one Tory backbencher, Robert Jackson, teased Milburn that he was 'facing exactly the same charges about privatisation and two-tierism as we did'. The minister responded that 'support from the hon. Gentleman is about as welcome as myxomatosis in a rabbit hutch – although I hope that it does not have the same deadly consequences'.[49] Jackson clearly didn't take that too personally – he defected from the Conservatives and joined Milburn's party just a couple of years later. But Tory support was definitely not something the Labour health reformers wanted; it would have made it even harder for them to face down the accusations from their own side that this was about privatisation.

Gordon Brown was opposed to the policy. He didn't like the overall principle, but made the fight about the money because that was where his power lay. Milburn had wanted foundation trusts to be able to borrow without that debt appearing on the government balance sheet. His fear was that if these organisations went broke, it would be the taxpayer who'd have to pick up the bill. The stand-off quickly became public: Brown had a furious row with Blair about it at the Labour Party conference in 2002. The to-and-fro forced Milburn to delay a conference for trusts interested in becoming the first to gain foundation status. And Brown won the battle; borrowing would stay on the balance sheet. Every trust would get a cap on its private patient activity, to assuage some of the privatisation-by-stealth accusations. He also forced changes in governance to encourage people from the local community to join the trust as members who could elect the board of governors. Brown was back on board, but many MPs still weren't.

In the middle of the row with his party, Milburn quit his post. His reason – that he wanted to spend more time with his family – had become rather hackneyed in British politics as a euphemism for hiding from a scandal or differences with a party leader. But in Milburn's case it was true: he'd grown weary of missing time with his young son and having to drive through the night to try to balance school meetings with Whitehall engagements. His replacement as Health Secretary was John Reid. Reid was a Glaswegian with a dry sense of humour who was drenched in Labour traditions. 'If you went and had a discussion with him about foundation trusts, he could find a quote from Keir Hardie arguing for them,' jokes Corrigan, who stayed on in the department.

Corrigan and the ministers he worked with held more than 400 meetings with MPs – with some backbenchers requesting multiple sessions before they saw fit to support the policy. The way to sell it to MPs turned out to be to appeal to the party's history, likening these new public benefit organisations to co-operatives rather than straightforward private companies. Many Labour MPs were also members of the Co-operative Party and owed much of their thinking to the idea of ownership by membership.

The strategy worked, but at a cost. There were big rebellions. At the second reading of the foundation hospitals bill, sixty-five Labour MPs rebelled against their party whip. When it reached its final stage in the Commons, fewer rebelled but the policy passed with a majority of just thirty-five (Blair's working majority at the time was 164).

In February 2004, thirty-two NHS trusts applied to be the first to get foundation status. This was whittled down to ten, who got their new freedoms the following year. There was some surprise at the names in this elite group. It wasn't dominated by the big prestigious teaching hospitals that everyone associated with NHS success and which came in later waves. The non-household names were instead: Basildon and Thurrock, Chester, Doncaster and Bassetlaw, Bradford, Homerton, Peterborough and Stamford, Royal Devon and Exeter, and Stockport. Moorfields Eye Hospital and the Royal Marsden were the two biggest names on that list.

The difference that the chief executives of these trusts and those in the ensuing early waves receiving foundation status found was that they were now able to get on with their jobs rather than having Whitehall breathing down their neck constantly. Being a foundation trust was soon something every hospital trust wanted – not just because of the freedoms, but also because it was a badge of prestige. And the problem with this was that not all trusts were up to it – or even up to the approval process itself. Their governance was weak and their leadership made poor decisions in order to game the system, ticking boxes to meet the strict criteria on finances, for instance, at the expense of safe staffing. It wasn't long before the scandals began to emerge.

One of Milburn's motivations in creating foundation trusts was to stop the Secretary of State from being responsible for every scandal in every hospital. But it should be very clear by now that this just isn't how health and politics interact. Even if politicians could escape the wrath of the public when something goes wrong in the health service, it's not clear whether many of them would be able to resist the temptation to meddle anyway. It's not just that the NHS is one of those organisations so complex that there is always *something* a minister can change to make their mark. It's also that healthcare is by its very nature hugely emotive. Dropped bedpans are one thing, but many decisions and mistakes really do have life-and-death consequences, and regardless of how much power and influence a minister has within legislation, the public don't care: it always ends up being the government's problem.

The National Institute for Clinical Excellence is one example of how easy it is for the public and politicians to get stirred up about healthcare policy. Given that Beveridge and Bevan's original assumption (that the health service would end up costing the taxpayer less as need was eradicated) was so wrong, the question of what the NHS could and should reasonably offer – both in moral and money terms – has been a hotly contested one. As treatments became more advanced and personalised, they were costing more. Pharmaceutical companies of course play a role in the huge costs of the drugs to the health service: as businesses they want to make money, and a number of them have been fined for inflating costs to the NHS. But it also costs a great deal to bring a drug to market, even before the question of profit arises. Either way, wonder drugs can also cause despair: there are not unlimited resources to pay for them. Should trusts offer unlimited rounds of IVF to patients with fertility problems? Should doctors be allowed to spend hundreds of thousands of pounds on prolonging the life of one dying patient, at the expense of life-saving treatment for someone else in the same hospital – maybe even the same ward?

In 1999, the government tried to remove political accountability for these sorts of rationing decisions, and set up the National Institute for Clinical Excellence (NICE), which served England and Wales. The quango's purpose was to set guidelines for treatment, including the use of medicines and technologies for specific illnesses. The basis on which it did this was whether a treatment represented value for money for the NHS. The idea, explains Rudolf Klein, was to allow 'the experts, not the politicians, [to] take the difficult decisions'.[50] Its job was partly to be controversial, so that politicians couldn't make decisions motivated by short-term thinking rather than the long-term good of patients and the health service. As a result of this, it even became part of the furious debate in the US over 'Obamacare', when Barack Obama was trying to reform the system of health insurance. Far from being the 'envy of the world', the NHS was used by Republican opponents of the reforms as a salutary tale of what happens when the state gets too involved in healthcare. Obama was, they said, trying to set up 'death panels' along the lines of NICE, where officials decided who was allowed life-saving treatment and who wasn't. One conservative advert told voters that $22,750 was a sum that, 'in England, government health officials have decided [is] how much six months of life is worth'. NICE contested the description, with its chief executive Andrew Dillon saying this was not 'the way in which we're perceived in the UK even among those who are disappointed or upset by our decisions'.[51]

By this point, NICE had disappointed and upset a lot of people with its decisions, as was only to be expected. Perhaps equally as predictable was that politicians haven't always been able to leave it alone to do its job.

One of the most controversial examples of political meddling came in 2000, when drug company Roche launched with enormous fanfare a 'holy grail of cancer treatment' called Herceptin. This breast cancer drug was designed for the 25 per cent of patients diagnosed with a high level of HER2, meaning they have a more aggressive form of the disease and are often young. It was, said one NHS oncologist at the time, 'the first targeted treatment for breast cancer' and 'represented a whole new era of cancer care'.[52] It also represented a whole new era of cost pressures on the health service: it cost around £25,000 per patient per year for early-stage breast cancer.

NICE approved Herceptin for use in 2002, but only for patients whose cancer had metastasised – or spread – from the breast. But word spread quickly, not least because of the marketing tactics of Roche, which worked with – and gave money to – campaigning charities to push for its use in early-stage cases. In 2005, a group of seven women from North Staffordshire who had HER2-positive early breast cancer started lobbying their local primary care trust (PCT), North Stoke, to be allowed Herceptin. The trust refused; it would cost hundreds of thousands of pounds. Moreover, it was still not licensed for this use, and so the patients' campaign became more and more vociferous, with national broadcast interviews and photocalls outside the door of Downing Street. Their stories were, of course, deeply moving: these patients wanted to live, and they feared that without the drug they would die.

The Health Secretary by this point was Patricia Hewitt, and she made a personal intervention in the row. She ordered that the drug should be 'fast-tracked' by NICE and that breast cancer patients should get tests to see if Herceptin could help them. In a speech to mark Breast Cancer Awareness Month, she said: 'PCTs should not refuse to fund Herceptin solely on the grounds of its cost'. Accepting that this would be costly for some PCTs that were already under financial pressure, she stuck to her guns, saying, 'I believe it is the right thing to do'.[53]

A few days later, Hewitt ordered a meeting with North Stoke PCT and the local strategic health authority, which was responsible for implementing health policy in the region, after the PCT refused Herceptin for one of the seven women: 41-year-old mother of four, Elaine Barber. The minister demanded 'the evidence they have used as the basis of their decision not to fund Herceptin'. A *Panorama* investigation on Herceptin early in 2006 found evidence of 'arm-twisting' by the government, who continued to talk a good game about local decision-making and decentralisation.[54] It also raised the question of whether health policy was being directed by the patients who made the most noise. It wasn't the fault of those women who were desperate for Herceptin that their cases had got so much attention, and nor was it their fault that Hewitt had felt it was politically expedient to intervene. But the whole affair showed politicians weren't really prepared to depoliticise decisions about treatment, regardless of what they claimed.

There was also a more immediate and practical worry about Herceptin. A number of PCTs – which at this stage were responsible for commissioning primary and secondary care from providers – were operating with deficits, and despite Hewitt's insistence that they should be able to manage the funding hit over two years, they were concerned that the mighty cost of this drug would impact on treatment of other patients. In November 2006, a team of doctors at the Norfolk and Norwich University Hospitals NHS Trust and the University of East Anglia warned that, because NICE had provided no extra funding when it ruled on the prescribing of Herceptin to early-stage patients, they would face dropping treatment for others to 'balance the books'. They calculated that they would have to find £1.9 million a year to cover the cost of the drug for the seventy-five eligible patients under their care.

New Labour was sufficiently ambitious and at times naive that it left a legacy involving a number of cock-ups.

The private finance initiative (PFI) was one of the messes most popularly associated with the Blair years. It wasn't a Labour brainchild – the Conservatives had introduced it – but Labour saw the value in continuing it. Nicholas Timmins explains that 'Labour had adopted the Tory private finance initiative to get around the lack of capital spending'.[55] In short, it allowed the private sector to pay for the upfront costs of building and maintaining a hospital, with the health service repaying that money annually over a set period – usually around thirty years. It allowed Labour to boast that it was running the 'biggest hospital building programme in the history of the NHS'. And it did mean more hospitals: between 1997 and 2003, thirty-four hospitals were built – compared to just seven between 1980 and 1997. By 2017, there were 127 NHS PFI schemes, with the total capital value coming to just under £13 billion.

From the beginning, there were concerns about the quality of the buildings, with Sir Stuart Lipton, head of the government's advisory group on buildings, warning that this building programme could make the same mistakes as the Hospital Plan in the 1960s. He told the BBC in 2001: 'They can get it right and the hospitals will be uplifting, efficient, or they can become blots on the landscape – the tower blocks of the '60s. There is not enough attention to detail, not enough care, not enough commitment.'[56] Trade unions representing health workers were unhappy too: in 2003, public service union Unison published a report complaining that the deals were failing patients and staff, with all the first-wave hospitals short of beds and some having to use Portakabins and old buildings to cope. It reported one union rep at the Edinburgh Infirmary saying: 'We have had several roof collapses so far and we are not even a year in.'

The first PFI hospital to open under Labour, Cumberland Infirmary, saw its pathology lab 'flooded three times in 18 months, twice with raw sewerage', according to a union official there. The union produced a number of reports on Cumberland's PFI, claiming in one that 'the scheme is only made affordable by selling land, cutting capacity (beds and services), cutting the services budget, and diverting income from other NHS services'.[57] The new hospital building replaced a 1960s tower block and opened in June 2000 at a cost of £87 million, and was immediately plagued with problems. The maternity unit flooded and the glass atrium – the centrepiece of the flashy new hospital's design – regularly overheated, reaching more than 40 degrees Celsius.

But it was the long-term financial implications that really made PFI hospitals notorious. It cost some trusts a staggering amount. Barts Health NHS Trust's PFI was worth more than £1.1 billion, and it was spending around 10 per cent of its income annually on repaying it. The Barts contract was for a new building for the Royal London Hospital, which had 845 beds in 110 wards. The Treasury estimated that the £1.1 billion private-sector outlay would end up costing the trust £6.2 billion by the end of the contract. Sherwood Forest Hospitals NHS Foundation Trust was spending 16 per cent of its total income in 2016–17 on repaying its PFI.[58] In 2013, the Department of Health announced it would be supporting seven organisations it believed were paying excess PFI costs, including Peterborough and Stamford Hospitals NHS Foundation Trust, which was paying £40.4 million that year, meaning the trust's estate costs were 22 per cent.[59] In 2019, the centre-left think tank IPPR warned that all trusts with such loans were being 'crippled' by PFI and still had £55 billion due in repayments before the end of the final contract in 2050. It found that the initial £13 billion invested by private companies would end up costing the health service £80 billion overall.

When the Conservatives came back into power in 2010, they banned the NHS from using PFI for future contracts, and regularly derided Labour for the scheme, especially when being accused of wanting to privatise the NHS. They also attacked Labour's GP contract, renegotiated in 2003 by John Reid, as 'disastrous' for the working of the health service. Perhaps a warning sign was that the contract was very popular with the GPs, with 79 per cent of the doctors balloted by the BMA backing the new deal. One of the reasons for this was that Reid ended up stuffing the GPs' mouths with gold: the new contract contained a 'substantial' pay rise for GPs from £65,000 per annum on average to £80,000, and an end to evening and weekend working. For the first time in the entire history of the NHS, individual GPs would no longer be responsible for 24-hour cover for their patients; now practices could opt out of out-of-hours working. The majority did indeed opt out, with the local PCT providing out-of-hours care instead. Many have since attacked the contract for leading to increased pressure on A&E. Timmins argues: 'The replacement services that the PCTs commissioned proved not only expensive, but from the patient's point of view too often deeply unsatisfactory. Their poor quality contributed to year-on-year rises in the numbers attending accident and emergency departments for matters that should have been resolved out of hospital.'[60] One thing that is clear is that the contract was even more expensive than expected: it cost £1.76 billion more than had been planned for.

Patients' relationships with their GPs were changing anyway. The introduction of NHS Direct, a telephone triage line set up in 1998 and rolled out nationally in 2000, meant people could speak to a nurse-led service about symptoms that worried them but which didn't seem to be an emergency. Geoffrey Rivett says the helpline 'responded to consumerism, doing what cash machines had done for banking, to offer a more accessible, convenient and interactive gateway', and points out that 'the commonest reasons for calls were rashes, abdominal pain, dental, tooth and jaw pain'.[61] Then there were the walk-in centres, often operated by private companies such as Care UK and based in shopping centres and hospitals. Their opening hours were supposed to target people who couldn't make it to a GP, usually 7 a.m.–9.30 p.m. and open at weekends, too.

The role of the nurse changed dramatically during the New Labour years, partly as a result of walk-in centres and NHS Direct and partly because nursing was now moving to being something taught in a higher education setting rather than in an individual hospital's own school of nursing. At the end of the 1980s, Project 2000 became the nursing education programme for the NHS in England, making training more knowledge-based rather than practical. It led to regular complaints from hospitals that their newly qualified staff did not have the necessary experience to perform the job. Doctors in particular disliked what they saw – though there did seem to be an element of professional gatekeeping. One medic complained privately to me at the time about 'the arrogance of these nurses who actually turn up wearing stethoscopes and think they're doctors'. In 2009, the Patients Association argued that 'since the introduction of Project 2000, which shifted training from the bedside to the classroom, nurses have lifted their eyes to the personal prizes of nurse specialisms and been allowed to ignore the needs of their sick, vulnerable and often elderly patients'.[62] But the Royal College of Nursing had supported the reforms, and continued to argue that they were necessary to ensure nurses could work in an increasingly complex health landscape.

The RCN has not played as dramatic a role in this book as the BMA. But its members weren't above roughing up a Secretary of State who they felt deserved it. In April 2006, Patricia Hewitt, now the Health Secretary, walked on to the stage at the RCN conference in Bournemouth. 'It's a real pleasure to be here today,' she began, not entirely convincingly. It was not a pleasure, and she knew that the speech was not going to be easy. Within a few lines, the nurses had made their displeasure quite obvious: they were heckling, hissing and slow-clapping her. 'I know that you're angry about the possibility of redundancies,' she said, to more cries. As the speech went on, she protested: 'You can't win as Health Secretary: if I say you deserve credit, you shout at me; if I don't, you also shout at me.'[63]

Why was the RCN, not known as a militant health union, shouting at Hewitt? The reason was money, naturally, but in this instance it wasn't the regular complaint that the health service needed more. The NHS budget had gone from being something the government was proud of to a scandal. The New Labour years were known for a dramatic increase in spending, but as they trundled to an end, that spending wasn't rising because politicians had decided it would; it was out of control.

The extra money pouring into the NHS meant services were all expanding rapidly, to the extent that there was too much capacity requiring too much money. Trusts were employing more doctors than central planning had allowed for and than they could afford. They were spending much more on staff pay and – as we have already seen – on meeting NICE recommendations. A contract for consultants, negotiated by Milburn, had added around £90 million to hospital costs – far more than had been anticipated by the department. Trusts were going into debt, and it wasn't clear how they were going to resolve their deficits. Things were getting out of hand. Timmins reports it thus: 'So the NHS first exceeded its budget by £250 million, a sum that [Nigel] Crisp cheerfully assured everyone could easily be gained back, and then by £500 million. That meant that in 2005, as the department applied new government accounting rules, it was required to claw back £1 billion to repay the overspend and to get its "run rate" back on track.'[64]

On taking over from Reid, Hewitt was horrified to discover what was going on in the spreadsheets for the health service. It was, she said in an interview, 'a really shocking moment'. The civil servants tried to find ways of making it seem less awful, but Hewitt wasn't the right person to do this with. She liked spreadsheets. She liked trying to understand how organisations worked. And she quickly realised that, despite the investment and despite the relentless focus on delivery, this organisation wasn't working. 'As we dug into what was really going on, we discovered unbelievable inadequacies in the leadership, capability, and financial frameworks, and the discipline of the department and the NHS, in which the Treasury was also culpable.'

She wasn't that impressed with the way the system tried to deal with what she was finding, either: 'So Nigel [Crisp] and the rest of them – about 13 of them – all came into my room and sat down along my very long table, with me, my special advisers and private secretary on the other side, and it was a complete "Yes Minister" moment. It was the sort of, "Minister, we have a problem." And that was the overspend. That was a huge wake-up call and very nasty. It was later that I learnt from Ken Anderson, the commercial director, that there had been a series of pre-meetings about how they were going to gloss this problem to me!'[65]

Crisp eventually resigned in March 2006, moving to the House of Lords. Hewitt and Crisp's replacement as NHS chief executive, David Nicholson, had to work out how to bring spending back under control. They managed it, but not without the fury of healthcare workers, who saw the efficiency savings pursued as being a threat to their ability to do their jobs properly. It was just a few weeks later that Hewitt had to speak to the RCN. Many in the audience were wearing T-shirts emblazoned with the slogan 'Keep nurses working, keep patients safe'.

Hewitt was Blair's last health minister. When Gordon Brown took over as prime minister in June 2007, he reshuffled the government and brought in Alan Johnson. Hewitt's view is that 'the brakes got slammed on' at this point.[66] Johnson's brief was a phrase we will hear a great deal more of in the next chapter – no more top-down re-organisations of the NHS, less interfering, and improvements in the quality in the health service. To that end, Brown brought in a top surgeon, Sir Ara Darzi, as a 'goat'. A 'goat' was a member of Brown's 'government of all the talents' – experts in their fields appointed to key ministerial roles. Darzi became a junior health minister and wrote a report in 2008 called *High Quality Care For All*, which tried to move away from the focus on targets and on to improving what was actually being done. The speed with which someone was treated wasn't the only thing the NHS should care about; quality was now important, too. For the first time, hospitals and GPs would be held to account for the outcomes of treatment, including through the publication of performance data.

One of the more controversial proposals was for 'polyclinics', which would move more care out of hospitals and into the community. GPs didn't like what they saw as a rival to their services. The left didn't like the fact that private companies (with scary names like Virgin, as opposed to the comely but still privately contracted GPs who had been part of the health service since its inception) could run them. Some disliked both possibilities: a group of GPs on Teesside set up a campaign called 'Save Our Surgeries' and warned that poly-clinics were 'the first stage in dismantling of traditional general practice in this country'. Johnson was furious, complaining in the Commons that the leaflets produced by this group were 'scurrilous', and that they had the temerity to use the NHS logo without being allowed to. In the same debate, though, he had to listen to the complaints of his own side that this was the sell-off of the NHS everyone had been warning about since the service had been set up. One Labour backbencher, David Taylor, told the Chamber: 'No wonder firms such as Serco, UnitedHealth and Virgin Healthcare are lining up outside the Department of Health just outside this place, licking their lips at the prospect of extracting vast sums from the NHS.'[67]

Virgin's founder Sir Richard Branson didn't need to queue up outside the department, as it happens. Consultants from his business had been working with Labour ministers for years by this point, advising on the state of the health service. In 2000, Virgin produced a confidential report for Milburn on visits to hospitals, GP practices and minor injury clinics. The minister had commissioned this partly to rival a review set up by Brown into the long-term needs of the health service, which became known as the 'Wanless Review'. The Virgin report looked at the 'customer' experience of the NHS, and found 'long waiting times throughout', a 'tatty, scruffy, dirty' environment and 'an organisation under siege, lacking direction and leadership, pulled every way by initiatives, politicians and the media'.[68] And among its recommendations for change was a concept the report called the 'polyclinic'. Eight years later, Branson's Virgin Care was being accused of wanting to cash in on that as the suggestion became government policy.

What is the truth about the involvement of these big, iconic – in some ways infamous – companies in the NHS? They are so often the bogeyman, and in the years that followed the row about polyclinics, Branson managed to make himself a bogeyman in popular political discourse, too. Virgin tried to open a polyclinic in Swindon, before dropping those plans. In 2016, Virgin Care Ltd launched legal action against six clinical commissioning groups, Surrey County Council and NHS England when it failed to win an £82 million contract for children's services in Surrey. The company claimed there had been 'serious flaws in the procurement process', and the case was eventually settled out of court. But that wasn't before the case had become a political rallying point. Labour leader Jeremy Corbyn seized on it, replying sardonically to a tweet from Branson claiming he believed 'that "stuff" really does not bring happiness'. Corbyn's response read: 'Perhaps our NHS could have the money back from when you sued it?'[69] It received 121,000 likes, which for that particular era in Labour politics marked it out as a huge success. It also demonstrated one of the private sector's most important roles in the NHS, which is a cultural one. The threat of privatisation has hung over the health service ever since its inception, but has never been realised. Even in 2019–20, just 7.2 per cent of the Department of Health and Social Care's total revenue budget was spent on private providers.[70] The private sector largely functions to make patients feel grateful for the care they receive, because things could be worse: we could have a *privatised* system. This invariably carries connotations of American healthcare rather than any of the alternative systems closer to home in Europe.

The privatisation-by-stealth accusation is curious because, as has been very clear throughout this book, the NHS has never been a uniform, monolithic, state-owned service in the crude way it is sometimes portrayed. It is also angrily contested by those who have worked in the private sector. David Hare, who advised private healthcare providers during this time, argues: 'I think politically, certainly those that were around in the mid-1990s would say that a government that presides over very, very poor access to NHS care, whilst private patients can afford rapid access, is politically a more toxic and real issue than a perceived Americanisation, a privatisation of healthcare, which as far as I can see, has never and will never be on the cards.'[71] Indeed, the joke within the senior echelons of the health service and most former Health Secretaries is that if any political party really wanted to privatise the health service, they might have managed it by now. The New Labour government didn't do it. But what it did do was get the health service back on its feet again.

9. The biggest train set on Whitehall

Politicians are obsessed with the NHS, but not just because voters are. It's also because of the opportunity that the health service presents. Jeremy Heywood rose to become the most powerful civil servant in Britain, and on the way noticed something about how politicians interacted with the NHS. He told colleagues that they all wanted to get their hands on what he dubbed 'the biggest train set on Whitehall'.

By the time Labour left office in 2010, this train set had become used to existing in perpetual motion, bouncing from one reorganisation to another. There had been nine big changes to the structure of the health service over the thirteen years the party had been in power. Health economist Alan Maynard describes these rather more accurately as 're-disorganisations', as they tended to last about eighteen months before another politician tore things up again. One manager recalls having to reapply for the same job each time the organisation in charge of it changed – eleven times in total. This was becoming the norm, but it wasn't healthy for the NHS, as institutional memory was lost, people were distracted from what should have been the focus of their job by the administrative burden of starting up a new organisation all over again, and it was easy to evade accountability when things went wrong.

So when a politician from a different party – with a promise to do things differently and to stop pointless reorganisations – came along, his message seemed very attractive.

The Conservatives' not-a-reorganisation of the health service under the 2010–15 coalition government was a Magritte's pipe of an exercise. Their health policy was sold before the election as no top-down reorganisations. Even when in the middle of the reorganisation, leading figures insisted that this was *not* actually a reorganisation. The political row that accompanied this legislation, the Health and Social

Care Act 2012, would have fitted right into a Surrealist work of art, too. To this day, health experts are divided on whether the NHS effectively ceased to exist as a result of what happened. The Act certainly made a lot of political capital disappear overnight from the Conservative Party – to the extent that, despite remaining in office in the ensuing years, they refused to touch the health service for another decade.

At the heart of this not-a-reorganisation was a man called Andrew Lansley. A cerebral fellow who had worked for the Conservative Party for many years, he had risen to become the party's shadow Secretary of State for Health. He knew public services inside out and had an impeccable pedigree. Over the many years prior, he had been involved in some of the Thatcher government's biggest market-based reforms, including the *Working for Patients* White Paper that created the internal market. Colleagues described him politely as being 'slightly professorial'. Civil servants who encountered him when the Conservatives came into government were rather less complimentary. 'He was completely off the wall,' said one.[1] But one thing that no one, whether friend or critic, could doubt was Lansley's commitment to the health service.

It was deeply personal. His father had been a biochemist and had advised on hospital-acquired infections. Lansley himself had suffered a stroke aged just thirty-six, and his experience of receiving treatment for that shaped his view of the NHS still further: his then-wife, a junior doctor, had to badger the GP for an MRI scan after he lost his balance during a cricket game. What was initially diagnosed as an ear infection turned out to have been parts of his brain dying after a blood clot.

'Now it was true, and continues to be true, that if you have somebody who knows their way about, you can argue your way through the system,' he said in an interview in 2006.[2] How that system worked for someone who wasn't married to a doctor and who didn't have a father who could advise on tackling MRSA began to consume Lansley. He soon realised that it was very easy to get lost in the health service, and very easy for people to lose track of who was responsible for what. Shadowing Alan Johnson in the House of Commons, he would find himself repeatedly asking who was in charge. He recalls:

> I was continuously presented in the House of Commons as his oppos-
> ite number with things that had gone very badly wrong. And which,
> from Alan Johnson's point of view, he said was either the responsibil-
> ity of the management of the hospital concerned or, in relation to
> changes in the NHS like hospital closures, were the responsibility of
> the Primary Care Trust (responsible for commissioning care in an
> area).
>
> So what was perfectly obvious was that ministers were routinely
> finding a political reason to announce things. And the NHS was
> much given to the 'I've got a party conference speech coming up; I
> must have an announcement. What am I going to announce? So can
> you have a trawl through the NHS for what the next thing is?'

Lansley didn't like this political interference. In fact, Lansley wasn't really all that into politics, which as we shall see made the row about the reforms he then proposed so much more explosive. But in deep-est darkest opposition he had the space to think about reforms in a way that was entirely separate from politics. He soon worked out what he wanted: 'It was terribly simple. What the NHS should expect is to be given the independence to do its job properly.'[3]

There is nothing 'terribly simple' about any NHS reform, though. And no one who truly understood what Lansley was working on would have called it simple or indeed modest. When NHS chief executive David Nicholson was presented in June 2010 with the White Paper formalising the reform Lansley had spent years working on called *Liberating the NHS*, he remarked to colleagues that 'this is really, really revolutionary'.[4] He later said the plan was 'so big you could see it from outer space'.

For six years, Lansley had beavered away on his plans to reform the NHS while serving as shadow Secretary of State for Health. He was given a reasonable amount of freedom to do so by his party leader, David Cameron. Cameron was not dissimilar to Lansley in that he too had a deeply personal attachment to the NHS. He had spent a great deal of time in hospitals with his son Ivan, who was born with a rare condition called Ohtahara syndrome, which includes regular, terrifying seizures and severe developmental delay. Ivan was treated first at the John Radcliffe Hospital in Oxford, then St Mary's, Paddington, before being moved to Great Ormond Street. Cameron, at the time a backbench MP, found himself sitting on the ward in that hospital reading stories not just to his own son but to other children who were stuck in bed waiting for operations or dialysis.

Ivan died aged six at St Mary's. By this point, Cameron was the leader of the opposition. He later explained the impact his regular spells in hospitals had on his view of the health service:

> What happened with Ivan was, I just suddenly saw so much of the NHS at such a close-up picture, and it did make a really amazing impression on me. Obviously it was extremely difficult, but you saw this incredible personal attention, the way that nurses in those paediatric wards and intensive care, just how incredibly talented and caring they are.
>
> The other thing is the way, if you have a really ill child, you can sort of escalate through the system to Great Ormond Street, which is effectively one of the best hospitals anywhere in the world, and I think this sense that you've got a really ill child, you're having a really difficult time, but in the NHS it's all there for you and you can get the best care in the world and they're never asking for your credit card or your insurance record or whatever, and that I think has a very profound effect on you.

Cameron was particularly interested in the personal relationship that people had with their GPs and the way that this was often the point at which the British love for the NHS was at its strongest. 'I think the GP plays a very important part in that sort of personal connection we feel in the NHS, because hopefully we don't all spend all our time in hospital, but you do know who your GP is. That was part of what lay behind the thinking of our health reforms was that everybody knows and likes your GP, everybody knows what your local hospital is, whereas a lot of the bureaucracies were rather faceless and nameless.'[5]

Lansley very much agreed with Cameron's sentiments on this.

Indeed, not long after taking on the shadow Health brief in 2005, he gave a speech to the NHS Confederation, which represents commissioners and providers of NHS services, setting out 'the structure of the service for the longer term'. It was a typical Lansley address in that it could have easily been delivered by a real professor in a seminar for students of public services. Perhaps the students were all snoozing when he told the room that 'the time has come for pro-competitive reforms in public services including health and education' – or indeed when he said he wanted 'GPs, if they are budget-holders, to be able to purchase actively, including negotiating offers on quality or price that help them better to utilise their budgets for their patients'.[6] He wanted care such as cancer and stroke services to be commissioned by organisations who were not the same entity as the providers – that is, that the hospitals weren't just commissioning themselves to carry out jobs. He wanted budget-holding GPs to choose between different providers of primary care services, and for 'independent providers' to have a right to supply services, too. He also talked about the regulation of this competitive landscape.

By the time the Tories were in government, the reforms had changed a little, although not in size. According to his long-serving special adviser, Bill Morgan, Lansley had been forced into some of the changes by the desire of Cameron's office to announce – ironically, in pursuit of some interesting headlines about the health service – that the new leader wanted the NHS to be independent, like the Bank of England. The shadow minister and his adviser were dumbfounded by this: in what way was the health service comparable to the country's central bank? Morgan explains that Lansley went off to try to make this strange idea work: 'In the space of about two days, it morphed into this idea of an independent NHS commissioning board. He basically came up with that whole thing over a weekend and wrote it.' Others who worked with Lansley on implementing this plan agree – though with less sympathy – that the idea for the independent commissioning board seemed, in the words of one senior civil servant, 'to leap fully formed from his head without him actually talking to other people about whether it would work'.[7] And even though

Lansley was adapting his plans – which had been a good number of years in the making – at the behest of his leader, he did not stop to consider whether they should change in the light of the 2008 world financial crisis, which had come after he had first written them back in 2005.

What Lansley came up with – and this wasn't his choice – was that the NHS would be run on a day-to-day basis by the national commissioning board, rather than by the Health Secretary. Ministers would not have any powers of direction over the service, and would instead write a mandate every three years, which would prevent petty political interference. GPs would be the ones to commission care locally, including from non-NHS providers. The regulator, Monitor, would encourage more competition between providers of healthcare – and in doing so, according to Lansley, drive up standards.

It was an unashamedly pro-competition set of reforms. But this was not a radical change to the *direction* of health service reform, which is perhaps one reason why Lansley felt justified in insisting that he was not pursuing a real top-down reorganisation. Indeed, in his detailed account of the legislation, Nicholas Timmins points out that Labour health ministers over the previous decade had talked of trying to turn the NHS into a 'self-improving organisation' and moving from a 'politician-led NHS to a patient-led NHS'. Timmins writes: 'The shadow health secretary's big idea was to take that to its ultimate conclusion while fixing it all in legislation – producing, if you like, the final NHS reorganisation of all time, or at least one that would last many years and could only be changed by further legislation.'[8]

That was the policy, at least. But as is the case throughout this tale, the politics intervened.

Cameron knew that the Conservative Party did not have the automatic trust of voters when it came to the NHS. He had watched as his predecessors tried and failed to introduce reforms which were caricatured as 'privatisation', only for Labour to do the same without the same kind of fuss. Just a month after being elected party leader, in January 2006, he gave a speech to the King's Fund in which he used health policy as an illustration of 'how the Conservative party is changing'. He said: 'I want us to leave no one in any doubt whatsoever about how we feel about the NHS today. We believe in it. We want to improve it. We want to improve it for everyone in this country.' He dismissed those in his party who wanted him to fund healthcare using National Insurance, saying 'I will never go down that route'.[9]

He was speaking a little ahead of his party, but in the years that followed, the Conservatives finally came to accept that the NHS was here to stay and that there was just no point in debating alternative models of healthcare provision. The public hated that kind of discussion, immediately assuming that it meant ending up with something along the lines of the mess in the US, where healthcare is very very good for those with decent insurance packages – and a nightmarishly different story for the many without. So the task for Tories was not to have endless debates about something that would never happen, but to try to win back the trust of the electorate on healthcare.

They came very close indeed. By the 2010 election, Labour had fallen to its narrowest lead over the Tories on the question of whom voters trusted with the health service. In the January before polling day, the party produced a series of enormous – and much-mocked – posters with a picture of Cameron's face plastered over one half, and on the other half the quote 'We can't go on like this. I'll cut the deficit, not the NHS'. The leader of the opposition looked even more fresh-faced than usual – suspiciously so, in fact. He dodged questions on whether his photo had been airbrushed. Meanwhile, in election planning meetings, his colleague and close confidant George Osborne was doing a little bit of airbrushing of his own.

Osborne was worried that the Conservatives just couldn't go into an election promising reform to the health service. He felt it always encouraged the sort of anxiety about US-style privatisation described above. Lansley says Osborne – then shadow Chancellor – told him that he wanted 'radical change in education and "steady as she goes" in health'. Lansley agreed on the point about reassuring voters. But the programme for government was a different matter. Lansley explains: 'I said, "Well, we can't have 'steady as she goes' because 'steady as she goes' isn't happening in the NHS. We've had a 25 per cent increase in the administration costs of the NHS in the last year." The NHS management cadre fattened the NHS up for market. They knew we were going to cut. So, basically, left to their own devices, they would offer up 20 per cent management reductions and get themselves back to where they were in 2008. I mean, it was shockingly cynical. Shockingly cynical.'

None of this mattered to Osborne. He wasn't interested in what Lansley had to say about management. He had an election to win. So he overruled the shadow Health Secretary and made clear that the NHS reforms would not be part of the election campaign. They would feature in the manifesto. That document, which bore the pompous and meaningless title *Invitation to Join the Government of Britain*, promised in its opening lines to 'protect the NHS'.

Its detailed healthcare section was entitled 'Back the NHS' and made the claim that the party had 'consistently fought to protect the values the NHS stands for and have campaigned to defend the NHS from Labour's cuts and reorganisations'. It then promised 'a reform plan to make the changes the NHS needs', which would 'make doctors and nurses accountable to patients, not to endless layers of bureaucracy and management'. Patients would be able to choose any healthcare provider that met NHS standards and price caps. GPs would get more power as 'patients' expert guides through the health system', including running local healthcare budgets and commission care and being put 'in charge of commissioning local health services'.[10]

But the NHS didn't feature much outside the manifesto, save for repeated assurances that the Conservatives just loved it. In the televised leaders' debates, Cameron tended to focus on two things: talking about how 'special' the service was, and complaining about the spiralling numbers and costs of managers. He was upbraided for this by Nick Clegg, who was then busily positioning himself as the anti-politics hero of the moment, calling Cameron and Gordon Brown out for having a 'phoney debate' and mocking Cameron's warm words, saying: 'The easy thing is to say how much we all love and depend and rely on the NHS.' In between appearing above the petty politics of the other two leaders, Clegg actually did want to talk about the wiring of the health service. He told the first TV debate on 15 April that 'I want to see strategic health authorities, which is a layer of bureaucracy, stripped away altogether and use that money on the front-line NHS services which are so important to us.'[11]

Just a few weeks after this exchange, Cameron and Clegg stood side by side in the Downing Street rose garden and announced they would be working together in a new coalition government. In a cringingly couply session, the pair ate humble pie over their previous attacks on one another and promised a 'bold, reforming government' that took power away from politicians and gave it back to people. They did not mention the NHS.

The health service did come up in the 'Programme for Government' that was published a few days later. In the negotiations on this document, Conservative eccentric Oliver Letwin and Danny Alexander, a rather dry Liberal Democrat who hovered around the right of the party, had taken a look at the health reforms and concluded that they could go ahead. A foreword signed by both leaders argued that the two parties could gel very well on the health service:

> And in the crucial area of public service reform, we have found that Liberal Democrat and Conservative ideas are stronger combined. For example, in the NHS, take Conservative thinking on markets, choice and competition and add to it the Liberal Democrat belief in advancing democracy at a much more local level, and you have a united vision for the NHS that is truly radical: GPs with authority over commissioning; patients with much more control; elections for your local NHS health board. Together, our ideas will bring an emphatic end to the bureaucracy, top-down control and centralisation that has so diminished our NHS.

The Liberal Democrats appeared to have agreed with the Tories that these ideas did not represent a top-down reorganisation of the NHS, because the document promised to 'stop the top-down reorganisations of the NHS that have got in the way of patient care'. Right underneath this pledge, the two parties fleshed out what they meant by a non-reorganisation, which was a more detailed version of the points in the foreword. All seemed harmonious. All seemed simple.

But just as the coalition in practice was nothing like the strange love-in held by Cameron and Clegg in the rose garden, so the Health and Social Care Bill that started heading for the statute books in the first few weeks of 2011 had a passage – and a legacy – that was nothing like what Lansley, Cameron or the Liberal Democrats discussing it in their coalition meetings had envisaged. It wasn't just that it was so big a piece of legislation you could see it from space. The row accompanying it ended up being the size of a supernova.

An old proverb summarises the tale of a missing nail in a horseshoe, which led to the falling of a kingdom. For the want of a nail, the horse was lost, one version starts, going on to conclude that: 'For want of a battle the kingdom was lost. So a kingdom was lost – all for want of a nail.' The Health and Social Care Act 2012 would still have been an almighty upheaval for the health service without a very small mistake made by those writing the 2010 coalition agreement. But that apparently very small mistake was responsible in large part for the size of the political row that ensued. For six years, Lansley had been promising that there would be no 'pointless top-down reorganisations' of the health service. The authors of the coalition agreement didn't manage to repeat that promise verbatim. Instead, they wrote that the new government would 'stop the top-down reorganisations of the NHS'. Lansley had never said he wouldn't reorganise the NHS. He'd just promised he wouldn't embark on a pointless set of reforms.

For the want of the word 'pointless', a kingdom's worth of political capital was lost on these reforms. But not immediately. When the government published its White Paper *Equity and Excellence: Liberating the NHS* in July 2010, Lansley and his Liberal Democrat junior ministerial colleague Paul Burstow set out what they were up to, including scrapping primary care trusts – something the Lib Dems had insisted on. The White Paper itself didn't seem that controversial – or perhaps people just hadn't read it, which happened quite a lot with anything involving Lansley. The Health and Social Care Bill that was then published in January 2011 ended up being 550 pages long. Even then, it wasn't initially controversial politically.

That bill passed its second reading in the House of Commons 321 votes to 235, with all Tory and Lib Dem MPs voting in its favour. The Labour Party opposed it on the grounds that it was 'ideological' and would further open up the NHS to profit-making companies. Over the coming months, the opposition within the healthcare community to that lengthy piece of legislation grew louder. One by one, organisations in the health service establishment started to sound the alarm. Clare Gerada, the newly appointed head of the Royal College of GPs, came out with a threatening soundbite about the impact of the reforms, telling the *Guardian* in November 2010: 'I think it is the end of the NHS as we currently know it, which is a national, unified health service, with central policies and central planning, in the way that Bevan imagined.'[12] The BMA opposed the reforms. Even think tanks that tended to err on the side of caution, such as the studiously neutral King's Fund, warned the reforms were going too fast.

Inside the health service itself, alarm bells were ringing. Lansley and David Nicholson started to have increasingly tense discussions about what the former wanted to do. In one, Nicholson accused him of turning the NHS upside down for no benefit. Lansley turned to him and retorted: 'If you think I'm mad, you should meet Michael Gove.' Gove was Education Secretary at the time and embarking on an ambitious and controversial – but largely successful – set of reforms to schools. He served as the inspiration for many of his colleagues in government, but also managed to wind up people in the sector he was trying to shake up. He was ably helped in this by a man called Dominic Cummings, whom we shall get to know much better later.

Nicholson claims that in another confrontation with Lansley he asked, 'How does workforce fit into all of this? How will we know we've got enough doctors or nurses?' Lansley's response, says Nicholson, was that 'he genuinely hadn't thought of that. He just didn't think like that. He said, "The market will decide," and he did dismantle a whole load of workforce and still today I think we've not completely recovered from that.'[13]

Meanwhile, the Liberal Democrats were bleeding members. They were approaching local elections where they knew they would lose many voters. This was all punishment for the Lib Dems, formerly a protest party, committing the crime of going into government and making a U-turn on their election promise to scrap tuition fees. While Clegg and his colleagues knew there was nothing they could do about those two offences in the eyes of voters or indeed their own party members, they needed something to show that they hadn't been entirely subsumed by the Conservatives. As has so often been the case throughout its history, the NHS had the emotional sway with voters that meant the smaller coalition partner hoped it could use the health service as a way of sending a message both to the electorate and to its increasingly agitated activist base. For Clegg, there was a personal issue, too. He was on the right of his party, which had a vocal and unhappy left wing. Before becoming Lib Dem leader, he had given the sort of interview that only politicians who aren't worried about the impact of their musings would give: he broke the taboo around questioning whether the NHS should even exist. He told the *Independent*: 'I think breaking up the NHS is exactly what you do need to do to make it a more responsive service.'[14] He hadn't paid much personal attention to what Lansley was up to until this point, but his own credentials where the NHS was concerned were not strong.

It wasn't just within the junior coalition partner that nerves were building, though. In the months following the publication of the White Paper, the Conservatives started to pick up from private polling and focus groups that voters weren't impressed by the changes, either. Craig Oliver joined Downing Street as director of communications in early 2011, and along with the prime minister's pollster Andrew Cooper and political secretary Stephen Gilbert, realised very quickly that the NHS was becoming a toxic issue as the parties approached their first set of local elections. The trio went to Cameron and George Osborne with this evidence. Oliver recalls: 'It was an incredible pain in the neck. He was then like: "Do I really have to? All that energy and effort that went into that: am I really going to have to go and dismantle that?" But then I think he just realised, very practically, "Look, there's a double-decker bus coming down the road and it's going to flatten me. If I don't get out of the way of it, it's going to be a problem." '15

It was, he recalls, a set of 'awkward conversations' between Cameron and Lansley, not least because the latter had once been the prime minister's boss when the two were in the Conservative Research Department. And, as Lansley quite reasonably pointed out, the man who was now *his* boss had agreed to all this. 'In so far as people hated the Act,' he says, 'they hated it because it did the things that David Cameron asked me to do, not because it did the things he *didn't* want to have happen. That's the absurdity of it.'

What brought things to a head was a vote at the Liberal Democrat spring conference in March 2011, where activists demanded what they considered to be important changes to the bill. Clegg's ignorance of the detailed problems with the bill was ended with a jolt when one of his party's founding members and general national treasure Shirley Williams told him she would be leading the revolt. Unlike Clegg, Williams – by now a member of the House of Lords – had taken a week off to read through the legislation in its entirety, along with its accompanying documents. She didn't like what she'd seen, and found party members agreed with her. In particular, they didn't like the fact that the plans appeared to remove a legal duty for the Secretary of State to provide important services such as ambulances, maternity services and so on. Lansley, though, disagreed that this was the case. The Lib Dems were also vulnerable to the charge from the Labour Party that the changes would open the NHS up to EU competition law.

Lansley blames the insecurity of the Lib Dems for what then happened. The whole row, he thinks, was merely synthetic, because he had read through the changes that the party's members wanted and found them largely 'trivial'. 'The point was, my getting up and saying, "The Liberal Democrats have asked for the bill to be changed and I can do all that," wasn't enough for them. They needed there to be a big row. So they had the row.' He says Cameron turned to him in one of their private conversations and said: 'I have to show the Liberal Democrats that they've made us change it.' Lansley adds: 'He made it perfectly clear that, if it came to it – and of course in the event, it kind of *did* come to it – he would have to sacrifice me in order to satisfy Clegg and the Liberal Democrats.' Cameron accepts this: 'They needed to show some wins all the time, because the way the media was writing up the coalition was that it was sort of the Conservatives taking all the decisions and the Lib Dems were just sort of coming along in our wake, which was never really fair.'[16]

The prime minister now had to work out what to do. Clegg was adamant that he needed changes to the legislation. But Lansley was adamant that as the reforms had already started at a local level, they had to go ahead. Staff were already being made redundant at PCTs, for instance. And he had already been recruiting the GPs to lead commissioning. In the biography of the then permanent secretary of Downing Street, Jeremy Heywood, his wife Suzanne recounts what happened next:

> 'But what you could do,' Gus [O'Donnell, then the Cabinet Secretary] and Jeremy advised the Prime Minister, 'is pause the bill to give everyone time to think.'
>
> After some thought, the Prime Minister agreed with this – though he remained reluctant to criticise the changes. On 31 March he called Andrew Lansley and Nick Clegg into Number 10 for a private meeting, and when everyone else, including Jeremy, filed in an hour later, he said they were halting the legislation.
>
> Andrew was sitting on the sofa shaking his head. 'Surely you don't mean we should stop the next round of the GP consortia expressions of interest?' he said.
>
> Jeremy held his breath.
>
> 'I'm not sure I even know what that means,' the Prime Minister said, 'but yes, everything will stop.'[17]

On 4 April, Lansley told the Commons that there would be a pause in the legislation. It was a painful session. 'We recognise that this speed of progress has brought with it some substantive concerns, expressed in various quarters,' he told the Chamber, to sarcastic laughter from the benches opposite. 'Some of those concerns are misplaced or based on misrepresentations, but we must recognise that some of them are genuine. We want to continue to listen to, engage with and learn from experts, patients and front-line staff within the NHS and beyond and to respond accordingly.' The laughter mounted as he continued: 'I can therefore tell the House that we propose to take the opportunity of a natural break in the passage of the Bill to pause, listen and engage with all those who want the NHS to succeed.'[18]

Two days later, Cameron and Clegg dragged Lansley along with them to Frimley Park Hospital in Surrey. The Health Secretary, who was generally a placid fellow, had spent the past few days in a grump. A colleague had been surprised to see him kicking a door in the Department of Health in frustration. By the time the trio turned up to their press conference at the hospital to talk about what they would fill the pause with, Lansley had the look of a teenager who had been both grounded and forced to go on a long winter walk with his parents. His answers to questions from journalists were surly and muttered. He remembers:

> Of course I was cross. Of *course* I was cross. I would ask 'Why are we pausing? In order to do what?' But then all of them would think 'Oh, well, the trouble with Lansley is, he knows the policy but he doesn't know the politics.' The fact that I had won a general election [in 1992, while working for the Conservative Party under John Major] more or less against the odds when they were all wandering around like headless bloody chickens never seemed to occur to them. The fact that, in 2011, we were spending some of the capital on the NHS that *I* had acquired in the previous decade . . . It didn't happen mysteriously that we were trusted on the NHS.

But Lansley's humiliation hadn't quite finished. The following week, he trundled up to Liverpool for the annual conference of the Royal College of Nursing, where 99 per cent of the college's membership backed a vote of no confidence in him as Health Secretary. As he tried to allay their worries about the legislation, he unwittingly underlined how he had made the reforms even worse. 'I am sorry if what it is I am setting out to do has not communicated itself,' he told a room of baffled nurses.[19]

The legislation went into a pause for two months, during which time civil servants conducted a 'listening exercise'. Lansley and his team drew up a series of amendments that they hoped would satisfy the Liberal Democrats and get the bill through Parliament. Andy Cowper, a health policy expert who by his own admission had become totally fixated upon both the problems with the reforms and the general lack of understanding about what they entailed, described the pause as merely a 'vajazzling' of the bill. He explained further: 'What we have seen here is a J-turn. A J-turn means you travel down the long leg of the J, get flicked up a bit to the left, but basically end up (thanks to gravity) very, very close to where you were going anyway before the diversion.'[20]

That vajazzling ran thus: the regulator, Monitor, would promote integrated care, and would no longer be tasked with 'promoting competition', instead doing the apparently strikingly different job of 'tackling anti-competitive behaviour'. NHS services wouldn't be open to being run by 'any willing provider', because instead only 'any qualified provider' would be able to bid for them.[21] Some changes had a little more consequence: hospital doctors and nurses would be added to clinical commissioning groups so that GPs didn't entirely dominate.

Clegg was determined to notch this up as a victory, telling his MPs that eleven out of the thirteen demands made by his party's spring conference had been met. He told the next meeting of that conference a few months later that 'the Health bill was stopped in its tracks and rewritten' and 'it is not a Liberal Democrat health bill but it is a better bill because of the Liberal Democrats, a better bill because of you'.[22] Party members disagreed. They voted against the changes and instructed peers to oppose the bill when it moved to the House of Lords the following week.

The medical world was just getting going with its opposition to the bill. People who'd been with Lansley from the start began to turn on him. Dr Sam Everington is a pioneering figure in the world of general practice. His Bromley by Bow Centre practice in Tower Hamlets, London, was the place Lansley chose to give his first speech as Health Secretary, because its work showed the transformative power of a good GP. Bromley by Bow has led the world in 'social prescribing' – that is, not assuming that all the problems patients present have medical roots or solutions. Patients are referred to a centre which offers housing advice and debt counselling, alongside prescriptions for yoga, drama and other forms of exercise. Everington was delighted by Lansley's proposals to give GPs power over health commissioning in their areas because he believed GPs knew best what people in their area needed.

But what didn't make sense to Everington about the Lansley reforms was that they shook up the NHS too much for too little gain, and introduced procurement processes and an emphasis on competition that he just couldn't support. So, with an hour's notice to Downing Street, he released a letter which turned on the bill. On behalf of his clinical commissioning group, he wrote: 'Your rolling restructuring of the NHS compromises our ability to focus on what really counts – improving quality of services for patients, and ensuring value for money during a period of financial restraint.' He added: 'Your government has interpreted our commitment to our patients as support for the Bill. It is not.'[23]

The bill was now a wounded animal as it went through the Lords. But in the end, peers didn't kill it off – or really substantially reshape it. There were just two defeats, which Timmins feels 'were on relatively minor matters'. His verdict on the passage of the bill is: 'Fifty days of debate in Parliament had produced a piece of legislation even longer, more complex and in some areas – notably on the regulator's duties – appreciably less clear, than the original huge edifice; even if Earl Howe was to argue that "we have made a bill whose key principles command wide acceptance: more joined-up, clearer and, in certain aspects, less risky".'[24]

It was quickly becoming clear that very few people in the NHS, or in politics, really felt the Lansley Act was in any way a success. Everington explains that the legislation led to a mess in procurement for services: 'The standardisation of procurement processes led to some extraordinarily poor outcomes. Actually, people succeeded in procurement based on the paperwork they produced, not on their credibility or their commitment or their energy for any of those things. This led to some pretty major mistakes.'

The Tories certainly didn't want to talk about health reform any more, feeling they'd lost all their carefully stored political capital in the row. Bill Morgan reflects that 'the Bill was traumatic, obviously. But look back at 2003, at the foundation trust legislation. That was traumatic, too. Blair almost lost his majority. In 1990, that was traumatic: I mean, Thatcher sacked Ken Clarke and told his successor to rip the throat out of the reforms. So any time you try to do legislation in health, it's traumatic, because it creates oxygen to have all these almost first principles arguments again about how the health service should be. We walked into it in 2011 and we shouldn't have done.'

David Cameron has a similar view. 'What's so annoying about this whole issue is everyone is always endlessly questioning everyone's bona fides about the NHS. I mean part of the point of the reforms was to try and get away from that.' Instead, the Tories found themselves spending the next ten years trying to get away from the mess they'd made.[25]

While the Conservatives were licking their wounds, a wonderful distraction heaved into view. London was hosting the 2012 Olympics. Right up to the opening ceremony, there had been doubts in the media as to whether Britain was up to the job of running such a big sporting event. The military ended up stepping in to provide security after the outsourcing firm G4S realised it couldn't fulfil its contract. Nerves were running high about what kind of an image Britain would project to the world. A thousand commentators wrote pointless pieces mulling over what Britishness actually meant and whether it was possible to capture that in an opening ceremony. On the night that the Games began, they were shown up for their lack of imagination. Film director Danny Boyle put together a captivating show running through England's green and pleasant land, wars, literature, the London Underground, Mr Bean – and for a long and moving sequence, the NHS.

The health service was represented by a series of light-up beds, which first joined together to draw the world-famous logo of Great Ormond Street Hospital. Lights whooshed across the stadium to pick out a group of GOSH workers and their patients, waving from a grassy knoll on the set. With the sparkling sounds of Mike Oldfield's 'Tubular Bells', the beds – pushed by actors in traditional nursing costumes and occupied by children in pyjamas – moved again, spelling out the letters N-H-S in the darkened Stratford stadium. It wasn't so enormous you could see it from space, but it was a big statement about the relationship of the health service to the British identity. No other nation hosting the Games before or since has put one of its public services in such a prominent part of the opening ceremony.

Not everyone was happy with this. In fact, a few years after the Games, Boyle claimed that the government had tried to get him to cut the NHS section right down and that he had threatened to resign in order to stop this happening. He didn't name the minister responsible for the Olympics – Jeremy Hunt – but the implication was that the Culture Secretary was uncomfortable with the focus on the health service. Hunt's aides insisted he was only worried about the length of the ceremony as a whole, to ensure that spectators had time to get home safely afterwards. But some in government privately felt the worship of the NHS *was* strange and inappropriate given they were at that very moment working on inquiries into serious failings in some parts of the service.

It's worth recalling the full sequence. Boyle hadn't started it with a tribute to the health service as a whole; he had focused in on GOSH, an institution that is much loved within Britain. The NHS is better-known globally, but his decision to pick out a children's hospital that had been running for a century before the health service became operational suggests that the public's affection isn't as simple as politicians often tend to think.

A few weeks after those dancing nurses and singing patients, David Cameron reshuffled his Cabinet. To no one's surprise, he moved Lansley to the role of Leader of the House – often seen as a waiting room for politicians on their way out of government – and brought in Hunt to run Health instead. Hunt found a health service in chaos as its leaders tried to work out what to do with the hand they'd been dealt. What the NHS did manage to do with that hand is almost as important a story as what the Conservatives tried to do to the NHS.

Lansley hadn't got quite what he wanted when he set out to reform the NHS. He also didn't get quite what the legislation that he ended up with was supposed to create. By now, the health service had learned how to survive through feast and famine, from government to government, and how to pick its way through reforms that its leaders had decided just wouldn't do.

'There are the Lansley reforms as intended, the Lansley reforms as executed, and the third thing which is Lansley as the NHS chose to implement it,' Nigel Edwards, chief executive of the Nuffield Trust, explains. 'To some extent, from the publication of the bill, NHS England started developing workaround mechanisms to prevent things like foundation trusts failing, which the logic of his reforms would have allowed. Then by 2014, the health service published a "Five Year Forward View," which showed it was putting its emphasis on integration rather than competition. 2014 marked a shift away from procurement as the main mechanism for improving healthcare to a combination of more managerial methods and an emphasis on collaboration.'[26]

Some of those workarounds came from Nicholson, and others from his successor Simon Stevens. Nicholson's account of what he did is that 'we mitigated the worst excesses and that enabled Simon to essentially ignore [the Act]'. He ensured that the health service was able to control the way money flowed through the system, rather than politicians: 'Essentially, we took the money and ran, we brought it over here.' He also had the name of the 'NHS Commissioning Board' changed to 'NHS England', because it was 'it was not a technocratic body, it was a leadership board for the NHS and that kind of held the NHS together because most of the Lansley reforms essentially fragmented stuff'.

A grip on the system: something politicians think they have and clever NHS figures work out how to keep without anyone else noticing. When offered the job of chief executive in 2014, Stevens accepted it after a conversation with David Cameron where he complained that the Lansley reforms had been a distraction from the things patients cared about, which was how to improve services and outcomes. He then embarked on a series of workarounds which allowed the service to focus on what was important. The Tories were so scarred by what had happened that they agreed Stevens could do this, and largely left him to it.

Unelected bureaucrats secretly undermining the will of a government? Lansley had wanted the NHS to have autonomy, but he presumably hadn't meant it quite like this. Never mind: his colleagues were so sick to the back teeth of what he'd tried to do with the health service that they were willing to let Nicholson and Stevens do as they saw fit – so long as they didn't have to have any more fights about the NHS.

10. The fight for safety

When Isabella Bailey — better known as Bella to her friends and family — was admitted to Stafford Hospital in September 2007, she was relieved to be in the hands of the NHS. A hiatus hernia that the 86-year-old had developed over the preceding year was giving her increasing discomfort, to the extent that she was struggling to eat, drink or sleep. Her doctor decided that there was no point in continuing to fiddle with her medication, told her she needed to go into hospital, and promised her 'I'll make sure you get the best bed on the wards.' Her daughter Julie recalls her reaction: 'Mom was relieved, she was sure she would be in the best place for her. Both Mom and I were proud of the NHS, she had only had good experiences. We both respected doctors and nurses and had always felt that they did all they could to help others.'[1]

You can probably already sense the 'but' following these words. Julie and Bella had the same feelings about the NHS as most of the population – but what unfolded in the following months was so contrary to the good faith they'd placed in the institution that Julie's quote about the pride they felt comes at the start of an entire book recounting what is now notorious as the 'Mid Staffs scandal'. It is one of the darkest chapters in the life of the health service: not just because of the way individual patients were treated at the small Staffordshire district general, but also because of the way the organisations within the health service and then politicians responded to complaints. We have seen over the past few chapters how regularly the NHS embodies the values that make up the British identity. The next few pages will show that this is not always a given.

It was, though, still a given in Julie's mind as she arrived at the hospital on 26 September after her mother's second night in hospital. A kindly nurse on the night shift had suggested she go home and get some rest. 'The thought of going home and Mom being in pain worried me but the nurse assured me that she would keep an eye on her and give her painkillers as soon as she woke,' Julie writes. She did as the nurse suggested, and tried to get some sleep. She couldn't believe Bella's claim the next morning that no one had entered her room all night, and thought her mother must be mistaken until she found the hospital drug chart, which showed that no one had given her any medication overnight. 'She told me how she called out for the staff during the night and at one point she heard them shut the door, ignoring her calls. I tried to change the subject as I found it hard to believe that the nurses would do this.'[2]

Bailey still sounds disbelieving when recalling her experiences more than a decade later. It is hard, even at the end of her book, or at the end of the myriad reports into what happened in the Mid Staffordshire NHS Trust, to believe that patients were treated by healthcare workers in the way that they were. The vocation, the compassion, the humanity that drives people to take up far less well-paid jobs in the NHS than their abilities often merit had evaporated. When the barrister Robert Francis QC published the first of his reports into the standard of care at the hospital, he found that patients were regularly left sitting in their own faeces, that staff often failed to help them eat or placed food out of reach, that their calls for help were ignored so frequently and for so long that they would often try to get out of their beds or chairs without the assistance they needed and inevitably fell.

Francis wrote: 'Some of the descriptions I received of lack of continence care might have seemed barely credible if they had been isolated.' But they weren't isolated; he had many different incidents recounted to him by different families. The nurses often ignored buzzers from patients who needed help to go to the toilet, to the extent that these people had to suffer the indignity of soiling themselves. Then, they would find themselves waiting for hours for someone to come along and clean them up. Often, the only person who was around to do this was a family member, adding still more to the humiliation. One relative of an elderly patient told the inquiry that 'the nurses there weren't unkind to him, but they were overworked. We often felt that if we asked them if they would clean him up, it would be hours before they came back to clean him up, and in that time he was just lying in a dirty bed with dirty nightwear on, and didn't want me to go in the room, even. He would say: don't come near me, don't come near me, I smell; and he was a very fastidious man and he really was left lying in his own excrement.' Others described finding their parents covered in dried faeces which had obviously been there a long time.

Some patients who tried to make their own way around fell and injured themselves. One patient died after her third fall, with staff trying to keep her son away from her prone body. When he was taken to see his mother, he found her 'lying full stretch out on the grey Marley tiled floor'. There was blood 'smeared all over the floor'. A doctor was holding the patient's head in her hands, and the son told her: 'This is my mother.' Her retort was almost as disgraceful as the circumstances in which the woman had been left to fall. 'As cold and as calculated as anything, her retort as fast as anything was: I have got a mother too,' he said in evidence. 'There was no compassion in that woman whatsoever.'[3]

Julie's own experience when visiting her mother involved trying to look after other elderly, frail and confused patients whose calls for help were ignored, passing drinks to people who were so dehydrated that their mouths were 'covered in a white film and bleeding', and patients left in their soiled sheets. Early on in her mother's stay, Julie watched a member of staff shouting at a patient who she claimed had 'nothing wrong' with her. 'The woman curled herself into a ball on her bed and sobbed. It's horrible to hear people crying when you know comfort will not come. But I would have to get used to hearing it over the following eight weeks. I would hear it every night.' She watched another confused and dehydrated patient drink from a flower vase, and staff taking away food that patients hadn't eaten without acknowledging that they hadn't been able to reach the plate.

It quickly became obvious to Julie that she could not trust the nurses to keep her mother safe, let alone care for her properly. So she organised a rota with her family so that Bella was never alone. Some of the nurses seemed overworked to the point of being overwhelmed. Others appeared to have stopped caring about patients long ago. One night, a young healthcare assistant dropped Bella while trying to put her back into bed after a toilet visit. When a nurse attended to her the following day, she tried to persuade Bella, 'You slipped, didn't you, Isabella? You weren't dropped, were you?' But she had been dropped, and that injury caused a heart failure that led to Bella's death, in agony, seven days later. 'I saw fear in her eyes like I had never seen in anyone before. I never saw my Mom alive again and my last sight of her was in fear. They destroyed her. A strong, vibrant woman who they robbed of any dignity, left begging for her life.'[4]

Julie might have gone home and tried to forget what the end of her mother's life had looked like as she grieved her. But she didn't. She left the hospital that day knowing that 'it was the hospital that was responsible', and vowing to do everything she could to stop anyone else suffering in the same way. She had no idea quite how much she would have to do just for someone in power to take her seriously, let alone stop the suffering.

Over the following years, Bailey, a determined, forthright woman, started to gather up a campaign group she called 'Cure the NHS'. She found there were many people in the town who had witnessed similar shocking incidents when their family members had been hospitalised. She found too that when they had tried to complain, they often watched as the nursing staff appeared to punish the patient for raising a concern, or a manager in the hospital dismissed their points. The group held vigils outside the hospital, wrote to the local newspapers and tried to sound the alarm with the chief executive and board members. At every stage, they were treated as though they were merely a group of bereaved relatives who had been driven mad with grief, not people who were shocked that the NHS that they felt proud of had failed their families so badly. And it wasn't just the hospital management that turned a deaf ear to their complaints. It was the local MPs and press, who seemed wary of criticising the hospital, and professional bodies such as the Royal College of Nursing. The hospital was Stafford's largest employer, which explains some of the antipathy towards the Cure the NHS group. People were frightened that their campaign would lead to the hospital closing altogether. Many in the wider community turned against Julie, to the extent that she received threats, had 'BITCH' daubed over the windows of her café, and eventually decided she should leave the town for her own safety. More than ten years later, she had only returned once, wearing a wig so no one would recognise her. Bella is buried in the town. Julie cannot visit her grave.

Shaun Lintern saw first-hand how hard it was for Julie and her group to get anyone to pay them attention. He was a young reporter on the *Express and Star*, which covered the area. He was sitting in a district office of the paper one day when a colleague took a call. 'I overheard him saying something along the lines of "unfortunately people die every day". It was relatively early in my newspaper career and I asked him for the number of this person. I rang her back and effectively I said, "I know you've not had a great response from us, can we start again." We had a conversation and I wrote a very small news-in-brief story in which she expressed her concern and asked for people to come forward.' They did, and they kept on coming.

Over the years, Shaun wrote so many stories about different incidents at Stafford Hospital that at one stage he was taken off the beat in an attempt to get more positive coverage about the local NHS. 'There was clearly an attempt to minimise the complaints,' he says of the hospital's response. 'They attempted to dismiss them and there was the classic NHS apology of "we're sorry that they feel that something didn't go right".' He even interviewed the then chief executive Martin Yeates, who Shaun says 'effectively lied to me and the public' by claiming that the hospital had turned a corner from problems it had been having. 'What we didn't know at that stage was the hospital was under investigation by the Healthcare Commission, and when he gave me that interview, I've since learned that almost on the same day he had received a letter and an inspection from the Healthcare Commission effectively warning him that the A&E department was unsafe.'[5]

It wasn't just patients who were trying to warn the hospital hierarchy, either. Since 2001, Dr Peter Daggett had been complaining to managers about shortages of nurses in the emergency assessment unit, warning that 'those few that are available are run ragged'. He was met with what he described as 'a wall of silence'.[6]

Dr Chris Turner started work in the emergency department in October 2007, and was also so horrified by what he saw that he complained to Yeates and approached the Healthcare Commission three times to raise concerns. He'd been working in the health service for twenty-five years by this point, and the Stafford A&E was by far the worst he'd come across. It was, he told the inquiry into the scandal, a 'disaster', with bullying of staff and shortages meaning it was impossible to ensure safe care. The worst bit of his evidence was that staff – himself included – had become 'immune to the sound of pain'.

All healthcare professionals have to deal not just with the daily reality of very sick people in front of them, but also the fact that some of their care necessarily causes pain. Even basic observations such as testing someone's level of consciousness or treatments including inserting a cannula can cause pain, and a doctor or nurse cannot run away from that. It is for the greater good of the patient. But how can someone stop noticing pain, to the extent that they don't seem to care? Turner explains that the decision of the Mid Staffordshire Trust in 2006 to cut 150 jobs to save money (on top of around 150 posts that were vacant) had led to staff being so stretched that it was impossible for them to do their jobs on a daily basis. They simply could not keep up with the needs of each patient. 'The organisation became denuded of nursing staff,' he says. 'What that meant was that patients waited for longer to get their analgesia. So what happened is that we gradually became used to people not getting their pain relief for a prolonged period of time, not because we wanted it to be that way but because that was the only way it could be with the resources that we had available, and as an organisation that gradually became normalised in some parts of it.'

He is robust in his defence of the nursing staff in the emergency department, including a couple who were later struck off for their involvement in the scandal. 'To accuse the nurses who were there of not caring is to completely miss the point. The guys who worked there really cared, but if you put somebody into an environment where you literally cannot discharge your responsibilities, psychologically you have to somehow deal with that, otherwise you spend your whole time in distress and dissonance.'[7]

Two nurses, Sharon Turner and Tracey White, were struck off for – among other things – changing patient records so it appeared that they had not breached the four-hour waiting time in A&E. Chris Turner now runs a campaign called Civility Saves Lives, which aims to help staff and organisations understand how behaviour impacts performance, so that care improves and patients have better outcomes. He is still racked with guilt about what happened to the nurses, and his work today is informed by that. 'To strike them off in that setting is to not understand the astonishing pressure that was put onto them,' he says. 'We had middle managers who were coming down and screaming at low-level nurses, newly qualified band 5s [band 5 nurses are the most junior staff], and threatening them with things like "If you have any breaches today, you will lose your job, I will get you sacked." Truth was, that was normal within the organisation. Sharon and Tracey changed things, and I'll tell you, they are not unusual, I could show you nurses doing this in every single acute trust in the NHS because of the pressure they are put under.'

The incentives for these nurses were going in one direction: focus on meeting (or appearing to meet) the targets, even if the way you do so breaks the law, and keep your job. It was the same for doctors: Turner himself was twice called away from cardiac arrests because patients in the injuries section of the department were about to breach the four-hour target – but he refused to leave the arresting patient. And the reason these incentives were so skewed on the wards is that they were skewed not just throughout the hospital and its management structures, but for the health service more generally.

You will recall from Chapter 8 that the Blair government had a number of 'enforcers' whose job it was to pressure chief executives of poorly performing trusts to meet their targets. Targets, boxes, numbers: none of these things reflect the quality of care that someone like Bella Bailey should have expected without a second thought. When she was admitted to hospital, the Mid Staffs Trust was not holding regular meetings about how to improve care; it was trying to become a foundation trust. And the way in which applications for foundation status – with all the freedom that entailed – were assessed was by a hospital's ability to meet targets and keep its spending in check. The job cuts in 2006 were part of this. The way the trust dealt with the consequences of those cuts – to blame the nurses still on the wards for failing to cover multiple jobs – was also part of this: the culture in the health service had become one of blame and accusation.

It was therefore inevitable that when the scandal became a political one, the same culture would rear its head in Westminster. Who would get the blame? Who would get the sack? Who could politicians shout at the most?

The question of what each leader at Stafford Hospital knew about what was happening on the wards ran through a series of inquiries. There was the Healthcare Commission's investigation in 2008 into the trust's mortality rates, governance, and care of older patients. That inquiry led to a highly critical report, published in March 2009, which found 'appalling' failures of care, bullying, and a focus on targets at the expense of quality. It prompted an apology in the House of Commons by the Health Secretary, Alan Johnson, who told MPs: 'This was a complete failure of management to address serious problems and monitor performance . . . This led to a totally unacceptable failure to treat emergency patients safely and with dignity.'[8] His immediate instinct was to get rid of the chair and the chief executive, but officials quickly pointed out to him that as Mid Staffs had just become a foundation trust, he technically couldn't. Bill Moyes, head of the regulator Monitor, told Johnson he didn't have the authority. That had been part of the rationale behind FTs. But as should be very obvious by now, that's not really how health and politics interact in practice. Johnson's response was: 'Now politically it would be very nice if you could get away with it and say, "That's yours. That's your can of worms." But I told him, you know, "Piss off. I'm dealing with this." '[9]

After this, it depends on whose account you listen to as to what actually happened. The Conservatives say that the Labour government at the time tried to cover up what was going on at Mid Staffs and make it a local rather than systemic issue, resisting calls for a formal inquiry into the trust. Labour politicians disagree, and believe their account has been lost in a political narrative. The row that developed over the hospital and the inquiries that followed mean Mid Staffs is not just a byword for poor care. It is now also a reference to a time of yet more intense political fighting over the NHS.

Under pressure from Cure the NHS, Johnson's successor Andy Burnham commissioned the independent inquiry led by Robert Francis QC into the trust. The inquiry's report concluded in April 2010 that patients were 'routinely neglected by a trust preoccupied with cost cutting, targets and processes and which lost sight of its fundamental responsibility to provide safe care'. Burnham says he was forced to fight a 'very large battle' to get that inquiry in the first place, because the Department of Health 'did not want it reopened'. He produces an official submission from the department that advised him not to have a formal public inquiry. 'The department's line was "a public inquiry will sink this trust when it is trying to recover",' he says. In the end, Burnham and his ministerial colleague Mike O'Brien worked out a way of giving Francis the option to come back and ask for the inquiry to be upgraded to a full public one if witnesses were not coming forward. He announced the inquiry in Stafford, at which point another row, which has never been fully resolved, blew up. Bailey and Cure the NHS say Burnham refused to meet with them. Burnham says there was a misunderstanding, that he had only wanted to ensure that his meeting with patients was an open forum and that Cure the NHS had wanted to see him on his own.[10] Either way, from then on, there was a serious souring in the relationship between the patients and the Labour politicians dealing with the scandal.

The Conservatives then campaigned for a full public inquiry in the 2010 general election. After they formed the coalition government, the newly appointed Health Secretary Andrew Lansley set one up, giving Francis the power to compel witnesses under oath. That inquiry reported in a febrile political context.

Lansley had by now been replaced by Jeremy Hunt, who had come from his own bruising experience in another department. As Culture Secretary, he had been dragged over the coals in the Leveson Inquiry for his relationship with the Murdoch dynasty. He had just about survived a number of potentially career-ending Commons encounters, and had even hidden behind a tree at one point in the hope that journalists wouldn't spot him attending a drinks event with James Murdoch (they did).[11] By his own admission, he had not had much interest in the Health brief before being offered the job, but he accepted that 'you do what the Prime Minister asks you to do' and saw it as a fresh start.[12] So did David Cameron, but for another reason (the previous chapter set out what political pain the Lansley reforms had caused the prime minister). His brief to Hunt was simple: 'Turn the volume down.' He told him he wanted someone who 'speaks English' and that he had to neutralise health as an issue. It was a twenty-first-century repeat of Thatcher's instructions to William Waldegrave to 'calm them all down' after a time of political upheaval. Here was another glazier.

It quickly transpired that this glazier would not even be allowed to make new legislation because of the toxic legacy of the Lansley reforms, and even that he would not be allowed to talk that much about health policy in public. Craig Oliver was Number 10's director of communications at the time, and recalls 'spending half my time in arguments with Jeremy Hunt, who wanted to go out there and sing the praises of the government that was actually incredibly supportive of the NHS'. But Oliver's job was to tell him that 'the more you mention this issue, the worse it is for us'.[13]

Hunt found this 'incredibly frustrating', but was soon distracted by another issue. On arriving in the department in September 2012, he found the Francis Report 'hovering like a dark cloud'. He had a few months to get up to speed.

Hunt says he spent that time trying to work out 'how has health policy led us to something like Mid Staffs happening and what is the big lesson'. His conclusion was 'what happens in health policy time after time is that politicians and civil servants and NHS leaders come up with well-meaning policies to address the big issue of the day that have horrific unintended consequences'.[14] But elsewhere in his party, others were reaching rather different conclusions about what the Francis Report meant. A meeting took place in Number 10 to discuss how to approach it in Parliament. One of those present recalls: 'It was very clear from the start that this was the opportunity to bury the Labour Party in terms of their record on the NHS.'

And that's what unfolded. Cameron gave the first statement on the Francis Report when it was published on 6 February 2013. He apologised again 'to the families of all those who have suffered for the way the system allowed this horrific abuse to go unchecked and unchallenged for so long. On behalf of the Government – and indeed our country – I am truly sorry.' It was a dramatic shift in language in itself: the prime minister was making clear that this was an assault on the British values that the NHS was supposed to be a part of. He promised that he would honour the desire of Bailey and the other Mid Staffs campaigners for 'the legacy of their loved ones to be an NHS safe for everyone'.[15]

This was a prime ministerial approach to the inquiry, but in the weeks and months that followed, Mid Staffs became the subject of an intense political bunfight. The Conservatives decided to focus on what Burnham and other Labour ministers had really known about Mid Staffs. Why had he approved the trust's application for foundation status? Why hadn't he met Cure the NHS? Why hadn't he granted a full public inquiry? Labour fought back against a statistic that Hunt regularly used, which was that up to 1,200 people had died needlessly at the hospital.

Hunt began to develop two grand themes. The first was a political one, and was acted out in every Commons encounter he had with Burnham: that the Labour Party had lost its way on the NHS. Their fights in Parliament were some of the most visceral those reporting on it at the time had seen. Each blames the other for this. 'I can still hear Andy Burnham's voice in my mind today describing a "toxic mix of cuts and privatisation",' says Hunt, adding:

> The weird thing about that job is that you're really having to do two jobs at once. One is running or being responsible for the fifth largest organisation in the world, with all the complexity of how do you stop problems like this happening again, how do you improve on cancer care or maternity care or mental health and so on. And then you will go into Parliament and you're suddenly in a completely parallel universe where you're having an argument about all these things that you're not actually doing, like we weren't privatising the NHS and

we weren't actually cutting the budget, and so it was surreal, and you spent hours trying to build your defences to this completely bogus argument.

Basically, by the middle of 2013, because Andy Burnham's onslaughts were completely full on – he's a very effective and powerful politician – I decided that attack is the best form of defence, and I am going to go out and point out the things that Labour got wrong, and not least the fact that Mid Staffs happened on his watch when he was Health Secretary, and he refused to meet the Mid Staffs relatives. So it was a last resort because the barrage was so persistent, and that's not my natural style of politics to do that, but I just thought if he's inventing all this stuff about us then I'm going to have to hold him accountable for his time as Health Secretary, and obviously things became extremely bitter between us when that happened.

Burnham agrees that it was bitter, but naturally feels that Hunt was the cause of that, not him. 'It was awful, wasn't it?' he recalls. 'It got politicised and slightly personalised and it became unedifying, to say the least. It was awful, yes.'[16]

Burnham wasn't the only person in the firing line. The press soon became very interested in NHS chief David Nicholson, who had been head of West Midlands Strategic Health Authority when the scandal was unfolding. It didn't help that he had once been a member of the Communist Party, which didn't exactly endear him to the average Tory. Backbench Conservative MPs started calling for his scalp, and Nicholson found himself in a surreal situation. 'Craig Oliver and Jeremy Hunt sat down with me to give me some advice. That was I was never to be photographed, all the time I was to wear a tie and I was to say nothing. None of these things are my natural thing. So I did that and they said if you do that, we'll be with you,' he recalls. 'This thing about never being photographed, I managed to avoid it all the time but at one point I was in the back of a car with a carpet over me, lying down so I wouldn't get photographed coming out of a meeting.'[17]

Nicholson eventually stepped down as chief executive of the NHS, though once again it depends on who you listen to as to the reasons for his departure. He says he served for eight years in the post, and a fundamental disagreement with the Tories on their plans to tackle health tourism precipitated his decision to move on. Most Conservatives think it was because of his role in Mid Staffs. Like so many fights in the health service, this one will never really end.

In the middle of these political fights was a group of relatives who remained bewildered by what they were experiencing. Julie Bailey, a Labour member herself, had never set out to become an enemy of the NHS, but she found herself being accused of being a 'Tory stooge' by Labour activists who couldn't see that she was just trying to stop others suffering in the way Bella had. At one point she felt she couldn't carry on with her campaign. 'It became awkward for me, even more awkward than it had in the past because I was seen a little bit like a political pawn.' She has since pulled back from her work advising people who are trying to pursue health service complaints, because she realised that she has not yet had the chance to grieve for her mother properly, despite it being more than a decade since her death. Not only did the NHS deny Bella a dignified end of life, it also denied Julie the chance to grieve properly, as she was forced to fight so hard for justice over many, many years.

Julie Bailey's frustration with the way the system responded to her complaints led to Hunt's second grand theme, which was less about politics and has arguably led to a step change in the way people talk about the health service. His conclusion from Mid Staffs was that the NHS was not taking the safety of patients seriously – and that those who tried to raise the alarm were often treated abominably. Inspired by Michael Gove, who as Education Secretary had insisted on a focus on school standards – as well as a fair few dramatic fights with the teaching unions – he tried to badge himself as a champion of patient safety.

He put up a whiteboard in his office with a list of 'never events' on it. These were the sort of mistakes that should never happen in the health service: the wrong limb being amputated, the wrong dose of a drug being administered, and so on. Hunt soon started making calls to hospital managers to ask for more details about these incidents, and about missed targets. One of those party to the calls says they weren't threatening, but inquiring.[18] Indeed, Hunt's aim was not to replicate the shouty culture of the Blair years, but to normalise honesty about mistakes in the health service so that the system could learn and make the term 'never event' accurate in that the same mistake would not be repeated.

He soon found that honesty – or a lack of it – was one of the biggest problems in the service. As Dr Chris Turner had concluded about the culture in the Stafford A&E, the incentives were just not there for staff to speak up and admit they had made a mistake. On top of that, people often struggle to process a mistake because, in the health service, the consequences are so terrible. 'It's incredibly difficult because if a baby dies on your watch in a maternity unit it's very hard to persuade yourself that you made a mistake,' Hunt explains. 'You try very hard to persuade yourself that it was inevitable, your colleagues tell you it was inevitable and everyone closes ranks. It's amazingly traumatic of course for a doctor or any front-line professional to have to cope with that. And that was when I began to realise that there is a fundamental problem in the culture of modern medicine, not just the NHS, but around the world, which is that we don't investigate things that go wrong, we don't have a learning culture, we have a blame culture.'

A conversation with Sir Bruce Keogh, then the medical director of NHS England, brought this home to Hunt vividly. 'This was in the first six months of me being Health Secretary, so I was really hoovering everything up like a sponge. Bruce was a heart surgeon and he told me how he operated on a patient who died and he was very upset about it and his colleagues all said to him, Bruce, he had a very bad heart, the guy was going to die anyway, let's face it. And Bruce said, yes, but he wasn't going to die on Tuesday.'

Another case that underlined this – and brought Hunt to tears – was that of Joshua Titcombe.

Joshua was born in Furness General Hospital on 27 October 2008, almost exactly a year after Bella Bailey died. Like Julie, Joshua's father, James, had no previous beef with the health service at all. He was delighted when his son – his second child – arrived. He wrote of his feelings at the time: 'I know all parents must feel this way about their babies, but Joshua really is a perfect and beautiful little boy. All my worries are over – Joshua has been born and we have all the time in the world to get to know our baby son.'[19] But that time was cut short in the most appalling fashion.

James and his wife, Hoa, had been feeling unwell in the run-up to Joshua's birth, and had told staff at Furness General Hospital about this on arrival. Not long after the birth, Hoa fell very ill indeed, and needed antibiotics. James asked a doctor if the baby would also need treatment. 'The doctor gives me a nervous look, waves his hand dismissively and leaves the room.' The midwives also rejected his questions, insisting that 'we know Joshua is fine just by looking at him'.

Joshua was not fine. He died on 5 November 2008 at the Freeman Hospital in Newcastle, after being transferred there when it became clear he was seriously ill with the same infection that had hit Hoa. James had repeatedly tried to raise the alarm with midwives at Furness General about his son's increasingly lethargic state, but was repeatedly told Joshua was fine. Increasingly, he found he was being treated as an annoyance. After Joshua died, that escalated.

James knew something had gone wrong and that Joshua's death wasn't just 'one of those things'. He became determined to get to the bottom of the mistakes that had been made, but everywhere he turned, he found he was treated as though he was merely a father driven mad by grief, not someone who had a point. Like Julie Bailey, he spent years writing hundreds of letters to everyone he could think of – but got nowhere. Like Julie, he found himself the target of local abuse, from people who worked at the hospital or feared that its maternity unit might close partly as a result of James's campaign to find out the truth. And like Julie, he was right in thinking that Joshua had been failed by the people looking after him.

James's own investigations revealed a system that closed ranks against those who dared complain that the NHS may have failed them. It was not the mistakes that hurt the most, but the cover-up afterwards. James found this culture at every level in the health service. At a hospital level, staff had quickly tried to cover their tracks. Joshua's temperature chart – which showed he was registering the kind of low temperatures that are a warning sign for an infection in a newborn baby – mysteriously went missing. In a bundle of poorly redacted documents sent to James, he discovered an email from one of the midwives involved in the case, which dismissed the report she had been required to write for the Nursing and Midwifery Council's investigation into Joshua's care as 'NMC Shit'.

The hospital management were no better: a report by Dame Pauline Fielding examining five serious untoward incidents in 2008 – including Joshua's death – at the hospital described a 'dysfunctional' team, facilities that were 'not entirely fit for purpose', and that 'relations between different categories of staff and between management have suffered within an atmosphere which at times may have embodied a "blame culture".'[20] That report was bad enough, but James quickly realised that it had not been passed on to the relevant regulators, including the Care Quality Commission. Worse, he had a recording of a conversation between him and the hospital's chief executive, Tony Halsall, in which the manager had claimed: 'There is nothing the CQC don't know about our organisation, or that we have not shared with them completely and openly.'[21] Halsall would have known about the Fielding Report at the time, but had effectively lied to James, in the same way the Mid Staffs chief executive Martin Yeates had chosen to mislead reporters about his hospital.

James went further and further up the hierarchy. He found a whole list of organisations who could have done something, but didn't: the local strategic health authority, the Nursing and Midwifery Council, the Parliamentary and Health Service Ombudsman, Monitor, the Care Quality Commission – and the Department of Health. The NMC were the worst of all the organisations he came up against, and he described them as 'refusing to listen, absolutely treating me like dirt'. They even went through a phase of monitoring what he said in public and on his social media – and then paid nearly £250,000 to have a legal firm redact as much as possible from the documents mentioning Titcombe that it was forced to hand over to him. He was stalked online by people he believes are family members of some of the midwives involved in the case, with one even setting up an account pretending to be Hoa.

All of this, just to cover up the conclusion that James knew to be the truth: Joshua Titcombe's death was avoidable. James has to live with the knowledge that his son could have been here today, enjoying his teenage years, were it not for mistakes made by the staff. He discovered that other parents had been failed similarly – and treated as badly.

A review of care in the Morecambe Bay NHS Trust by Dr Bill Kirkup found 'significant or major failures of care' associated with the deaths of three mothers and sixteen babies – deaths which could have been preventable for one of those mothers and eleven of the babies. The inquiry uncovered a dysfunctional maternity unit where doctors were afraid to disagree with the midwives, and where an 'overzealous pursuit of the natural childbirth approach led at times to inappropriate and unsafe care'.

Kirkup, a softly spoken man in person, had some forceful words about the significance of what he'd found. He wrote: 'These events have finally been brought to light thanks to the efforts of some diligent and courageous families, who persistently refused to accept what they were being told. Those families deserve great credit. That it needed their efforts over such a prolonged period reflects little credit on any of the NHS organisations concerned. Today, the name of Morecambe Bay has been added to a roll of dishonoured NHS names that stretches from Ely Hospital to Mid Staffordshire.'[22]

There were political implications, too. Hunt met James Titcombe in August 2013. 'I told Joshua's story and he listened intently with tears in his eyes,' recalled Titcombe. 'After discussing patient safety and my experience in the nuclear industry I handed over a document I had written with eight suggestions for making the NHS safer. I have stayed in regular contact with Jeremy Hunt since this first meeting.' Titcombe started working for the Care Quality Commission as their national adviser on safety, while Hunt reformed the CQC so that it offered an Ofsted-style rating of each hospital (the Michael Gove influence again, there) and examined quality of care, access to care, and the money. 'Middle-class parents today are weighed to send their kids to Ofsted-rated outstanding schools, and so that was the model I had in mind,' Hunt explains. 'I saw Mid Staffs and I thought yes, this is like a "bog-standard comprehensive" and the first step is you call a spade a spade and you create a public rating of the problem, which forces the system to deal with it. By the time I left, three million more patients were using good or outstanding hospitals compared to when I arrived, so it has had I think a very important effect on quality.'

But Morecambe also revealed that NHS scandals do not just arise as a result of political decisions to do with funding and staffing. One of the elements in the disastrously poor care of those mothers and babies who died was the emphasis on 'normal birth'. This is a curious term, but until 2017 – nearly a decade after Joshua Titcombe died – it was an official campaign of the Royal College of Midwives. It refers to vaginal births, rather than delivery by Caesarean section.

The obsession with the phrase 'normal birth' in Britain came about as part of the pushback against the over-medicalisation of birth across the Western world that we read about in earlier chapters. But a well-meaning attempt to liberate women from the stirrups led to a vast overcorrection, which became tied up in an unscientific 'natural birth' movement. That movement in part arose from attempts in the 1940s Soviet Union to distract from a shortage of analgesia, in which doctors told women they could use breathing as pain relief instead. In her forceful assault on the natural birth movement, *Push Back: Guilt in the Age of Natural Parenting*, American obstetrician Amy Tuteur finds one problem with this approach: the women who were forced to try breathing instead of analgesia didn't find their pain lessened. Oddly, though, that small detail was overlooked by the largely male physicians across the Western world who started promoting it more widely. So the manipulation of women by a Communist regime that was failing to provide for their needs as they gave birth bled into a wider movement that claimed to prioritise women's needs – not ignore them. Prunella Briance, who we met in Chapter 4, was still campaigning for less intervention in birth even as the Morecambe scandal was unfolding. In a highly controversial letter to *The Times* in 2013, she wrote that her charity was 'based on the life-work of an English GP-obstetrician who proved that 97 per cent of mothers, accurately instructed, attended and encouraged, can give birth without any interference or medication whatsoever. The remaining 3 per cent are usually ill or damaged women who require skilled medical help and are grateful for it.'[23]

Even those who didn't accept the dodgy statistics Briance produced still embraced the 'normal birth' culture. But such a culture did not prioritise the needs of the mothers and babies in Furness General, and it similarly failed the families in the Shrewsbury and Telford scandal that started years before the Morecambe deaths – and continued well after the health service should have learned the lessons that Kirkup set out in his report. The Ockenden Review into Shrewsbury started with 250 cases, but widened that to a horrifying 1,862 where care may have been inadequate. There were thirteen deaths in eighteen years, stillbirths which could have been avoided – and, once again, an emphasis on 'normal birth', which meant staff refused to perform Caesarean sections, leading to severe physical trauma or even the death of the baby. Women were told the pain they were in was 'nothing' – as though this was a hospital operating in a country with shortages of anaesthetics, not the modern NHS – and were blamed for their babies' deaths. Kirkup had written that Morecambe must lead to a change in NHS maternity services. But he watched as Shrewsbury and Telford health chiefs considered his own report and dismissed its relevance to their trust. Two families had to mount their own investigations into what was going on after losing their daughters. Once again, the system waited for people in the worst mental anguish imaginable to get to the truth. It is not yet clear that the health service has learned these lessons.

What is clear is that, for the first time in the history of the NHS, patient safety became something politicians were interested in. It wasn't a niche within the health service: scandals such as the Bristol heart scandal (which saw high numbers of babies dying in the paediatric cardiac unit of Bristol Royal Infirmary, and led to a massive change in clinical governance and leadership following a public inquiry) and serial killer Dr Harold Shipman had already made safety an essential focus of many working in the service. Infection control was another area that had forced clinicians to think again about their work and the culture in which they operated. But Hunt was the first minister to take a lead on this, and get under the skin rather than call for heads to roll and bark instructions. And the funny thing is that a key reason he had become so interested in it was he had been given so little opportunity to do the things a minister normally relishes, like fiddling with legislation. He needed to find something else to focus on. It has been to the benefit of patients – and the NHS – that he was at a loose end.

Not long after this, though, NHS doctors found themselves wishing Hunt didn't have so much spare time on his hands. The man who became the longest-serving Health Secretary in the history of the service can reasonably claim patient safety as his high point. But what that focus led him to work on turned out to be his nadir.

The battle between the government and doctors over changes to their contracts ran almost as long as the 1980s miners' strike and saw the first-ever all-out strike from doctors in the history of the NHS.

Hunt had not set out to have this kind of incendiary confrontation with junior doctors. He had started his work as Health Secretary hoping to emulate Michael Gove, but he had thought he might be able to avoid mirroring his mentor's ability to pick unnecessary fights with the teaching unions – in no small part because he did not, as Gove had, employ Dominic Cummings as one of his special advisers. Cummings later became notorious during the coronavirus pandemic, but at this time he was known only in Westminster as a driven reformer who enjoyed scrapping with the education establishment who opposed his plans for higher school standards. Those who worked with Cummings found him brilliant, thoughtful and usefully stubborn. Those who worked against him found him infuriating, myopic and lacking the ability to know when to walk away from a confrontation. Hunt was not this kind of mercurial operator. He did not have these two stark sides to his character, but he did still possess a steeliness under his polite exterior. Some former colleagues in the Department of Health recall him as 'absolutely charming, but a man used to getting his own way', which made him 'difficult to work with'. And he became determined to get his own way through months of confrontations with one of the most trusted professions in the country.

It all started rather innocently. For a long time, figures inside and outside of the NHS had become concerned about weekend provision in the health service. Mortality was higher, training of junior doctors wasn't as good, and expensive facilities went unused. This was the view not just of Sir Bruce Keogh and medical directors of the strategic health authorities at the time; it was also something the Royal Colleges and the BMA agreed on, saying the first step should be improving urgent and emergency care at the weekends. Andrew Lansley had supported this, with the NHS England board approving new standards in 2013.

Hunt took the work on, becoming even more worried when he read analysis from Keogh and colleagues suggesting that people admitted to NHS hospitals at weekends were about 15 per cent more likely to die. But David Cameron was concerned that most people working normal hours struggled to get a GP appointment. This was in the run-up to the 2015 general election, and Keogh recalls getting a call from Number 10 saying: 'There's an election coming up and we don't really have a health policy.'[24] He shared the proposals signed off by NHS England for improving urgent and emergency care with Downing Street, but was shaken when Cameron then gave a speech and said: 'We're going to have a truly seven-day NHS.'[25]

That speech was the first of Cameron's election campaign. His argument was that he couldn't announce plans to improve urgent and emergency care at the weekends, because this would be an 'admission of failure' of the health service. The only way, as he saw it, that he could sell the policy was to say he was going to boost everything. And so, in the party's manifesto document – under the slightly threatening header 'We have a plan for every stage of your life' – was this promise: 'We will continue to increase spending on the NHS, provide 7-day a week access to your GP and deliver a truly 7-day NHS – so you know you will always have access to a free and high quality health service when you need it most.'[26]

This still seemed innocuous: indeed, there wasn't much reaction from people working in the health service. Keogh continued to see the reforms as being about formalising arrangements for consultants to come in at the weekend rather than the existing arrangements, which saw them giving time outside their contracted hours. 'I went to talk to the Doctors' and Dentists' Review Body and argued that the consultant contract needed to be changed and that kind of stuff. We didn't even touch on junior doctors. I mean, junior doctors were not even in the frame, in my head.'

By now, NHS England and the Department of Health were separate, so Keogh only heard belatedly when the department started negotiating a new contract with junior doctors. 'When I heard, I said: "That's not where the issue is." But they were too far in. I wasn't consulted. I wasn't asked. It ran completely against the plan and I took a load of flak for it.'[27]

'Flak' is a gentle description for the response to the renegotiation of the junior doctor contract. Not long after the Conservatives won their surprising majority in the election, Hunt lit the blue touchpaper. In a speech in July, he said he wanted to bring back a 'sense of vocation and professionalism' into the contract for consultants, which doctors read as a criticism of them rather than of the paper on which their employment was detailed. Then, in September, he announced changes to the proposed new contract for juniors. This would change the classification of normal working hours from 7 a.m.–7 p.m. Monday–Friday to 7 a.m.–10 p.m. Monday–Saturday. He argued that this was fair for doctors – and necessary for safety in the NHS. He claimed that 11,000 people died unnecessarily at weekends thanks to poor staffing. This was using data that doctors argued had been wilfully misinterpreted, because the original study said it would be 'misleading' to claim all the excess deaths were preventable, in part due to the fact that patients admitted at weekends are often sicker. The editor of the *BMJ* called on Hunt to withdraw this misuse of statistics. This poured petrol on the flames, and it took more than a year to put them out.

Junior doctors were horrified, arguing that these changes would lead to unsafe working practices, to many either leaving the profession or the country, and to a desertion of acute specialties in favour of those with more manageable working hours. Thousands of doctors took to the streets in protests in September and October, and the BMA junior doctors' committee announced it would ballot its members on the government's proposals. Initially, Hunt insisted that no doctor would see their pay cut, but at the end of October he was forced to admit this wasn't true: anyone working more than fifty-six hours would get less money. He told the BBC: 'There's a very small minority of doctors who will be working more than an average of 56 hours and at the moment they get paid what's called colloquially in the NHS "danger money".'[28] Neither the admission nor the reference to 'danger money' helped things. Doctors do have rather dark colloquialisms for many aspects of their jobs: the small amount of money they are paid to cover the time and responsibility involved in filling out a cremation form for a deceased patient, for instance, is known as 'ash cash'. But 'danger money' was a new one for most of them, and they once again felt their intelligence was being insulted.

No one likes it when their intelligence is insulted. But many people are far more used to it than doctors, who are generally top of their class at school – and rightly applauded by the public for the way they use their intellect and physical skills for the good of their patients. This is not lost on Hunt. 'Being a doctor and being a politician is very different,' he explains. 'When you're a doctor you are loved your whole life by your patients and when you're a politician you are hated by your opposing team and all their supporters for your whole life and so they are very different professions. But I think that many junior doctors really did believe that the Health Secretary didn't think they worked at weekends and wanted to cut their pay, and I think that was the heart of it and there was really nothing I could say that would persuade them otherwise.'

Doctors were indeed at great pains to point out that they did work weekends already. One set up a hugely popular hashtag on Twitter called #ImInWorkJeremy. It trended for days, flooding social media with pictures of healthcare workers wearing stethoscopes, theatre scrubs and ambulance uniforms while the rest of the world enjoyed their Saturdays and Sundays of leisure. It didn't just speak to the dispute over the junior doctor contract – or indeed the consultant one. It also spoke to the low morale in the profession. Many felt as though they were merely the playthings of politicians with an agenda that went far beyond looking after patients. They appeared on news programmes to explain their frustration and to give the public a glimpse of what their working lives were like. They sat in their cars at the end of lengthy night shifts and outlined how exhausted they were, to the extent that they weren't sure they could drive safely.

The dispute led to a bizarre cultural moment for the health service when an NHS choir from Lewisham and Greenwich beat Justin Bieber to become the UK's Christmas No. 1. The Canadian pop star had actually endorsed the choir on Twitter, telling his fans to 'do the right thing & help them win'. It is hard to imagine any other public service in the world getting close to the coveted top spot, let alone winning the backing of a music megastar.

The row also gave rise to a new form of literature: the junior doctor memoir. Public interest in the medical profession had always been high, with senior surgeons such as Henry Marsh captivating readers with accounts of operations and low points throughout lengthy careers. But now the war of words between politician and physician spilled into books by doctors at the very start of their working lives. Rachel Clarke and Adam Kay were two of the most high-profile authors, writing *Your Life in My Hands: A Junior Doctor's Story* and *This is Going to Hurt: Secret Diaries of a Junior Doctor*. Kay's book started life as a sketch at the Edinburgh Fringe, where he read excerpts from the diaries he'd kept while practising, in an attempt to tell the doctors' side of the story following the dispute. Clarke, who had been a journalist before going to medical school, had spent much of her spare time during the dispute explaining on television and in newspaper articles why the government was so very wrong to be pursuing these changes. She admits in her book that countering the ministerial spin machine became 'an obsession'. But her anger wasn't solely reserved for Hunt. She – and many other doctors – felt increasingly let down by their trade union, too.

The BMA had refused to accept the new terms offered by Hunt, despite the entreaties of organisations such as NHS Providers to do so. In November 2015, the union's ballot came back with 99.6 per cent in favour of industrial action that stopped short of a strike, and 98 per cent backing all-out strike action. Unlike many disputes between governments and unions, the turnout was very high, at 76 per cent. The first strike was planned for the following month, but was suspended after Hunt temporarily withdrew his threat to impose the contract without agreement. This was not, however, before Keogh had horrified junior doctors by writing a letter to the BMA's chair, Dr Mark Porter, in which he referenced the recent terror attacks in Paris and asked for clarification that doctors would return to work if there was a major incident. At the time, it was revealed that the Department of Health had 'strengthened' the letter, even though Keogh was supposed to be independent of government. But what hasn't been known until now is that he also sought assurances on what would happen if there was a major incident because another organisation had asked for it. That organisation was the BMA.

Keogh says he was initially instructed in a meeting with senior government ministers and members of the security forces – who were jumpy about the prospect of a copycat terror attack on London – to confirm his assurances with the BMA that junior doctors would be prepared to call off their strike in a civil contingency. He thought this would go without saying, but phoned Porter to discuss it:

> I said, 'Look, I've got to write you a letter to ask whether the junior doctors would call off their strike.' I said: 'So there are two ways I can phrase the letter.' The first option was that I was going to say, 'I have absolutely no doubt that in the event of a civil contingency or an emergency or something, that junior doctors would call off their strike.' I said: 'The other way is just to ask you, quite bluntly, that if something happened . . .' and he said: 'I think you should ask specifically, if there's an emergency, would the junior doctors call off their strike? Because I think there are some very rabid people in the junior doctors' committee who would not call off the strike.'

Dr Porter remembers the meeting a little differently. He says: 'I do not recall saying and indeed did not say that there were very rabid people in the junior doctors' committee who would not call off the strike. I knew from my regular attendance at the JDC, my many meetings with the committee officers and indeed from their presence at the meeting, that the junior doctor representatives in the BMA were responsive to the potential patient safety issues raised by industrial action and would respond appropriately in relation to their responsibilities as registered medical practitioners.' It is Porter's view – and that of many other doctors to this day – that 'it was the actions of the government that had needlessly provoked, insulted, attacked and angered junior doctors'.[29]

Bad feeling and mistrust were running high – but would soar still further in the coming months. Neither side was prepared to back down: the doctors continued to insist that their pay could be cut by as much as 40 per cent under the new contract and that it would be unsafe for patients. Hunt was still determined to get his own way. He also had the might of the government machine behind him; despite needlessly offending doctors with his comments about 'vocation and professionalism' and his slapdash use of statistics, he was seen by colleagues as someone holding out for all of them. In Cabinet meetings, other ministers encouraged him to stand firm because they feared that if the government folded on the doctors, then industrial action from teachers, police officers and other public sector workers would swiftly follow. David Cameron was happy to defend his minister, too, despite him failing to meet the original brief of 'turning the volume down' that he was given when he started the job. The volume was to rise still higher.

When the talks did not reach an agreement by the BMA's deadline of 4 January 2016, the unit announced that the strike would go ahead. On 12 January, junior doctors took to the picket lines, withdrawing all work save emergency care. And then on 10 February, doctors held another strike in routine care. Around 3,000 elective operations were cancelled as a result. Two months later, on 26 April, the junior doctors withdrew all routine and emergency care in protest at Hunt's announcement that he would impose the contract without agreement. Never in NHS history had this happened. Many doctors felt deeply uncomfortable with the action, but blamed the government.

It seemed as though ministers and medics would be locked in stalemate for ever, but for a twist that still leaves a bitter taste in the mouths of many of the doctors involved. A month after that all-out strike, the *Health Service Journal* received an explosive leak. Shaun Lintern, who had done so much to expose Mid Staffs, had now moved to the specialist publication and he was handed a cache of WhatsApp messages between members of the BMA junior doctors' committee. The messages revealed 'a strategy that tied the DH up in knots for the next 16–18 months'. And while the committee were saying publicly that the problem was safety, not how much doctors would be paid, members agreed privately that pay was 'the only real red line'. They also criticised Porter for, as they saw it, letting down their cause and being too willing to negotiate.[30]

The BMA folded that month and accepted a new contract. Its members were not happy: 58 per cent voted against the new wording, and it was imposed on them without agreement. Clarke, who had found the picket lines of the preceding months emotional and stirring, wrote of her deep disillusionment with the body supposed to represent her. The WhatsApp discussion about pay being the real 'red line' left her 'incandescent': 'This was simply not true. My red line was drawn at the threat to my patients and, frankly, to my own sanity of the government trying to eke out a seven-day service from a workforce barely fit for five. To be misrepresented by the government was one thing, but to discover that my own union had so misjudged its members' concerns was devastating. I had gone on strike in good faith – voiced my safety concerns in good faith – but now I felt undermined by my union, which had made its own members look untrustworthy.' She was bitterly disappointed that the union then accepted a contract that 'exacerbated gender pay gaps, left doctors with weakened protections against excessive hours and made it cheaper for hospitals to spread us more thinly'.[31]

This was not the end of the dispute. In fact, it wasn't until January 2020 that the stand-off really finished, when Hunt's successor Matt Hancock signed a new agreement with the BMA, which the union said 'brings a £90 million investment for junior doctors over the next four years'.[32] The new Secretary of State was rather baffled on entering the department to discover that Hunt hadn't even needed to have this stand-off.

That year of disputes and strikes has left many scars in the NHS workforce. It is still the cause of a great deal of bad feeling between many medics and the government – and a source of low morale in the profession, too. But in January 2020, as the doctors on the union's committees finally filed away their negotiating papers, something else was looming that would leave scars far, far deeper.

11. Fighting to breathe

The doors of the hotel swung open and two figures in hazmat suits came wading in. The staff on reception watched nervously as they approached and explained what they were doing, before disappearing to the first floor. Among the staff, the word started to spread: this might not be a false alarm – one of the guests staying there had flown in from Wuhan, China. They never saw that guest or the paramedics again. The group had slipped out of a fire exit and into their ambulance. The first confirmed UK cases of coronavirus were on their way to hospital.

It was inevitable that a disease first described over the new-year holiday period was going to reach the UK at some point. What was more of a surprise was where it turned up. The infectious disease doctors at Castle Hill Hospital, Hull, certainly hadn't expected to be receiving any patients any time soon: they were at a retirement dinner for a colleague when their phones started to ring. Patrick Lillie was one of them. He and the other doctors were largely interested in what the disease would look like if the patients tested positive for it – but they didn't expect this to happen. Being infectious disease specialists, they were quite used to the steps they had to take in order to examine and treat the two patients: isolate them, and don and doff personal protective equipment as they came in and out of their rooms – a fifteen-minute job at either end. On 30 January, they received the test results for both patients: a 50-year-old woman who had developed a sore throat and dry cough, and a 23-year-old man who then went down with a fever and a dry cough, too. They were positive.

The coronavirus pandemic which started in 2020 represented the greatest peacetime challenge for the world so far. In the UK, it was when the NHS became more a part of our lives and thinking than ever before, and when appreciation for the health service became a weekly ritual. It could also prove to be the event that most endangers the health service in the coming years.

In the early days of January 2020, doctors were not sure what they were facing. It was a disease that at this stage only affected infectious disease units. Those first two positive tests, the results of which Lillie received in the small hours of the morning on 31 January, activated something called the NHS England Airborne High Consequence Infectious Disease (HCID) network. It was time for Lillie and his team to transfer their patients to a special unit in Newcastle, set up to deal with these kinds of HCID cases. Ashley Price was one of the consultants waiting for them.

Dr Price, like most infectious disease doctors, found Covid academically fascinating. That's one of the reasons people like him work in this discipline, after all. 'It's a really interesting area of medicine,' he explains. 'You've got the ability to cure people. And the other thing is that interplay between pathogen and human is just so vast and so interesting.' Initially, he followed the pandemic in China through Twitter. 'It rapidly became a big deal. I was on the train back from Newcastle to where I live, and they announced that it was a pandemic. That was shortly before we received our first patients.'[1]

The whole department at Newcastle was, by its nature, ready. This was what it was set up to do. The health service had also been doing preparation exercises for a pandemic: in fact, before Covid struck, Britain was scoring highly in the league tables for pandemic preparedness. It had the relatively recent experience of dealing with swine flu in 2009–10, and had come through that pretty well, too. This was just the next in a series of global diseases – right?

'The problem with those exercises,' explains Price, 'is that they don't actually tend to prepare you for what is to come, because each pandemic is very different. You're thinking about the flu. Last time we had it, it wasn't that bad. And I think that was probably a bad thing, for the NHS and for the world: it kind of led us into a false sense of security that actually things will be alright and it will be easily dealt with.'

It was when the first patients died of the illness that Price started to really worry. The first UK patient died with Covid on 5 March

2020. At this stage, just 116 positive cases were in the country – though the testing capacity was also very small, with just 20,000 people receiving tests. 'This was when we realised that we couldn't manage this as a high-consequence infectious disease. We had to get down from that, and it had to become a general management thing,' Price recalls. 'I was on call the first weekend that we had patients die, and that was the weekend that it really hit me. I was having sleepless nights. I really was sleeping maybe three hours a night because I was trying to help the trust with the response. There were a lot of meetings, we were making sure that we had enough oxygen as we knew that was necessary. We were making sure we had PPE. We were making sure that we were ready for what was about to happen, and we knew it was going to be bad.'

It *was* going to be really bad – in many ways much worse than anyone could have expected. The UK government's response to Covid deserves an entire book – and plenty already have been written. This chapter is not a poor attempt to look at everything – the travel restrictions, the decision to go into lockdown, the Downing Street parties held by the very people who had written those lockdown rules – but instead to cover how the NHS coped with what it was given, in terms of resources, the peaks of the virus and its leaders. It is one of the most devastating chapters, but also the one with the greatest sense of heroism within a health service that, if not set up to fail, had not been helped by its political masters.

By early 2020, the health service had not only maintained its salience in political debate, it had become even more of a political football than before. In 2016, the famous blue lozenge had been plastered all over a red bus that toured the country claiming that if Britain left the European Union, £350 million a week that was being sent to Brussels could instead go to the NHS. One of the passengers on that bus was Boris Johnson. At the time, he was coming to the end of his term as Mayor of London and was a thorn in the flesh for David Cameron, who had assumed that he would win the referendum he had granted his unruly backbenchers to try to stop them, in his words, 'banging on about Europe'.

The NHS logo on the bus was the idea of an adviser called Dominic Cummings. Also a thorn in Cameron's flesh, Cummings had worked for Michael Gove when he was Education Secretary, but often worked against anyone else in government he felt was getting in his way. Cummings had an ability to pick up on what ordinary voters beyond the 'Westminster Bubble' cared about. Tim Shipman's magnificent account of how Britain voted for Brexit, *All Out War*, recounts one ally saying Cummings had 'found that Europe was deeply unpopular, but that if you wanted to reach people you had to talk about immigration and the NHS'.[2] Cummings rapidly realised that the attraction of saving the money sent to the European Union – which loomed in the public consciousness as a bigger spending black hole than the NHS had ever done, even in the minds of the most parsimonious Chancellors – could be coupled with that desire for the NHS to get more money, to devastating effect. Shipman reports that the happiest a fellow Vote Leave strategist ever saw Cummings was 'on the morning he told the team to put the NHS logo on the side of Vote Leave's bus: 'He was literally jumping around saying, "We're going to use the NHS logo and they're going to hate it." '[3]

They did hate it: Jeremy Hunt, still the Health Secretary, sent a legal warning to the campaign when they put the logo on their leaflets, which was hardly surprising given the trouble even NHS organisations find themselves in when they use that precious brand in the wrong way. It became such a controversial point in the Brexit campaign that Johnson himself spent months afterwards feeling browbeaten about where the £350 million a week for the NHS was now that Britain had voted for Brexit. For the first time in his political life, he started to take a keen interest in the health service as a way of proving to his critics that he hadn't been hitching a ride around the country in a bus with a big lie emblazoned on the side. A friend recalls Johnson's state of mind in the year after the referendum: 'He took the accusation that he'd been lying really, really personally. He would go on about it, and build himself up to making some kind of intervention to prove he really thought the money would go to the NHS, then someone would advise him not to.'[4]

Johnson was made Foreign Secretary in the brutal reshuffle that

Theresa May carried out when she took over as prime minister in July 2016. Some assumed this was a joke – an attempt to expose Johnson for the lightweight May thought he was. The job was quite plainly not very much to do with the NHS, but his obsession with being proved right on this did eventually lead Johnson to demand that the Brexit cash to go to the health service. He bowled up to a Cabinet meeting one Tuesday in January 2018, having carefully briefed the media beforehand that he was going to make a pitch for a £100-million-a-week 'Brexit dividend' for the NHS. Cabinet discussions are supposed to be confidential, and certainly not briefed before they even take place, so this put colleagues' backs up even before they'd entered the Cabinet room in Downing Street. May herself gave Johnson what one minister present described as a 'bitch slap', by reminding ministers of the need to keep their discussions private – while Jeremy Hunt also complained about the pre-briefing.[5] In the end, Johnson didn't even make the pitch he had told journalists he was going to. Later, Chancellor Philip Hammond told reporters very pointedly that Johnson was the Foreign Secretary, not the Health Secretary. But while this plea was all about Johnson's own personal psychodrama and not the policy itself (a pattern to be repeated in the years to follow), it wasn't unhelpful to the cause of the actual Health Secretary.

By now, Hunt was about to break a record and become the longest-serving Health Secretary in the history of his department. He had been doing the job for long enough to have wearied of going regularly to the Treasury, cap in hand, to try to get more money that the NHS urgently needed. The Treasury, of course, had already been wearied of this for about sixty-nine years. When Johnson started his own NHS funding campaign, Hunt was in the middle of a particularly bad NHS winter crisis and was also trying to negotiate a longer-term funding settlement for the health service, so that he wasn't trailing back and forth to the Treasury so often. He had already refused to be moved in a reshuffle that May had carried out earlier that month. When I asked May about it, she reflected, with a slightly grim laugh, that it was 'difficult, when you're doing a reshuffle, and you'd got this huge board with people moving here, there and everywhere, and if somebody says, "Actually, no, I don't want to move," then that causes you issues'.[6]

Hunt's reasoning was that he felt responsible for this winter crisis and didn't want to abandon the health service right in the middle of it – and he wanted to make sure he'd got the long-term cash. May asked him to go and sit in a side room in Number 10 while she tried to work out how to resolve the 'issues' Hunt had caused. While she was doing this, the Cabinet Secretary, Jeremy Heywood, put in a call to the head of winter-crisis planning Pauline Philip, who told him 'this is a terrible time to change the Health Secretary and it really won't help you'. Heywood fed that back to May, who called Hunt back in. Before this reshuffle, Hunt had also suggested that his department – presumably led by someone one else – take over Social Care: the minister responsible for that, Damian Green, had just resigned for his own 'issues' (lying about having porn on his work computer, if you were wondering). May, meanwhile, was politically weak: a stronger leader who hadn't recently squandered their own majority in Parliament might have been able to tell Hunt where to put his ambitions. She didn't, Hunt stayed, and his department gained the 'and Social Care' in its name that he'd suggested. When he entered Downing Street on the morning of the reshuffle, Hunt had taken a selfie in the White Room of that building, assuming he'd be on his way out of government. When he left, he had an even bigger department.

A few weeks later, Hunt, still in the job, pitched up to ITV to complain that the health service needed more certainty. 'There's no doubt that NHS staff right now are working unbelievably hard and they need to have some hope for the future, but their real concern is this rather crazy way that we have been funding the NHS over the last twenty years, which has basically been feast or famine.'[7]

May was also under public pressure from NHS chief executive Simon Stevens, who had pushed the independence of his job far beyond what ministers had expected, and was lobbying the government for a more sustainable settlement. Stevens, too, had seen that the Vote Leave NHS line could now be quite handy for him. He had always been as good or better a political operator than the politicians he'd worked with, but by this point he had figured out how to out-smart them on a regular basis. He was not the sort of NHS chief executive who would end up hiding under a carpet in a taxi; he was more likely to encourage a politician to do it and leave them thinking it was their own very good idea. He was only going to get better at this by the time the pandemic hit.

After Stevens published a 'Five Year Forward View' for NHS England in 2014, which made clear how much money the health ser-vice needed, in November 2015 he forced then Chancellor George Osborne to stump up an extra £3.8 billion. Stevens had threatened that if Osborne didn't agree, he would brand the money going to the health service as 'not enough'. Osborne was, at the time, also very politically weak, as he was under fire for planned cuts to tax credits. Now, with May as prime minister and Hunt in a strong position, Stevens saw the opportunity to tie things down. He continued to make things extremely difficult for ministers. In January 2017, he gave evidence to the Health Select Committee of MPs, saying it was 'stretching it to say the NHS got more' money than the £8 billion it had asked for in the most recent spending review – a direct contradic-tion of the prime minister's own claims. He said the 'austerity' imposed on the health service and all other areas of public spending from 2010 onwards had been 'placing huge pressure' on the NHS, and pointed out that day-to-day funding for the service was coming at the expense of the capital budget. In his view, this was 'robbing Paul to pay Paul'. It is putting it mildly to say this did not go down well in the corridors of power.

So, in June 2018, May announced that there was going to be a five-year funding settlement for the NHS, alongside a ten-year long-term plan. The money would include a £20.5 billion (3.4 per cent) increase between 2019/20 and 2023/24 – a significant change from the serious squeeze that had been put on the service from 2009/10 onwards, when funding only rose by 1 per cent a year in real terms. The ten-year plan would set out how the money was going to be spent, and ministers made very clear that productivity had to grow at a rate of 1.4 per cent a year – something that was going to be extremely challenging for the NHS.

How much of an influence the Brexit bus was on this pledge depends on who you talk to. One minister familiar with May's thinking claims: 'The bus and the £350 million weighed much more on Theresa May's mind than on Boris's. She felt the need to prove the value of Brexit more than he did because she had been against it.'[8] From May's perspective, it was the regular pressure for more money from Stevens that was the key factor, not the Brexit pledge:

> It wasn't really part of my thinking. It so happens that we put more money in than the Brexit campaign said it was going to put in, but that wasn't what drove the extra cash boost. And the ten-year plan was this realisation that year after year, we were having to deal with this whole question of NHS funding . . . And the ten-year plan was there to say, right, this isn't just a whole load of money that now you've got it you can just go off and spend it how you like. You've got to show what the priority is going to be, what the differences are going to be, and what this is going to actually deliver. And within that, encouraging them to look at genuine efficiencies.[9]

That last line was a particular reference to the frustration felt by – you've guessed it – the Treasury, that the NHS was continuing to suck up money without anything to show for it. By contrast, the NHS was in fact on the receiving end of the longest funding squeeze in its seven-decade history. Philip Hammond was now the Chancellor, and like most of his predecessors, had very little time for these endless pleas from the health service. He was also resentful that the NHS top brass hadn't pushed back against the £350 million claim on the bus and had instead welcomed the pledge as a recognition of the need for extra money. In fact, he tried to stop the money and the ten-year plan, arguing that he didn't believe that Stevens would ever deliver the targets that Hammond wanted in exchange. He felt a ten-year plan was irresponsible as it was impossible to know what would be happening in the wider economy over that period. He also thought the deal was deeply one-sided: ten years of guaranteed increases for the NHS, with an option to reopen discussions in Stevens's favour if circumstances changed, such as rising inflation. Stevens refused to do what he saw as selling the NHS down the river, and it turned into another stand-off between the NHS and the Treasury. But May could see where this would go politically. One of her former colleagues remarked: 'Stevens is a total snake. I don't know why successive PMs haven't forced him out. He never delivers on his side of NHS reform. Every time they say, "You can have this cash if . . ." and he says "Yes", but the "if" never happens.'[10] The feeling was mutual. For their part, NHS leaders felt that the Treasury had failed to deliver its side of the earlier reform bargain. The NHS was increasingly being left to pick up the pieces from collapsing social care, with clapped-out hospital buildings and equipment, and a complete Treasury refusal (until Jeremy Hunt became Chancellor) to agree a workforce plan to train the nurses and doctors the NHS would need. Ultimately Hammond was overruled by May, having got Stevens to promise to welcome the eventual deal in public. Stevens duly did. But that a Chancellor had to stipulate this for a public servant shows quite how far Stevens had pushed the boundaries of his role.

A month later, May carried out another small reshuffle. This was prompted by Boris Johnson resigning over her Brexit deal. He holed himself up in the Foreign Office with a photographer who took a series of 'candid' portraits of the outgoing Foreign Secretary writing his resignation letter on a point of principle, while missing a conference he was supposed to be opening with the Balkan states. Hunt couldn't refuse the Foreign and Commonwealth Office, a great office of state. So off he went, having chalked up just over six years in the job.

Hunt's replacement was a young, very ambitious minister called Matt Hancock. Hancock had been an aide to George Osborne before being elected as the MP for West Suffolk in 2010. Shortly after being rewarded for his ambition with his first promotion into government in 2012, Hancock described himself to my *Spectator* colleague James Forsyth as having 'a huge affinity for Disraeli'.[11] By 2018, the media-savvy minister was Secretary of State for Digital, Culture, Media and Sport, a job he adored – though he did complain to one colleague that he wasn't getting enough chances to go on the *Today* programme. His new role in Health would lead to a greater level of exposure than Hancock could possibly have imagined when he accepted it.

Hancock's initial priorities were the digital transformation of the NHS and mollifying a very grumpy workforce. The first was a personal enthusiasm: Hancock came from a tech family and couldn't contain his interest in it. He had even launched a 'Matt Hancock app' on people's phones, which served the dual purpose of updating his constituents on his political activities and giving the inhabitants of Westminster a good laugh. Sadly, the reshuffle deprived them of a second laugh because it meant Hancock no longer had a real reason for appearing as a hologram at his party's annual conference later that year. The second priority was obvious to everyone, whether hologram or human, because the contract rows of the past few years had taken their toll across the NHS workforce, with GPs leaving at a record rate. Hancock wanted to lovebomb staff, and encourage them to stop using the fax machines that, while obsolete in the wider world, were still a feature of life in NHS hospitals and surgeries.

Hancock, now serving under Boris Johnson as prime minister – first heard about the cases of an unusual pneumonia emerging in Wuhan, China, on New Year's Day 2020. On that day, the World Health Organization went onto an emergency footing to deal with the outbreak, which at this stage involved no deaths. On 5 January, the WHO sent an email notification warning of 'cases of pneumonia of unknown etiology [unknown cause] detected in Wuhan City, Hubei Province of China'. There were forty-four patients, with eleven who were severely ill. The WHO's notification, which was aimed largely at the scientific and medical communities, added: 'National authorities report that all patients are isolated and receiving treatment in Wuhan medical institutions. The clinical signs and symptoms are mainly fever, with a few patients having difficulty in breathing, and chest radiographs showing invasive lesions of both lungs.'[12] Within a week, Hancock was having meetings in government about this mystery illness, with the assumption being it would be like the swine flu outbreak that the NHS had managed to deal with in a reasonably routine way in 2009–10.

By the end of that month, the government was holding a Cobra meeting on the threat of the virus, which was now spreading across the world. Cobra has a mythical status in British politics. It is an anticlimactic acronym, standing for 'Cabinet Office Briefing Room A', a room in Whitehall with a long table and large screen set up for briefing officials and ministers on the government's response to unfolding and serious events. Hancock chaired that meeting: Johnson didn't attend this or any of the subsequent four Cobra meetings in the early stages of the pandemic. His aides insisted that it is normal for a prime minister to delegate chairing such meetings to the Secretary of State responsible. There was also anxiety within government that anything agreed at a Cobra meeting would be undone by Nicola Sturgeon, who had a tendency to ignore the instructions for the four nations of the UK to move as one at the same time, and would announce her own Covid measures shortly after the latest Cobra meeting had concluded. '[Sturgeon's behaviour] destroyed the trust in the room,' says one official who was present. 'Instead Boris was being briefed in these side meetings that took place with him, Chris Whitty [the Chief Medical Officer] and Dominic Cummings.' But it also showed how unconcerned Johnson was about the unfolding pandemic. He didn't attend any Cobra meetings until 2 March. There also seemed to be precious few warnings coming from the meetings that did take place to make him pay any more attention, anyway. Hancock, meanwhile, was energised. One colleague rather pithily remarked that 'Matt was someone who quite liked the pandemic in a way, because it meant he was in the middle of something important'.[13]

Initially, though, Hancock didn't ascribe a great level of importance to Covid. The first Cobra meeting concluded with the minister telling the press that the risk of what was now being called coronavirus 'remains low and the chief medical officer will be making a full statement later today'. Whitty's statement said much the same: 'We all agree that the risk to the UK public remains low, but there may well be cases in the UK at some stage. We have tried and tested measures in place to respond. The UK is well-prepared for these types of incidents, with excellent readiness against infectious diseases.'[14]

The confidence behind that last statement was based largely on something called Exercise Cygnus. Held in 2016, this simulation exercise lasted three days and involved nearly 1,000 officials, medics and ministers practising what their responses would be to various scenarios involving a pandemic flu. The scenario they were working on involved between 200,000 and 400,000 deaths. It didn't go well.

The report into the exercise concluded that: 'The UK's preparedness and response, in terms of its plans, policies and capability, is currently not sufficient to cope with the extreme demands of a severe pandemic that will have a nationwide impact across all sectors.' It found that there was poor working between organisations when the 'scenario demand for services outstripped the capacity of local responders, in the areas of excess deaths, social care and the NHS'. A key line in the secret report was that 'local responders also raised concerns about the expectation that the social care system would be able to provide the level of support needed if the NHS implemented its proposed reverse triage plans, which would entail the movement of patients from hospitals into social care facilities'.[15] The failure to learn that lesson alone would lead to tens of thousands of deaths involving those very patients.

Dame Sally Davies, the Chief Medical Officer at the time, told an international health summit a few days later: 'We've just had in the UK a three-day exercise on flu and on a pandemic that killed a lot of people. It became clear that we could not cope with the excess bodies, for instance. It becomes very worrying about the deaths, and what that will do to society as you start to get all those deaths, [including] the economic impact. If we, as one of the most prepared countries, are going through an exercise and find a lot of things that need improving just on the internal bit, add to it the vaccines and then the global traffic and the lack of solidarity . . . a severe one will stretch everyone.'

She described one of the problems they'd found: 'If you don't know you've got a new disease then you don't isolate people. There was overcrowding in the emergency room, inadequate ventilation, family and friends going through. That could happen in any of our countries.'[16] Sir Ian Boyd, then the chief scientific adviser to the Department for the Environment, Food and Rural Affairs, described being 'shattered' by how badly the practice exercise had gone, and reflected that the lessons that were learned from it were then not implemented.[17] The government was supposed to ring-fence the money to cover the improvements the NHS needed to make in order to get ready for a pandemic. This didn't happen. In their study of how Britain's response to Covid went wrong, *Failures of State*, Jonathan Calvert and George Arbuthnott report an anonymous Downing Street adviser admitting that most of the recommendations from Cygnus were ignored, largely because everyone was distracted by the looming prospect of a no-deal Brexit: 'All the blood was flooding to the Brexit planning and we never picked it up.'[18]

There was another problem: Cygnus had gamed the UK's response to flu. But this new virus wasn't influenza; it was part of a different group. Davies had suggested that the government also test dealing with severe acute respiratory syndrome-related coronavirus (SARS-CoV), which was the virus that had devastated many Asian countries between 2002 and 2004. 'I felt as chief medical officer that we should practise a number of things,' she told the *Telegraph*. 'I did ask during a conversation in my office in around 2015, should we do SARS? But I was told no, because it wouldn't reach us properly. They said it would die out and would never travel this far. So I did ask, but it was the Public Health England people who said we didn't need to do it, and I'll say that to Parliament. That advice meant we never seriously sat down and said: "Will we have a massive pandemic of something else?"'[19]

Jeremy Hunt, who took part in Cygnus, says the government was suffering from groupthink which led it to take the wrong decisions when Covid hit. Many of those decisions, such as whether and when to lock down, are out of the scope of this book. But, of course, they had a huge impact on how many cases the NHS had to deal with – and how long the pandemic went on for.

So the UK might have been one of the most prepared countries in the world – but that didn't mean it was well prepared. It was when it became clear, as Ashley Price put it, that this new virus wasn't just going to be a concern for infectious disease departments but the whole health system, that the weaknesses very quickly became apparent.

By March 2020, the initial optimism of the infectious disease community that this was merely going to be a disease that tested pandemic preparedness – rather than a serious crisis – had faded. There was another teleconference between government officials and medics from infectious disease units across England on 3 March, and it dawned on the doctors on the call that the system was already under severe strain. 'We call it the Teleconference of Doom,' says one of those party to the discussions. 'You had units dialling in saying they could take three or four patients. And then we had the chair of the meeting, say, okay, so we've got sixteen new beds, and we've got sixteen cases. And you just heard this intake of breath from around the country. We'd already filled the extra capacity. Then in the background, you heard someone else shouting out "Actually, I've got another six cases just come through." That was the night the system broke.'[20]

The system breaking at this stage meant that it was no longer possible to take all positive patients and isolate them in infection diseases units in hospitals. Instead, patients who were reasonably well could stay at home, and the rest were going to have to take any bed that could be found. What this meant across the country was different: initially the outbreak seemed to be at its worst in London and the south-east, but Patrick Lillie's team in Hull, for instance, went from caring for twelve beds to fifty by the end of the month.

On 5 March 2020, the first death of a confirmed Covid patient was announced. The woman, in her seventies, had been in and out of the Royal Berkshire Hospital, a district general in Reading, with other health problems. The day before, Chris Whitty had told MPs that the UK was now in the second stage of its pandemic response, moving from a strategy of trying to contain the virus within China to delaying the peak of cases in the UK 'into a time when there is more capacity to respond'.

At this stage, there were two images of Covid in other countries that were arresting the British public's attention. The first was of the mega hospitals that China was managing to build almost overnight, in order to deal with the increasing numbers of cases. The Huoshen-shan Hospital in Wuhan, for instance, went from bare construction site to opening in just ten days (according to the Chinese authorities) at the start of February. A time-lapse film showed the buildings rising up like mushrooms from the ground.[21] The second image was rather closer to home. In Lombardy, Italy, the Covid outbreak had got going in late February, and by mid-March the hospitals in the region were in meltdown. They were full, and could not admit any more patients. Seriously ill people lined corridors, meeting rooms, any space available, with plastic bubbles over their heads to try to equalise the air pressure in their lungs; and doctors and nurses rushed between them trying to stay on top of the alarms from machines that were working to keep them alive. These health workers were exhausted, working non-stop, in tears and begging international camera crews to film what they were describing as an 'apocalypse' – to warn the rest of the world what was coming.

These images had a profound effect on the British public, and also on policymakers. What they inspired, though, did little to help the NHS as it tried to survive the pandemic.

The Lombardy images were at the forefront of most NHS workers' minds as they wondered how their own health service was going to cope. At the time, they didn't know how badly Cygnus had gone, or that its major lessons hadn't been implemented: all that was locked away in classified documents that were only released after an outcry in the autumn of 2020. They also didn't know whether Boris Johnson was as scared as they were. On 3 March, at a press conference at Downing Street, Johnson had been in an ebullient mood, smiling as he told journalists: 'I was at a hospital the other night where I think there were a few coronavirus patients, and I shook hands with everybody, you will be pleased to know.' It was almost as though Johnson thought coronavirus was a misunderstood disease with a huge stigma, like AIDS, and he was just an extremely unkempt twenty-first-century Princess Diana.

Just sixteen days later, the prime minister gave another press conference at Downing Street, standing behind a lectern with 'Stay Home. Protect the NHS. Save Lives' written on it. That slogan was in part borrowed from the 'Stay Home, Save Lives' messages in other countries, but Johnson's communications director Lee Cain had suggested adding 'Protect the NHS', given the affection in which the health service was held, and given the general horror at the images emerging from Lombardy. It was a tremendously powerful slogan. It was popular in government – but not universally so. In fact, one of its greatest critics was Simon Stevens. Stevens wasn't on the calls where Cain and others came up with 'Protect the NHS', and initially he complained in private that it gave the impression that the public was there for the health service – not the health service being there for the public. Being the operator he was, he soon had no compunction about criticising it in public, too, writing in the *Spectator* later that year that: 'Rather than say "Protect the NHS", health service staff prefer to say: "Help us help you".'[22]

Either way, the focus quickly became about the importance of 'protecting the NHS'. But there was never a clear definition of what it was being protected *from*. The most obvious fear was that Britain's hospitals were going to end up being like the ones in Lombardy, with trolleys of dying patients lining the corridors. That was a tangible expression of the collapse of a health system – but it wasn't the only one.

Within the NHS, the initial focus was on freeing up enough beds for the influx of Covid patients when it came. The big fear was that the intensive care capacity of hospitals was going to run out very quickly. The modelling by Public Health England suggested that NHS intensive care was going to be overwhelmed by the end of March in London, and then in the rest of the country a couple of weeks after that. The first big – and disastrous – step was to clear the wards of patients who were 'medically fit for discharge'. This is the internal NHS phrase for those who are popularly – and demeaningly – called 'bed blockers': patients who do not need treatment in a hospital any more but who for various reasons, can't yet go home. 'Medically fit for discharge' is a phrase that strikes fear into the hearts of teams working on wards in normal times. The longer it is applied to a patient, the more complicated the reasons for them not leaving are: generally there is no care package and therefore no assurance that they will be safe as they recover in the community. As well as keeping the bed from use by another patient who still needs treatment, there is a risk to the 'medically fit' patient, too: with every day that they stay in hospital, there is an increased risk that they could contract hospital-acquired pneumonia or another infection – which would not only mean they end up staying for longer, but that they could die when the problem they were admitted for was eminently treatable. Now, with a wave of Covid cases looming, it was even more urgent than usual to get these patients out. And for once, the Treasury stumped up the cash to make it happen.

On 17 March, Stevens wrote to chief executives of all NHS trusts, officers in clinical commissioning groups, GPs, and providers of community health services. His letter was entitled 'Important and urgent – next steps on NHS response to COVID-19', and included the instruction to 'free up the maximum possible inpatient and critical care capacity'. He stated that the NHS in England needed to free up at least 30,000 of its 100,000 general and acute beds by: postponing all non-urgent elective operations; block-buying capacity in independent hospitals; and urgently discharging all hospital inpatients who were medically fit to leave. We will deal with the impact of that first instruction later. The third point was little remarked on at the time, given the general maelstrom of restrictions and cases. But it involved emergency legislation, which would ensure that there weren't unnecessary delays to discharges. The letter predicted that these discharges alone could free up 15,000 acute beds.[23]

In the event, hospitals managed to discharge 25,000 patients. Matt Hancock's view looking back is that it 'was an indicator of how many people need to be in hospital', and a lesson for the long term about improving the discharge process.

The very big short-term problem was that there was no requirement for any of these patients who were coming out of hospitals to have a Covid test. By this point, it was becoming clear that people were infectious for a while before their symptoms started – if they showed symptoms at all. So a medically fit patient might nonetheless have the very disease the NHS was preparing for. Inside Downing Street, there was confusion about whether patients were being tested or not, and Cummings would claim in his testimony to MPs in 2021 that 'we were told categorically in March that people would be tested before they went back to care homes' and that 'we only subsequently found out that that had not happened'.[24] Hancock denied he had ever given that assertion. Either way, within the Department of Health it was well understood that there wasn't going to be testing. Helen Whately, then the care minister, was anxious about what this would mean for care homes who would have no idea whether the patients coming into them had Covid or not. She pressed colleagues repeatedly about the absence of testing in the admissions guidance that had been published by the NHS. The sector itself was anxious, too: Ian Hall from the Association of Directors of Adult Social Services contacted NHS officials on 18 March to warn that care homes were concerned about the lack of testing for discharges. But there was a strange complacency among some of those officials and ministers, who seemed to think that because there wasn't much data showing Covid was spreading within hospitals at this time, there wasn't a problem with sending patients out without a test. Even at the time, this didn't make much sense: the reason there wasn't much evidence of Covid spreading among patients was precisely that there wasn't very much testing going on. And so it was impossible to say where the infections were coming from. It wasn't until 15 April that the government mandated testing of all patients coming into care homes from hospital, and of all symptomatic care home residents and care home staff. The damage, though, had been done.

Discharging so many patients in this blind manner was just what the NHS needed – but it was devastating for the care sector. Between March and June 2020, 20,000 people in care homes died with Covid. By April 2022, the government was the subject of a court case from relatives of two of those who had passed away. Cathy Gardner and Fay Harris argued that the policies in place at the start of the pandemic represented 'one of the most egregious and devastating policy failures in the modern era'.[25] When it heard the case, the High Court found that there had been a failure – not so much in that people weren't all being tested, but that there were no measures that dealt with the absence of testing. Its judgement sympathised with the government's concern that the NHS was on the brink of being overwhelmed, and said there was 'nothing unlawful' in the discharge policies issued between 17 and 19 March. And the court also said it was 'hopeless' to expect that every patient could have been tested prior to discharge when there were only 5,000 tests available each day by 18 March. But it added: 'However, there is a separate question as to how those discharged from hospital to care homes should have been treated and cared for. The fact that discharge was necessary to preserve the capacity of the NHS to provide in-patient care to those seriously affected by Covid did not eliminate the need to consider the best way to manage those discharged.' It also criticised the discharge policy for failing to require newly admitted patients to be quarantined for up to fourteen days, arguing this should have been in the March discharge policy, and 'could and should' have made it into the guidance issued on 2 April. The court concluded that the claims the pair made against the Secretary of State for Health and Social Care and Public Health England were correct: 'The policy set out in each document was irrational in failing to advise that where an asymptomatic patient (other than one who had tested negative) was admitted to a care home, he or she should, so far as practicable, be kept apart from other residents for 14 days.'[26]

In the rush to protect the NHS, there was scant attention paid to how the care sector might be protected. Hancock claimed at a press conference on 15 May 2020 that 'right from the start, we've tried to throw a protective ring around our care homes'. He kept using that phrase during that first summer of the pandemic, even though that ring turned out to be little more use than an inflatable armband would be in the middle of an Atlantic storm.

The other way in which the government initially tried to protect the NHS was to emulate those super-speedy Chinese hospitals. On 24 March 2020, Hancock announced at a press conference that a series of temporary 'Nightingale' hospitals were going to be set up around the country, starting with the London Nightingale in the ExCel convention centre in London's Docklands area. This was lying empty, and in the days before the announcement, NHS staff and members of the military visited the site to work out how to set up a hospital there. Members of the armed forces helped plan and build two enormous wards, each capable of treating 2,000 people. A week later, it was ready to take its first 500 patients.

The hospital – described by one figure involved in its development as a 'critical care barn' – was vast, and used many of the materials which normally make up the stands in the exhibitions the ExCel hosts. The beds sat within cubicles, with a wide carpeted thoroughfare for the staff to move around in. Two of its ventilators came from the set of the BBC's hospital drama *Holby City*. In all, there were seven Nightingales set up across England. In Glasgow, the NHS Louisa Jordan was similarly set up in the SEC Centre in Glasgow, and was ready by 19 April 2020. The Principality Stadium in Cardiff was converted into a temporary hospital with 2,000 beds, opening on 11 April. There were also smaller temporary hospitals in North and South Wales to increase bed capacity. The staff were a mix of NHS workers seconded from other trusts, members of the armed forces, and airline staff who were grounded due to the travel restrictions in place at the time.

As the staff readied themselves for their first patients, there was an air of anxious expectation, both among those in the buildings and among the general public. The NHS was ready for what was going to happen. But what did happen?

In the event, the Nightingales, which cost around £530 million, were never packed to the rafters, or indeed to a level that even came close to the initial wave of beds built for their opening. By May 2020, the London Nightingale had only treated fifty-four patients, which turned out to be the total number it ever received through its doors as an intensive care facility. At its peak, there were just thirty-five patients in the facility. All fifty-four of its patients went onto ventilators, and twenty died at the hospital, with a further six dying in critical care units near their homes. It was a similar death rate to other intensive care settings in conventional hospitals, but what was markedly different was how long the patients stayed in the cavernous exhibition centre. The Nightingale couldn't give tracheostomies, a procedure whereby a tube is inserted into a patient's windpipe, which may have affected the way staff were able to care for these patients.[27]

An inquest into the death of one of those patients, Kishorkumar Patel – a 58-year-old London bus driver who was one of the first patients to arrive at the London Nightingale – also heard that staff at the hospital were stretched. Patel died of multiple organ failure and Covid-19 pneumonitis, but had also suffered a cardiac arrest after the wrong filter was fitted to his ventilator. He had been transferred to the Nightingale from Northwick Park Hospital in North London after the intensive care unit there ran out of spaces for more patients. This was precisely what the Nightingales were supposed to do: take patients from hospitals that were in danger of being overwhelmed. But in Patel's case and that of Kofi Aning, who was also treated at the Nightingale in April 2020, there was a serious mistake made in their care. Coroner Nadia Persaud issued a serious incident warning about the 'widespread' confusion about which filters to use on ventilators, making clear that they were 'not confined to the Nightingale, emergency provision, hospitals'.[28] But the inquest that followed the report also heard evidence of staff working 'leanly'. There was plenty of evidence of that elsewhere in the health system, too.

Initially, though, the small number of patients meant that staff could do things differently. One of the Nightingale's doctors, Gareth Grier, had last been in the ExCel centre to watch a triathlon. Now, the emergency medicine consultant from Barts Health NHS Trust was having to work out how to treat patients in a dignified way, rather than the whole institution feeling like a 'warehouse'. He described what it was like in the early days: 'The Nightingale was a clean slate for us. We know in many places family are not getting calls and we said let's work to a gold standard we would like to achieve.' The staff tried to ensure that families could visit their dying relatives – something that was not allowed in many permanent hospitals. But it was easier to do this with such a small number of patients – Grier was well aware it was unlikely to be maintained if admissions rose dramatically.[29] They never did. By May 2020, the discussion was about how to mothball the Nightingales. Some had a second life as vaccination centres; others as recovery units for patients who had left the danger zone of intensive care but who were still too sick to leave an acute environment.

One of the problems that all the Nightingales faced was that it is much easier to make a flat-pack hospital than to create staff out of thin air. Where would the staff come from if they weren't going to be taken from the very institutions these field hospitals were supposed to be relieving? At one stage, the London Nightingale had aimed to recruit 16,000 staff.[30] It never needed that many, anyway, but it would have struggled to find them. The pandemic exposed a problem that had been well known within the health world, but largely ignored by politicians: the NHS was in a workforce crisis, with more than 100,000 vacancies before the pandemic even got going. The King's Fund concluded that 'the Nightingales experience also unfortunately highlights the folly of having a chronically under-staffed health service'.[31]

When ministers and officials were planning these hospitals, they kept getting stuck in the same argument. The line from senior NHS figures in meetings was: 'The problem isn't the buildings, it's the number of people we have.' The response from Hancock was that the number of people wasn't the problem if you stretched the ratios of staff to patients. Staff were going to have to look after more people, he insisted. Instead of a hospital saying it was full, it had to stretch the ratios. Unsurprisingly, this turned into a big row between the minister and the NHS. Hancock won that battle, and in late March, acute trusts were told to flex their ratios so that there would be one critical care nurse for every six patients – as opposed to the 1:1 ratio recommended in normal times. There would be one critical care consultant for every thirty patients, up from a maximum of 1:15.

This applied to all hospitals, not just the Nightingales, and meant that existing trusts were able to double their own ICU capacity through sweating their existing critical care staff, redeploying others from different specialties, and repurposing wards. It was also not sustainable. Within a month, the Faculty of Intensive Care Medicine was pushing for a return to the old ratios, with its dean, Alison Pittard, warning that the health system 'cannot sustain' the level of pressure it was putting on its staff.[32]

But in the short term, what all of these measures meant was that the National Audit Office, the powerful government spending watchdog, was able to conclude that: 'Between mid-March and mid-April, the NHS increased bed capacity for Covid-19 patients in NHS trusts in England, meaning that the number of patients never exceeded the number of available beds.'[33] Johnson himself ended up in one of those beds when he was admitted to intensive care at St Thomas's Hospital, where it was at one stage '50:50' whether he would make it through. Jenny McGee was one of the nurses who cared for Johnson, and described him as looking 'very, very unwell', adding: 'He was a different colour really.'[34] McGee kept vigil by his bedside overnight, along with another nurse, Luis Pitarma. Johnson gave his son Wilfred, born just seventeen days after the prime minister was discharged from the hospital, the middle name Nicholas in honour of the two doctors, Dr Nicholas Price and Dr Nicholas Hart, who treated him. The system had responded to the prospect of a surge in the best way it could, and Lombardy was not repeated in the UK.

There are two narratives around the small number of patients who ended up in the Nightingales. There's the argument that these field hospitals could never have admitted any more people for the reason set out above: they couldn't get enough staff. And so, this first narrative goes, the Nightingales didn't help an overwhelmed system that did need them. Then there's the second one – that the temporary hospitals were only ever set up as an insurance policy that wasn't needed to the extent that policymakers, moving as fast as they could in one of the most uncertain periods in British peacetime history, anticipated. This is the line that Hancock, who was one of the architects of the Nightingales, takes: 'They were a massive insurance policy.' And it was a triumph of the NHS, rather than an exposition of its weaknesses, that they were never used.

The truth is the NHS simply didn't have enough staff, and the way it dealt with that was to sweat the ones it had to prevent the system from being overwhelmed. The empty Nightingales, therefore, are a red herring. The real sign that the system wasn't working properly came in a less eye-catching form, which was a nurse rushing between six beds of seriously ill patients rather than working at just one.

One of Hancock's other big battles was to get to a self-imposed target of 100,000 Covid tests a day by the end of April 2020. When he announced it, this seemed impossible given that at the time there was only capacity for 12,000 daily tests in England. He explained his thinking to MPs in June 2021: 'We got to 2,000 a day by the end of February and it was still rising, but by the middle of March it was not rising fast enough, we were not doing enough to bring in private sector capacity, so I took personal charge of it, and then, a couple of weeks later, set the 100,000 target. That 100,000 target was essential in galvanising the whole system and building a diagnostics organisation and ecosystem in this country, and now we are doing about 6 million tests a week and I'm very proud of that.'[35] But as we have seen in earlier chapters, targets can galvanise systems in the wrong way. The New Labour years showed how targets do create a focus on a particular problem within the NHS, but also create incentives for gaming the system. And that's exactly what happened with the Covid testing. By May 2020, Hancock was delighted to announce that 'we have met our goal. The number of tests yesterday, on the last day of April, was 122,347.'[36] He seemed visibly relieved, almost out of breath from the personal effort it had taken. And indeed, meeting the target had required a great deal of effort. But not always in the right place.

The *Health Service Journal* revealed that the Department of Health and Social Care had started to include within the number of tests any that had merely been sent out to people to take at home, rather than tests definitely taken and with a result from a laboratory. It wasn't even clear that the people who were definitely being tested needed to be either. Dominic Cummings later complained that it distracted Hancock from the more important task of building a proper testing infrastructure.[37] Jeremy Hunt, by now watching from the sidelines as chair of the Health and Social Care Select Committee, was unimpressed by the way the testing system was set up, writing in his book *Zero*: 'As intended, the new target galvanised the system. Huge numbers of people were dragooned into getting tested. One of those happened to be my brother, who was in hospital for cancer treatment. He was suddenly told he would be tested for Covid-19 alongside every other inpatient – just two days before the 100,000 target was due to be hit.' Hunt believes that 'the national testing target then became a classic example of what is now called Goodhart's Law: the British economist Charles Goodhart argued that when a measure becomes a target it ceases to be a good measure and starts to distort outcomes and behaviour. So it proved: NHS laboratory managers were ordered to rush out meaningless antibody tests ahead of the deadline.'[38]

The opprobrium Hancock received for gaming the system to get his target paled in comparison to the reaction to the 'NHS Test and Trace' system. I use quotation marks for this advisedly, because part of the furore surrounding it was over whether it was really an NHS service or whether it was merely using that precious logo – in part to cover for its errors.

NHS Test and Trace was set up in May 2020 to notify people of their Covid status, and trace the contacts they had made in the days running up to their positive test. It is by far the biggest part of the NHS spend from Covid – something critics of the healthcare system seem to forget when they use the rise in spending as part of their argument for scrapping the NHS entirely. It spent £29.5 billion within two years (an underspend on its £37 billion budget), of which the vast majority went to the tests themselves. Even though a much smaller amount – around £900 million – was spent on contact tracing, it was this part that was controversial. The influential cross-party Public Accounts Committee, which scrutinises whether the taxpayer is getting value for money from government spending, concluded in October 2021 that 'NHST&T has not achieved its main objective to help break chains of Covid-19 transmission and enable people to return towards a more normal way of life'. The committee discovered that the system had lost trace of the majority of its lateral flow tests, and it was at risk of 'wasting public money' over the way it used labs and contact centres.[39] Anecdotal evidence had emerged early on that contact tracers were being paid a whole lot of money for doing a whole lot of nothing: one, speaking to the BBC anonymously, claimed she had worked thirty-eight hours but had yet to make a single phone call to trace contacts and had spent her time watching Netflix.[40]

The anger about the use of 'NHS' in NHST&T was largely related to the fact that some of the tracing was contracted out to Serco, one of the large – and largely unaccountable – outsourcing giants that hoover up public sector contracts. Outsourcing was supposed to improve standards and lower costs through competition, but it has often led to near-monopolies presided over by a handful of enormous companies, including Serco and G4S, who have the ability to bid for contracts successfully and a more mixed record of delivering on them. This should be a source of frustration to the right, but has largely ended up being an obsession of the left, to the extent that misleading claims were regularly made during the pandemic about the role of Serco in Test and Trace. In March 2021, for instance, former Labour leader Jeremy Corbyn claimed that 'if £37 billion can be found to pay Serco for a failed track and trace system, the money must be available to pay NHS staff properly'.[41] Serco would have been less of a giant and more of a behemoth if it really had been paid £37 billion, but as we have already seen, the majority of that budget was not spent on the Serco contract but on the tests.

The other point of controversy was that the head of NHST&T – or 'NHS TAT', as it became nicknamed within health circles – was Dido Harding. A Conservative life peer and former boss of TalkTalk, Harding did not have a brilliant digital track record outside the health system, and failed to impress within it: the app that NHSX, the digital arm of the health service, tried to develop was abandoned after endless glitches. Hancock tried to defend Harding, to the extent that at one point she was his favoured candidate to take over from Simon Stevens as NHS boss. Others within government felt that, given her notoriety, this would be a very silly way of spending political capital.

One of the mistakes Harding and her colleagues made was to focus on the infrastructure for testing and tracing, rather than working backwards from the question of what it would take to get someone to stay isolated at home for two weeks after being identified as a close contact. 'That should have been sick pay,' explains one official. 'But Sunak blocked that, and there were lots of good reasons for that in terms of stopping there being a precedent for putting up sick pay more permanently, but what it means was that they spent all this money on this vast infrastructure but not on the thing that would actually work. So we had these outbreaks in places like garment factories in Leicester where people just needed to be paid enough to stay at home.'[42]

There was significant frustration among those running the NHS that Test and Trace was supposed to stop the second wave of infections. Because the sick pay issue was never sorted, people didn't self-isolate, and that wave came in September 2020, meaning doctors like Lillie and Price were once again stretched – just as they were hoping for a breather from the first wave.

NHS workers were pushed to the limit by Covid, working shifts that even they, with their general Stakhanovite ethic, were unused to. Patrick Lillie, who has a jovial manner that doesn't fully disguise the fact that he's seen a little too much in his job, had still not had a proper chance to wind down more than two years since his first Covid case. Asked if he'd had a break, he replied 'define a break' with a wry smile, and explained that he'd taken a week or two off here and there, but that wasn't anywhere like the amount of time he or other colleagues would need in order to process the relentless two years of working beyond their limits and dealing with traumas that even they weren't used to. He added: 'My wobbly bit came early on in the pandemic when we had our first death, because it was someone I had diagnosed, and I told them, and I could tell they looked absolutely shit-scared. And at the time, we couldn't do anything for them. The health service got bent quite badly in terms of the human cost to staff. We've certainly had a few people who've had pretty bad PTSD and breakdowns, and people who still struggle with that.'

Ashley Price described what it was like for him: 'The intensity of it was massive. And I don't think people really understood how intense it was because when you were doing it you were surviving on adrenaline. We dropped everything else to be able to do this. It was overwhelming, there were lots of people dying. I was working from eight o'clock in the morning to ten o'clock at night, it was just very, very, very, very busy.' It was when the more seriously ill patients started coming into his ward that the enormity hit him. 'I think what really upset me, and actually one of the first times I've ever cried in front of junior doctors as a consultant, was speaking to those first few families about what was going to happen, because they were at home, and they weren't able to come in and see their families. It really brought it home to me. The impact that this was going to have not just on those families but on the communities, and how this was going to be disastrous.'[43]

It wasn't just disastrous for the people outside the hospitals, though. On 28 March, the first front-line NHS worker died of Covid. Amged El-Hawrani was fifty-five when he tested positive for Covid. He was an ear, nose and throat specialist at Queen's Hospital, Burton. He was very well liked by his colleagues and known for what one of them described as a 'very high workload'. 'He never complained,' wrote his colleague Adrian Thompson in the *BMJ*. 'He cared deeply about his patients and always strived to do the best for them. He was very popular around the hospital, with a rare skill to engage and talk to people of all ranks and backgrounds. He had time for everyone. He was full of energy, with an excellent memory for detail, yet sometimes had an endearing flight of thought and scattered malapropisms, to his colleagues' amusement.'[44] He died after three weeks in critical care.

NHS workers – particularly those working in specialties like ENT – were naturally more exposed to the virus than the rest of the population, most of whom were staying at home. But many of them were clear that, in the first few months of the pandemic, they were being left even more vulnerable because they were not being given the protections that should have been available. A poll by the Hospital Consultants and Specialists Association in March 2020 found that 80 per cent of hospital doctors did not feel safe, and 69 per cent were not confident that the guidance issued at the time by Public Health England for wearing masks only around patients who were suspected of having or confirmed to have Covid was sufficient. Just over a third claimed their own employers were not following that guidance anyway.

One of the reasons the guidance and its implementation seemed to be insufficient was that, in the initial stages, there was a shortage of personal protective equipment across the NHS and social care system. The infectious disease wards had a good supply as they were always operating with this equipment. But there was a procurement problem: the NHS had been told by the Department of Health at the start of the pandemic that 'just in time' PPE was being ordered, but due to a perfect storm of Covid closures in Chinese factories and a spike in worldwide PPE demand, it took a very long time to arrive – and the existing stock was going out of date. Some crates of new PPE turned out to be lace gowns, which weren't much use either. Another problem with the stock that was already available was that it was impossible to get it out of the warehouse quickly enough. 'It was in this warehouse with a door that wasn't big enough to get it out. So the rate-limiting factor on distributing our PPE stockpile was this fucking door. You had to be doing loads of packing and unpacking to get it out of one lorry-sized door. In the end we had to send in the military just to manage the flow. Maybe we should have just ripped down the wall instead.'[45]

The supply problem quickly translated into shortages on the front line. This is the account of one anonymous GP in Coventry in June 2020: 'My GP surgery that I work with is currently struggling with stock of surgical face masks for PPE. Recently we had a day where there were none for patients or staff to wear, and at the moment we've had to stop giving them to patients because of low stock for staff . . . We've barely had any from the Clinical Commissioning Group – I was told we were given one box only and requests for more had been ignored or delayed . . . Our practice has been buying their own but running out of suppliers with stock now.'[46]

One intensive care doctor told the BBC in April 2020 that she and her colleagues were 'having to put bin bags and aprons on our heads', and that 'the respiratory protection face masks we're using at the moment, they've all been relabelled with new best-before end dates. Yesterday I found one with three stickers on. The first said, expiry 2009. The second sticker, expiry 2013. And the third sticker on the very top said 2021.'[47]

Trusts rushed to procure sufficient PPE as quickly as they could. Ministers did the same, leading to endless stories about crony contracts for businesses that had never seen the inside of a hospital prior to the pandemic but which were owned by mates of ministers. The problem was one of procurement, but Hancock managed to offend anxious workers by saying: 'We need everyone to treat PPE like the precious resource it is. Everyone should use the equipment they clinically need, in line with the guidelines: no more and no less.'[48] Given the amount of time it takes to don and doff full PPE, it was a strange idea that NHS staff might be overenthusiastic in its use.

Then there was the line from Priti Patel when asked whether she would apologise for the lack of PPE provided to front-line workers. 'I'm sorry if people *feel* that there have been failings,' she said. 'I will be very, very clear about that.' It was the ultimate sorry-not-sorry apology: conditional on people 'feeling' that things had gone wrong rather accepting that there might be hard evidence for it. Inside government, there was a blame game under way about whose fault this was: ministers felt it was a collapse in the privatised NHS supply chain (SCCL), itself overseen by DHSC, not the department's emergency procurement work. This is one of the many areas in which accusations of lying started to fly around. Many ministers and officials felt the other side lied to them, with Dominic Cummings being the main figure who went on the record to accuse Matt Hancock of lying about PPE – and many other things. He also revealed text messages where it appeared Johnson was accusing the Health Secretary of a 'disaster' on PPE, and suggesting that Michael Gove, then the Cabinet Office minister, might have to take over some of Hancock's responsibilities.

Once again, even though the formal responsibility for PPE was clearly with the Department of Health and Social Care and not the NHS, everyone was busy blaming each other. At one stage DHSC ministers tried to point the finger at Stevens and the NHS. 'He went to ground on PPE,' complained one senior figure. 'The NHS centrally basically ducked and did not want accountability for this, Simon refused to engage. It was woeful.'[49] Though the DHSC was responsible for the supply of PPE, this source was claiming there was enough but it was just that the NHS wasn't distributing it properly. Boris Johnson and Stevens went way back, but this was the biggest test of their relationship, to the point that the prime minister had to ask him if he'd accidentally muted himself on a Zoom call when Hancock tried to blame Stevens on PPE. Others on the call remember Stevens going quiet, but largely to avoid dropping Hancock in it by publicly contradicting him.

By June 2021, Hancock told MPs that more than 1,500 health and social care workers had died with Covid-19: 639 in the NHS and 922 in social care. They kept going to work despite the risks to themselves. In some cases, those risks were greater than they needed to be.

The sacrifices that NHS workers were making were enormous, and were underlined every time someone used the 'Protect the NHS' slogan. That and the new life the general population were having to adjust to, involving curbs on their liberty that went far further in many cases than those seen in the Second World War, led to an emotional outpouring towards the health service on a scale not seen before, even in NHS-besotted Britain.

Clapping for carers wasn't actually a British idea. As Covid spread across the world, and as people were locked down in their homes, many countries saw spontaneous events where healthcare workers were applauded from balconies, front doors and on Zoom calls. In London, Annemarie Plas saw videos of people clapping in the Netherlands, where she was originally from, and she posted an image suggesting a British clap at 8 p.m. that Thursday, 26 March. It went viral, and on that night and in the weeks to follow, many were surprised by how loud the clapping was in their streets, where neighbours had lived alongside one another for years but had barely looked each other in the eye until they were banned from going near one another. The Queen described it in a national address in April 2020 as 'an expression of our national spirit'. She also praised another spontaneous cultural expression: the appearance of rainbows drawn by children in the front windows of their homes. Many of them remained for years after, with the colours rather faded, and the sentiments perhaps a little different, too.

These rainbows weren't initially about the NHS; it was something promoted by schools as a way of keeping children busy and hopeful in a bewildering time, when many of them were out of the classroom and learning at home. There were local challenges for children to spot as many rainbows as possible in the front windows that they passed on their daily walk outside. Again, this wasn't a solely British idea: other countries had their own rainbow windows. But in

Britain, the message of hope started to merge with other notes posted in windows such as 'Thank you NHS', to the extent that many businesses started to add decals to their vehicles and buildings with a 'Thank you NHS' or 'Thank you key workers' under a rainbow motif.

In the early days of the pandemic, people needed that sense of solidarity and hope as much as they needed to thank the NHS workers. Not all workers were that happy with the clapping, though. Many remarked that they felt deeply uncomfortable with the level of adulation directed at them for doing what was their job. One complained that it was 'encouraging the God complex in some of my more egotistical colleagues'.[50] Others felt it quickly became politicised, with ministers including Boris Johnson making a point of clapping for the cameras while at the same time failing to ensure adequate supplies of PPE, and so on. It also gained menacing overtones in some communities, where WhatsApp groups discussed those who had 'failed' to clap – including NHS workers themselves, who weren't outside their doors because they were, er, doing the work that was allegedly being applauded. Health service managers were also sceptical about what would happen as the pandemic wore on. Caroline Clarke, the chief executive of the Royal Free, warned her colleagues that the British love of the NHS was going to be tested like never before, as patients found the services they were used to disappearing.

Perhaps more sincerely moving were the claps in NHS wards as patients who had recovered from Covid took their first steps home. Many would have long rehabilitations ahead of them. Some were unlikely to ever return to the health they had enjoyed before the illness struck, with permanent damage to their lungs, hearts and mental health. The same description of long recovery and even permanent damage might also apply to the NHS itself.

As the pandemic continued, the claps started to fade, but popular expressions of appreciation for the NHS didn't: they just changed. Getting a Covid vaccine became – for many members of the population – part of the membership of the society of doing your bit, which had helped many through the darker times of the pandemic. Now you could, at the first possible opportunity, get your dose of the vaccine, and wear a sticker or change your social media profile to prove it. Politicians were all too keen to talk about this part of the pandemic response: the government used the vaccine programme to regain a great deal of the political capital it had lost in the early days of the pandemic. This really was – unlike many of the other programmes set up in response to Covid – world-beating, and the way the NHS was structured was an important factor in its success.

The centralised nature of the NHS provided what Oxford vaccine creator Sarah Gilbert described as 'the backbone of the NHS' for the success of testing the jab and then rolling it out. Hancock says: 'The NHS's responsibility wasn't procurement or creation of the vaccine but deployment. And they were brilliant. I gave them a reasonable best-case scenario that we'll be ready by the 1st of December. And lots of people in this system didn't believe this would happen, but they kept on track and delivered the first jab on the 8th. They were absolutely magnificent at it.'[51]

On 8 December 2020, ninety-year-old Margaret Keenan was the first person in the world to receive the Pfizer jab at University Hospital Coventry. She was given her first dose at 6.31 a.m. by May Parsons, a matron who had worked in the NHS for nearly twenty years after moving to Britain from the Philippines. She was already a dab hand at jabbing, clocking up 140 flu vaccines a day as one of the leading members of the hospital's flu programme. Parsons was the embodiment of the NHS's ability to get going as soon as a vaccine was ready. The system already knew how to roll out vaccination drives because it had been doing these for years. The Covid vaccine was, of course, of a far greater magnitude, requiring volunteers, temporary sites and national booking systems. The volunteer recruitment was, according to insiders, easy – 'because this was the NHS, something that's part of the community ties that bind: people wanted to be involved'.[52] The NHS recruited more than 71,000 people to volunteer with the vaccination programme. More than 10,000 of those have since joined the health service in paid employment.

The UK became a world leader in the roll-out of the vaccine. This wasn't just down to the health service: there was a government task force set up by the Department of Health, which was chaired by pharmaceutical venture capitalist Kate Bingham. With members picked by Bingham and chief scientific adviser Sir Patrick Vallance, it was designed to ensure the UK got a strong supply of the right vaccines as quickly as they became available for use. It was not an NHS-heavy group – though NHS figures argue that this was because it was a job for the Department of Health, not the health service specifically. When it started out, it didn't have anyone from the deployment side of the NHS on it at all. It was also, however, not a Department-of-Health-heavy group. That was because Downing Street figures in particular had tired of the chaos within the department on PPE procurement and on testing. In his explosive and lengthy testimony to the joint inquiry that the Health and Science Select Committees held into Covid, Dominic Cummings claimed that it was only when he and Vallance decided to take testing and vaccines away from the 'horror' of the Department of Health that things started to improve: 'I have got a text from Patrick Vallance, when he texted me directly . . . where he says explicitly "I want to set up a vaccine task force, and do it outside the Department of Health and Social Care." '

But the roll-out of the vaccine was very much within the NHS itself. One of the key figures alongside Stevens was Emily Lawson, the chief commercial officer for NHS England, who had been trying to fix the PPE crisis and get enough ventilators to hospitals. She was an organisational genius, and also someone who tried to understand what might work best – rather than jumping in with preconceived confidence about the set-up. She read the World Health Organization's report on what makes a successful mass vaccination programme. She told the King's Fund that every part of the programme had to be 'operationally excellent because if people are nervous about a new vaccine, a brilliant operational experience gives them confidence in the programme, and they tell people about it, and that feeds back to people's perception of the vaccine itself and the programme'.[53]

The NHS deployed the vaccine through three routes: GPs, hospitals and mass vaccination sites. The last route got the most attention, in part because of some of the locations. Salisbury Cathedral was a vaccine centre. Lord's Cricket Ground was another. Epsom Downs Racecourse, the Royal Highland Showground, the Royal Horticultural Halls and my local scout hut all became places where people got their latest dose of the jab. But the GP centres were also an important part of it, not least because many elderly and infirm people found the mass centres daunting or difficult to get to.

Johnson saw that a well-run programme delivering a vaccine that was going to restore normality for people had rather a lot of political opportunity for him. He became obsessed with pushing the NHS as hard as he could to get as many vaccines out as quickly as possible. 'It was the most energised and focused I've ever seen him,' says one Cabinet minister. 'Everything was "Why can't we do that, no, go away and find out whether you can do it better." It was infectious and gave the rest of government a sense of purpose too.'[54] The prime minister did, though, have to be persuaded that some of his ideas didn't make practical sense. He was keen for vaccination centres to be open 24/7, and was egged on in this by Tony Blair, who announced that he would happily queue in the middle of the night if it meant he got his jab (this amused Blair's former colleagues, who pointed out that the former prime minister had probably last queued for anything in the mid-1990s). It was the job of Stevens and others to argue that while some people might like the *idea* of a round-the-clock service, in reality it would be difficult to fill the slots in the witching hours, particularly when the roll-out was focused on older and more vulnerable members of the public who wouldn't be very keen on a 2 a.m. appointment. In the end, a handful of centres did do some 24-hour drives, which seemed to satisfy the prime minister.

The Treasury was, once again, not very helpful. 'It took months for them to sign off anything, and so they [the DoH and NHS England] had to ignore them and get on with spending the money anyway,' says one insider. Kate Bingham covers the exhausting and baffling process her task force was required to follow in her book, complaining that it took three months for the Treasury to endorse the Vaccine Taskforce's business case and budget, and then they didn't sign off on it until September. The Treasury's view of it is that it was a much quicker process than three months. Nevertheless, the permanent secretary of the Department of Health and Social Care Sir Chris Wormald told a committee of MPs that: 'One decision that Simon Stevens and I took – as I say, this one got retrospective approval – was to approve the vaccine roll-out ten days before the business case was approved. I do not think there is anyone in the country who would not have taken the same decision.'[55]

Bingham was unimpressed that the forms her team had to fill in required them to answer questions that were just not relevant to a vaccine programme, and took no account of the value of saving lives. She complained to Boris Johnson about the delay in signing it off, and the prime minister challenged his Chancellor on what was going on in the Treasury. 'Rishi had no idea,' she writes. 'This was my first inkling of the power of officials, who get to decide exactly what they show to their ministers for approval and decisions. Vaccines had clearly not been high on the list of priorities for the Chancellor's office.'[56] She blames the officials. Another senior figure involved in the vaccine programme blames Steve Barclay, then Chief Secretary to the Treasury, who was the lead minister on the Vaccine Taskforce: 'He was a total dick, a total control freak but also not very good at it. He refused to sign off the vaccine programme for ages, saying "Is it value for money?"' Barclay disputes this, saying he took 'significant risk and acted early'.[57] Either way, the processes and culture in the Treasury militated against the programme. By the time the money for the resources had gained official approval, the NHS had already vaccinated close to a million people.

The Department of Health and Social Care has – as we've seen – often been regarded in the rest of Whitehall as a bit of a basket case. That view goes beyond the Treasury. But it is often the case that the NHS was bundled in with it. In this instance, Stevens was very keen to put clear water between his organisation and the department, pointing out to anyone who would listen that the success of the vaccine roll-out showed the importance of having a programme within the NHS, rather than trying to do it outside it – as had happened with the testing system. NHS England was in charge of this programme, and that's where the credit should lie, went his reasoning.

Others who worked on the strategy within government take a slightly more nuanced view: they say that part of the reason everything got moving so quickly was that they told GPs that pharmacists would also be able to vaccinate patients and would receive a payment for this. 'That bit of competition got them going,' chuckles one minister.

In fact, the way Stevens responded to the vaccine roll-out became the source of much frustration among the politicians he had to work with. 'Suddenly, he was *everywhere*,' complained one minister. Another insider said that until the vaccines were on the horizon, 'He was nowhere and that was driving them wild, and it was a case of "you *will* do some bloody press conferences", "you *will* come out and talk about this".' Stevens and senior NHS doctors had let it be known they were concerned about the 'Protect the NHS' messaging used at the government press conferences, worried that it was putting people off coming forward for non-Covid care. However, as Covid cases once again began to increase in autumn 2020, Stevens did appear alongside Johnson at a succession of press conferences. Then, when the vaccine hove into view, ministers complained that it was difficult to get a word in edgeways with Stevens. It's almost as though they were jealous that a non-politician had managed to out-operate them so deftly. It was also a bit rich to complain, as Stevens and the NHS had explicitly been given responsibility for delivering the vaccine roll-out – at a stage where it wasn't clear if it would be a success. A colleague of Hancock's pointed out that Stevens was only ever as good as the Health Secretary he had to manoeuvre around: '[Hancock is] the wrong person to deal with Simon Stevens as he's just interested in his media image and Simon is just constantly blindsiding him. Simon is not my favourite person: his office is like a black hole, but Matt has never learned how to work him properly and that's the problem.' It may not come as a surprise, then, that Hancock was involved in legislation in the form of the Health and Care bill, which was intended to hand back a great deal of power from the NHS England hierarchy to the Secretary of State – nor that Stevens was careful to make clear in public that he didn't support these ideas.

The vaccination programme wasn't the only NHS triumph. A less well-publicised way that the health system responded to Covid was the RECOVERY trial. The name stood for 'Randomised Evaluation of Covid-19 Therapy' and the trial started in March 2020, just days after the first Covid death. On 19 March, the trial enrolled its first patient – the first of 47,000 to take part in research to find effective Covid treatments. It found four: dexamethasone, tocilizumab, Ronapreve, and baricitinib. It also ruled out many other drugs, including hydroxychloroquine and aspirin. RECOVERY was run by Oxford University researchers, and relied on the NHS for its patients. One doctor involved in the trial described the health service as 'turning the engines on big time' for recruiting patients: in the end, 15 per cent of all Covid patients in UK hospitals took part. It was easier to recruit, thanks to the National Institute for Health and Care Research cutting a great deal of the bureaucracy normally associated with clinical trials because there simply wasn't time to spare.[58] The NHS provided the perfect recruiting field, and gained a great deal from the trial too – as did health systems across the world. But at the same time as it was pioneering Covid research, the health service was also falling behind with its other work.

For a man interested in media exposure, it is fitting that Matt Hancock lost his job after rather too much of it. In June 2021, photos of him in a rule-breaking 'clinch' in the Department of Health and Social Care with his adviser Gina Coladangelo were splashed over the front page of the *Sun* newspaper. He resigned, realising that he had flouted restrictions that he himself had been energetically promoting. But he had been busily working on the reopening of the health service – and the backlog in treatment that had built up.

If the NHS wasn't overwhelmed, it was in part because it shut down a great deal of its normal functions. It would become clear that the knock-on effect of cancelling elective surgeries and of having to reopen in much smaller ways due to social distancing and infection control requirements could be the thing that *really knocked over* the health service, not the pandemic itself.

It wasn't just the operations that the NHS knew it would have to carry out once it opened up, or indeed the more complicated surgeries resulting from a delay in which someone's condition continued to deteriorate. It was also that for a significant period of time, people avoided going to their GP or to hospital, either because they were told not to or because they were too frightened to. This meant that patients were presenting later with illnesses which were much more advanced than usual. It meant that the health service simply did not know the size of the backlog that it was going to have to deal with as it returned to 'normal'. And the new normal wasn't like the pre-2020 era, because as well as being in short supply as they were before the pandemic, NHS staff were by now exhausted, traumatised, and in many cases sick themselves, as a result of their herculean effort over what turned out to be two long years.

By March 2022, the NHS England waiting list for surgery and other hospital procedures had reached nearly 6.4 million, with some projections suggesting this would be more like 10 million by its peak. NHS emergency services were under severe pressure, with twenty-four NHS trusts declaring a 'critical incident' in their services in the first week of January 2022 alone. This meant they could not guarantee urgent or safe services. The ambulance services, often seen as the canary in the coal mine for the emergency sector as a whole, went into a crisis from which it would take years to emerge. In May 2022, the nursing director of the West Midlands Ambulance Service, Mark Docherty, warned that patients were 'dying every day that shouldn't be dying every day'. He told the *Health Service Journal* that ambulance delays were as long as twenty-four hours as they waited outside hospitals to hand over sick patients.[59] The Royal College of Emergency Medicine warned that there was a 'serious patient safety crisis' in A&E, blaming this not on Covid but on a long-term decline in the number of beds, with the health service losing almost 25,000 since 2010. Its president Adrian Boyle claimed in January 2023 'somewhere between 300 and 500 people are dying as a consequence of delays and problems with urgent and emergency care each week'.[60]

Compounding this is, of course, the NHS workforce crisis, which politicians have continued to pay lip service to, without any evidence that they will address it. In 2022, the Health and Care Act made its way through Parliament, with repeated attempts in vain by Hunt and

Stevens (now in the House of Lords) to amend it and require Health Education England to produce independent forecasts of the number of doctors and nurses that would need to be trained in order to keep the health service running in future years. It sounded so sensible to most people, but to Treasury ears it sounded like a huge long-term spending commitment and a political stick with which opponents could beat a government. So it never made it out of the starting blocks.

The result of these pressures is not just that the NHS continues to operate at a pace and level of stress that it simply has not seen in its entire history, but also that patients are starting to lose faith with it in an unprecedented way, too. The NHS itself continues to be the institution that British people hold in the highest esteem and affection: in May 2022, a poll by YouGov put the health service at the top of a list of the best things about Britain. It had a 62 per cent approval rating, above the countryside (61 per cent), Britain's history (37 per cent) and even the monarchy in its Platinum Jubilee year (just 34 per cent). But beneath that continuing adoration of the system lay a deep worry about its service. The British Social Attitudes Survey in the same year found public satisfaction with the NHS at its lowest since 1997 – just 36 per cent, which was a record-breaking fall of 17 points since 2020. Back in 1997, the worry was that the middle classes, whose support was so important for the health service at its inception, would turn to private medicine just to get seen in a timely fashion. Now, people are looking to the private sector again, even though they would like to stay committed to the NHS itself if they can.

But it's not just the middle classes who can afford private medical insurance who've started to turn away from the NHS. It's also people who cannot afford it, for whom the NHS should be there in place of fear but is unable to be. The data journalist John Burn-Murdoch discovered that in the five years to 2022, the number of people in the UK who were setting up crowdfunders to cover medical expenses had risen twenty-fold. Some were fundraising for treatments that have never been available on the NHS, but others were trying to get enough money together for operations that they had been told wouldn't happen for a year or more, leaving them in unbearable pain for that time. These crowdfunders were to cover what is known as 'self-pay' medicine: where a patient isn't covered by private medical insurance and has to pay all the costs up front. One of the biggest independent providers in the UK, Spire Healthcare, saw its revenue from self-pay patients rise 80 per cent in the final three-quarters of 2021 as compared to 2019. A new private hospital run by the US-based Cleveland Clinic opened in London in March 2022, to respond to the demand for private treatment.

It isn't just the elective treatment backlog that is damaging the NHS now, though. Another part of the NHS which had to change the way it operated very quickly was general practice. Like all parts of the NHS, primary care was under instructions to reduce contact unless absolutely necessary. NHS England issued instructions in March 2020 for GPs to move to a system called 'total triage', whereby every patient who wanted an appointment had to be triaged first, before being offered a remote consultation either by phone or video call. GPs were still seeing patients in person when necessary, but often found that a problem could be resolved remotely anyway. It forced an extraordinary change in the way GPs operated: the Royal College of GPs carried out a survey in July 2020, which found that where just 5 per cent of practices had the necessary equipment for remote consultations before the pandemic, 88 per cent were now able to hold them. There was even an argument that this way of working drove down A&E attendances – though the Health Foundation analysis of this points out that people were generally avoiding emergency departments at this time for fear of getting infected or unnecessarily burdening the health service. Either way, the damage was done, with the lowest satisfaction scores on record for GP services in the 2021 British Social Attitudes Survey – at just 38 per cent. When asked what the top priorities should be for the NHS, making it easier to get a GP appointment came out top at 47 per cent, followed by improving waiting times for planned operations at 47 per cent, and increasing the number of staff in the NHS, also at 47 per cent. Once again, patients started to vote with their feet: in May 2022 a poll for *The Times* suggested that 1.6 million people had used a private GP for the first time in the last two years.[61]

On one level, it doesn't matter if people who can afford it opt out of the system for a bit so that the NHS is under a little less pressure. That was the argument that Margaret Thatcher and her ministers made back in the 1980s. But it ignores the point that a lot of the people trying to raise money for medical bills are the ones who can't afford it, who should be able to rely on the NHS, and who can't. Private medicine also recruits from the same pool as the public health service, meaning some doctors and nurses who have become exhausted by the demands of an overstretched NHS are lured away from it by better working conditions. The health service celebrated its seventy-fifth year in an existential crisis. If this is protecting the NHS, it hasn't worked.

12. The last battle?

Will it still be here in another seventy-five years? It's a question we obsessively ask about many of our big British institutions – not just the NHS. The monarchy, the BBC, even the established Church are all regularly in a sufficiently precarious position for commentators to wonder if things are drawing to a close – if the NHS, or the royal family, has had its time. It is quite hard to imagine our culture without any of them, but that doesn't mean they have a god-given right to exist. And just because a national health service was inevitable by the time 1945 came along doesn't mean it will inevitably survive.

The NHS opened its seventy-fifth year in what looked like its last battle: ambulances waiting for hours outside packed emergency departments; patients on trolleys or even dying on the floor, soaring waiting lists, patients turning to the private sector, and another debate in the political classes about whether it was time to let its life come to a close and move on. But to a certain extent the survival question is less important or interesting than one about the form in which the NHS *will* survive – and whether it will be a service that still performs its founding task of removing fear from people's lives. The backlog, which was exacerbated by the Covid pandemic, and queues of ambulances outside A&E departments, has meant that fear has crept back into people's thoughts about their health. If they have a heart attack, will the paramedics make it to them in time? If they find a lump, will the operation to remove it be cancelled repeatedly?

It is highly unlikely that we will see the end of the National Health Service any time soon, but what is more likely is that it struggles to return to a level of service that the public find acceptable – and so, as explored in the previous chapter, many start to turn elsewhere while continuing to support the principle of the service. This could, of course, have an impact on the readiness of voters to pay higher taxes to fund the NHS – but then again, the only real impact would be on the political fortunes of the party in power. There are also questions about what services the NHS can continue to offer patients, or whether it will have to scale back its ambitions in coming decades in a way not seen in its history so far.

The scale of the crisis that the health service faces has renewed the calls from its critics to consider an alternative model. At this stage, the 'NHS as a national religion' is wheeled out as the key reason why there hasn't been a proper debate about retiring an increasingly senile service and replacing it with something that is better suited to the modern day. It was Nigel Lawson who said: 'The National Health Service is the closest thing the English have to a religion, with those who practise in it regarding themselves as a priesthood. This made it quite extraordinarily difficult to reform.'[1]

But he wasn't the first to make these theological comparisons. Bevanite Barbara Castle described it in similar terms, saying: 'Intrinsically, the National Health Service is a church. It is the nearest thing to the embodiment of the Good Samaritan that we have in any aspect of our public policy.' It is worth pointing out that she was praying in aid of her policy on pay beds, adding: 'What would we say of a person who argued that he could only serve God properly if he had pay pews in his church?'[2] And a lot of the cultural behaviour around the health service is reminiscent of organised religion – right down to the cover-ups when things go wrong. There are some aspects of the British love for the NHS that are very hard to explain to outsiders: Justin Bieber helping a choir get to No. 1 being a recent example. But insiders don't always appreciate the strength of sentiment. Remember the discomfort that the carers who were being clapped during the pandemic felt – and I encountered a striking number of senior figures across the service who privately described some of the 'I Love the NHS' sentiment to me as 'a bit creepy'.

The problem with the NHS-as-religion argument is that it overlooks quite how many times it *has* been reformed since Lawson made that observation. It is more of a Church of England model of religion, where most adherents don't want things going too far, rather than strict Brethren. There are still certain lines that can't be crossed: the underlying model is not one the Brits seem willing to contemplate changing. Threats to local hospital services, however poor-quality, are almost always met with fury from the local population and from political representatives. In the 2004 Hartlepool by-election, Labour found itself under pressure in the seat it was defending, as rumours started to spread that the local hospital would close. So great was the threat that Tony Blair gave an interview to the *Hartlepool Mail* where he pledged: 'There is no question of the hospital closing or being run down. I hope people understand there has never been any question of the hospital closing. We are there to improve it and not run it down.'[3] Behind the scenes, the Labour campaign team in Hartlepool had asked John Reid to endorse the future of the hospital so they could 'save' it. His response was: 'Well, they will have the worst hospital in the country. But OK, we will do it.'

Labour already had experience of what would happen if a hospital wasn't 'safe' in an election. In the 2001 general election, Labour MP David Lock had decided to do what he thought was the right thing and support the downgrading of emergency services at Kidderminster General Hospital. He lost the Wyre Forest seat to a single-issue campaigner, Dr Richard Taylor, who beat him with a majority of 18,000. It served as a salutary warning to anyone who thought it was a good idea to try to reason with voters about the value of centralising certain services.

What Lawson really meant was not so much that the public don't like reorganisations – though they *don't* like them either, as it happens – but that they will not stomach a change to the model of the health service. The British suffer from exceptionalism in many quarters, but particularly on the notion that the NHS is the best in the world. In 2021, the Commonwealth Fund put the NHS fourth in its rankings of healthcare systems, below Norway, the Netherlands and Australia.[4] That's not a bad ranking, and the details of the study showed that the UK came out top for affordability of care. But then again, the UK was near the bottom for healthcare outcomes – at ninth, and above only Canada and the system everyone likes to scare people with, the US.

The high-ranking countries contain other models of healthcare provision that show it is not a binary between the highly centralised, taxpayer-funded, free-at-the-point-of-access National Health Service in the nations of Great Britain and the chaos of the United States. Norway is funded by a mixture of general taxation, contributory payments by employers and employees, and 'co-payment', which is upfront charges for certain services and products. Australia offers tax incentives for people who take out private health insurance on top of its universal taxpayer-funded public health insurance programme, and also makes far greater use of the private sector to provide services. In the Netherlands, which follows the Bismarck model of care, everyone is required by law to buy a basic package of health insurance covering GP care, hospital care, maternity, prescriptions and some mental health care from private companies, and the government oversees healthcare at arm's length. That last provided some inspiration for Andrew Lansley's ill-fated reforms, which among many other things have underlined that it is very difficult in British political culture for a Health Secretary not to end up taking a detailed interest in bedpans in individual hospitals, regardless of what the legal structures say they should get involved in. It might be worth asking politicians who argue for social insurance models whether they could bear to let go of the big train set that they so enjoy playing with – or whether the electorate would let them.

On the other side of the debate are those who excuse every failing of the NHS as merely being the result of underfunding. It is true that the health service has often run on the goodwill of its staff, which is one of the reasons the public hold it in such affection. It is also true that the UK has a bizarrely low capital spending budget for health, which means the equipment that can improve healthcare outcomes is often missing from practices and hospitals. But we have seen that toxic cultures can grow even when the spending taps are wide open. The New Labour era led to huge improvements in the quality of NHS care. It also contributed to a bullying culture that still hangs over the health service like a bad smell today.

The health service has had to move with the times, but often there has been resistance to that. It hasn't just been an internal, institutional resistance, though: some of the most vicious battles we've covered have been entirely political, and often fought over what different groups think was Bevan's vision, or whether that mattered at all. Even the battles which were about preserving the health service in a time of existential crisis often involved a great deal more internal party bickering than they did convincing the health service itself that it needed to change.

Modern healthcare – and that is not confined to the NHS – has been so successful in treating many illnesses that it now faces entirely different ones: a diagnosis of cancer now doesn't always mean time to start planning the funeral. It might yet mean you live long enough to develop dementia instead. Dementia, incidentally, did 'exist' back in 1948, and the arrival of the NHS allowed people who had been stigmatised for senility to get care. Today, people are living longer, and not only is dementia currently regarded as an inevitability of that, it is also often part of a complex package of conditions which the health service has to try to join up its many moving parts to treat in just one person.

Of course, the NHS is only responsible for the treatment of illness, rather than the long-term care of those in the population who have dementia. This book has not exhaustively covered the repeated failures to ensure that the social care sector responsible for the care of elderly and vulnerable adults works and is properly funded. Those failed reforms have stretched back decades. Today, local authorities have a legal obligation to provide care for those deemed to need it, but there is so little money available to finance the often complex, demanding and lengthy care packages that it can take weeks to set something up that is regarded as vaguely safe for a patient ready for discharge from hospital. The chronic crisis in social care places a severe financial burden on the health service, as patients stay in acute settings for longer, return to them more often and risk catching infections while they wait, to the extent that any politician today who talks about the NHS needing to be more efficient needs to take a long hard look at themselves and ask why they aren't helping it become more so by getting on with proper social care reform.

Even the claim by Boris Johnson's government to have 'reformed social care' was entirely false: it merely made an attempt to deal with the aspect of the care conundrum that most exercises Conservative voters, which is the risk of selling one's home to cover the costs of care. The Health and Social Care Levy introduced in April 2022, and then scrapped later that year, was ostensibly part of this plan to 'fix' social care by bringing more funding from a rise in national insurance contributions. But that money was earmarked for the NHS backlog to begin with, meaning the cash-starved care sector once again came second to its more politically salient relative and had to wait. The Johnson government did absolutely nothing to overhaul the system of social care so that more patients who are medically fit for discharge can leave hospital safely, with a local-authority-provided care package that offers more than a harried, underpaid carer charging in for fifteen minutes to try to wash, feed, talk to and dress an often socially isolated older person, before rushing off to their next visit.

One of the problems that all governments who have tried to reform social care have bumped up against is that people tend to think that it *is* part of the NHS already, or at least that it is already free, which means that any discussion of how to fund it, whether through taxation or through upfront costs, ends up frightening those who don't realise what the current upfront costs are. Theresa May came up against this in 2017 when she presumed she was going to win such an enormous majority in the snap election that she'd called that she could be honest with the electorate. It turned out that being honest wasn't such a good plan, especially not with a policy that was only half thought through at best. When I interviewed May about her time as prime minister, she explained: 'Social care wasn't going to be a key part of the campaign, but the key issue of the campaign was about being honest with the voters. And that's why the social care arguments came out in the way that they did, and on reflection of course, though we had done a lot of work on thinking about this, the timing meant it hadn't been possible to sort of socialise that and get more discussions with people going on that. So I recognise now that it rolled out cold to a lot of people.'

The annoying thing for May was that her plan – which involved people paying for their own care using the value of their home, until the last £100,000 worth of assets – wasn't the worst idea, even so far as the Labour politicians publicly campaigning against it were concerned. Many who I spoke to privately during that campaign admitted that they respected her for doing something, and for being honest – before saying that this wasn't going to stop them going out and branding it a 'dementia tax'. It was in part revenge for the 'death tax' label the Conservatives had given Andy Burnham's own attempt to reform social care just under a decade before. All's fair in elections – but May's shock loss of her majority made it even less likely that politicians would attempt genuine reform of the sector in future.

The impact on the NHS of a care sector that is on its knees is impossible to exaggerate. Every night that a medically fit patient spends in an NHS bed while the haggling over their care package continues costs hundreds of pounds to the health service, while other patients cannot be admitted or their surgery scheduled if there is no bed for them to move to. But if someone is given an unsafe discharge, they are likely to end up back in hospital again, often with far more serious needs.

The Health and Care Act 2022 was in part an attempt to address the dysfunctional interaction between social care and the NHS, and the change in the health of the population. It created 'integrated care systems' (ICSs) between primary and secondary care, mental health, social care and local government. The idea is that the partnerships within these systems will ensure the NHS is managed for the reality of twenty-first-century health, which generally involves one patient having a number of conditions and ongoing care needs, rather than one illness which needs to be dealt with by one silo of the health service. It is hard to accuse Bevan of creating a flaw in the health service that wouldn't address the needs of the population seventy-five years from its foundation. But the health service has *had* to change from his design, and to treat the 1948 set-up as sacrosanct would fail the very people he was most interested in helping. That's not to say that ICSs are necessarily the correct solution, by the way: it's just that for once the health service has largely been on board with the legislative changes rather than bracing itself reluctantly. But until social care reform actually happens, the NHS will never be able to function properly.

Has it ever functioned properly when it comes to mental health? From the very early days, Bevan was concerned that there was going to be a scandal in the long-stay psychiatric hospitals. By the late 1960s, there was one: at Ely Hospital in Cardiff. The *News of the World* reported whistle-blower allegations about mistreatment of the patients, and staff stealing from them at the institution – which had started out as a Poor Law school, converted to a workhouse, and joined the NHS in 1948. The 69,000-word report into conditions at the hospital was as much about the wider system of care for the mentally ill as it was about Ely itself. It found individual acts of cruelty, but also a system that made it impossible for those in the hospital's 'care' to have any dignity: just three doctors, only two of them full-time, were responsible for more than 660 patients. Some of those patients, generally the most vulnerable, were isolated even within the cut-off institution, and subject to rough treatment by the nursing staff. Incidents were regularly covered up. The report led to better inspection of hospitals, and contributed to the movement of closing long-stay institutions in favour of care in the community. Ely remains a landmark case in the NHS.

It is unfortunately not clear whether the service has changed that much for many acute patients. Indeed, after the scandals on patient care at Mid Staffs and the multiple maternity failures, the next big NHS scandal was in mental health. In March 2022, an independent inquiry into deaths in mental health units run by the North Essex Partnership University NHS Foundation Trust (NEP) announced it was probing 1,500 cases of patients who had died either while inpatients or within three months of discharge, but by January 2023 that number had grown to 2,000. The inquiry was set up to cover deaths between 1 January 2000 and 31 December 2020. Richard Wade was one of those who died. He was thirty years old and had been admitted to the Linden Centre in Chelmsford in May 2015. It was his first inpatient admission. Within twelve hours he had tried to take his own life, and his parents were there when staff found him. He died four days later. An internal investigation discovered Richard had been left with a number of items with which he could have harmed himself, despite staff knowing he was being admitted because he was suicidal. A report into his death and that of Matthew Leahy, who also died at the Linden Centre, by the Parliamentary and Health Service Ombudsman found that 'year after year there was a repeated failure to recognise the seriousness of the ongoing risks to the safety of people using NEP's acute adult inpatient service', and that the trust was not learning the lessons of incidents.[5] Richard's father, Robert, told the inquiry into his death: 'They didn't care. They didn't care for him, they didn't seem to care for their professionalism, the consequence was he paid a big price.'[6]

At the outpatient level, things are little better: the NHS has never really universalised care, let alone the best care, for people with mental illnesses. The health service has been committed for the past decade to something called 'parity of esteem', which means it aims to – in the words of its constitution – 'improve, prevent, diagnose and treat both physical and mental health problems with equal regard'. The 'Five Year Forward View' that Simon Stevens published in 2014 said 'we have a much wider ambition to achieve genuine parity of esteem between mental and physical health by 2020'. That was not achieved – not even close. Since the pandemic, the NHS England mandate – the instructions from the government to the health service – has promised merely to 'treat mental health with the same urgency as physical health'. By the time that period in the 'Five Year Forward View' came to an end, a third of its goals on mental health had not been met. It had set targets for improving treatment which were both ambitious and pathetic – tiny levels of access to treatment which were nonetheless still very hard to reach. One was that, by 2020/21, 25 per cent – around 1.5 million – of people who need therapy for anxiety and depression should be able to access it. The modest level of this target alone shows how poor access was prior to 2014. But that target was still too ambitious for the health service to meet: by 2020/21, the Improving Access to Psychological Therapies (IAPT) programme had missed its target by a whopping 32 per cent.

The IAPT target was for two of the more user-friendly illnesses. Anxiety and depression can be totally debilitating, life-threatening illnesses (I should know: I suffer from both conditions myself). But they are still better understood than conditions with psychotic symptoms such as bipolar disorder or schizophrenia, or the 'personality disorder' group of diagnoses, which within the health service seem to load extremely vulnerable and traumatised patients with the stigma of being 'manipulative'. The NHS is so underfunded when it comes to eating disorders – the most deadly mental illnesses – that sufferers are often told they cannot be treated unless they have lost more weight. The government pledged to end the practice of transporting patients out-of-area for a bed by the end of 2021, but there were still 660 inappropriate out-of-area placements in England. Out-of-area doesn't just mean taking someone into a nearby county, but often hundreds of miles across the country to the first available bed – and therefore hours away from their family and support network. Child and Adolescent Mental Health Services (CAMHS) are in an appalling state. Between April 2020 and March 2021, one in five young patients waited more than twelve weeks for a follow-up appointment.

Does the NHS really exist in any meaningful sense for mental health, when access is this poor? If the health service was set up to end the fear of having to find the money or languish without treatment, it has demonstrably failed when it comes to mental health. Despite the efforts of many ministers – including Enoch Powell – there has not really been a National Health Service for mental health in its seventy-five-year history, and there may not be a proper one come the centenary either.

The real missing piece in the health service today that was present in the original visions for the NHS, and that remains as relevant now as it was at its foundation, is prevention. The NHS is often described by its critics as a National Sickness Service, and it manages illnesses with varying levels of success. But it has done far less in the preventive field.

When he wrote *In Place of Fear*, Bevan argued that 'the victories won by preventive medicine are much the most important for mankind. This is so not only because it is obviously preferable to prevent suffering than to alleviate it.'[7] The trouble is that as soon as someone starts talking about the importance of prevention, everyone else nods in recognition of this worthy topic before their eyes glaze over. We don't view preventive healthcare as being interesting or important in the British health service. One of the key differences between the UK and other developed nations on health policy is that our health spend is heavily weighted towards hospitals. It's easy to see that just from this book, which has covered battles largely fought over acute care, not outpatient or preventive care – meaning the NHS tends to make contact with people once they are sick, not before.

We saw in the early years of the health service the struggle that scientists had to make ministers – and doctors – pay attention to the mounting research that smoking was killing people. That cost the NHS dearly in the treatment of lung cancer, emphysema, heart problems and other illnesses: when the government finally outlined the 'Smoking Kills' plan for cutting down on the prevalence of smoking in 1998, it was costing the NHS in England an estimated £1.4–1.7 billion. The NHS's belated work on cutting down smoking has paid off: it has fallen in prevalence from 20 per cent of adults in 2011 to 14 per cent in 2019. But the lessons from that extremely long period between understanding the risks and really doing something about them have not been learned for another preventable health problem which is already costing far more.

Obesity was not something Bevan needed to worry himself with, not least because at the time he was working on his blueprint, food was still being rationed to the population. Now, it is a major concern. In 2019, 64 per cent of adults in England were overweight, with 28 per cent obese and 3 per cent morbidly obese. People living in deprived communities are far more likely to be obese: the gap for women between the most and least deprived areas is 17 percentage points, while for men it is 8 percentage points. It is a complex, emotive subject, as it often leads to suggestions that someone who is obese is at fault for burdening the NHS. But if obesity is viewed less at an individual level and more as a public health failure of one kind or another, then it is difficult to justify inaction in tackling it. One million hospital admissions in 2019–20 were linked to obesity. The cost to the service is expected to reach £9.7 billion a year by 2050. Obesity was discovered to be a major factor in whether someone developed serious, life-threatening Covid. Successive governments have tinkered with 'obesity strategies', most of which have been watered down or poorly implemented. Much of the anti-obesity work is cross-government, but it would be wrong to say the NHS has no role in preventing it, whether in equipping primary care practitioners to offer proper evidence-based nutrition advice, or in the social prescribing of group exercise such as parkrun, or in the sort of surgical interventions that often get the most media attention, such as bariatric surgery.

A hugely significant moment in the preventive agenda came in 2008 when Ara Darzi, a pioneering colorectal surgeon, published a review for Gordon Brown's government. Entitled *High Quality Care for All*, this report tried to move the NHS away from merely aiming to meet targets fast and towards a focus on improving care and outcomes. Darzi's role as a 'goat' (a member of the 'government of all talents') was eye-catching, and was the sort of smart-sounding idea that could easily shatter on contact with the reality of political life. But in Lord Darzi, Brown and his Health Secretary Alan Johnson had found a really good goat.

Darzi had made his name in robotic and other minimally invasive forms of surgery, and his report included a great deal on how advances in technology could improve quality of outcomes and of life more generally for people who came into contact with the NHS. Darzi's professional life involved him working with patients for whom things had already gone very wrong, and whose illnesses he wanted to treat. But he was also fascinated by prevention, not least because of the strong tradition of public health in Britain. 'Queen Victoria would have been the best public health doctor that this country has ever seen,' he told me. 'But we haven't kept up with that. Population-based interventions are important, and we need to move into a more sophisticated way of doing them. I'm not talking about the classic public health work, which is about giving everyone a vaccine in winter. I'm talking about identifying those at the greatest risk so that we can actually intervene firstly to prevent their illnesses.' In Darzi's eyes, technology is the key to preventative healthcare. It's hard not to catch his excitement about it.

Artificial intelligence is something politicians like to mention when they're trying to sound in touch with the times, along with 3D printing, without necessarily understanding what it is or what it is already achieving in fields such as medical science. In 2020, a team which included researchers from Imperial College London wrote up a study of an AI model they had created to detect breast cancer from mammograms. It was more effective at spotting cancer than one doctor working alone, and was as good as the current labour-intensive system of two radiologists assessing each mammogram. Given the workforce crisis in the NHS, AI could make clinicians' workloads much more bearable. In three major London hospitals – Barts, the Royal Free and University College Hospital – another AI tool saves doctors thirteen minutes per patient as it analyses heart MRI scans and spots heart disease.

Big data – a term that sounds as evil as Big Pharma and all the other Big Nasties that allegedly ruin the world in insidious ways – can, if used responsibly, allow a health system to personalise treatment to the patient, rather than run it through standardised protocols. It can predict who is most at risk of a certain illness *before* they become ill – thus allowing interventions to be targeted, less costly and more effective. It has already helped the health service with its waiting lists: a pilot of the Foundry system run by the not-uncontroversial US tech company Palantir at Chelsea and Westminster Hospital helped cut the waiting list there by 28 per cent. Its dashboard allows entire teams to work out which surgeries are the real priority, and which operations are possible when – according to who is on the rota and which theatre is available.

But there is a problem. Not all parts of the NHS are currently capable of using these whizzy technologies. In June 2022, Health Secretary Sajid Javid attracted some ridicule when he told the Cabinet that this country has a 'Blockbuster healthcare system in the age of Netflix'. It didn't help that he was speaking the morning after Boris Johnson had survived the vote of confidence in his leadership, which nevertheless revealed that 40 per cent of his party didn't support him. It also didn't help that Netflix is a service people pay for that has nonetheless struggled to make money. But what Javid was aiming at was clear: he told colleagues that 'large-scale changes were needed in areas such as the use of technology and data to help front-line workers deliver the high-quality service the public expects'. This was not a ridiculous statement to make: less than a year prior to this, the newly appointed chief executive of NHS England, Amanda Pritchard, told MPs on the Health and Social Care Select Committee that a large section of the NHS was lagging behind the modern world: 'About a fifth of trusts in the NHS are still largely paper-based. We have some that are absolutely at the other end, but that is a very important thing to be able to fix if we are to achieve some of the interconnectivity we were talking about earlier.'[8] Even within trusts that weren't paper-based, there have been astonishing failures of technology. One recent health minister described walking into a flagship NHS hospital and being impressed by a nurse in charge of the emergency department, who was directing operations from behind two computer screens 'like a city trading desk'. It turned out, though, that the reason this nurse had two screens was that 'two of the different hubs within that emergency department had different computers that wouldn't talk to each other. So somebody came into resus and then went into majors once they'd been stabilised, and he would then have to type the details from their entry and transcribe it from one screen to another'.[9]

The NHS itself accepts that it needs to move with the times, but often fails to do so. Part of this is down to capital funding, part of it is down to the siloed way in which different branches of the service operate. Either way, as Pritchard made clear, the benefits to health-care from exciting technological advances are only going to be felt if the system is managing basic digital functions, too.

When the doctor assisting Edna Thomas in her labour on 4 July 1948 told her to hold on, he created a moment's peace at the end of the fighting that was necessary to create the National Health Service.

What a lot more fighting there will have to be for the future of the NHS to be secure. And those battles will be even bigger and harder, to ensure that this future is a strong, effective one where the British love of the principles of the health service doesn't outstrip what the NHS can actually deliver. It should be clear by now that, despite the rainbows, dancing Olympic nurses and choirs, the story of the NHS is in fact a story of a lot of fights: from pugnacious Bevan having an almighty battle with the doctors and his own colleagues; to the patients and relatives fighting for better care during the worst times of their lives; and to the NHS staff fighting for our lives – and theirs – during the pandemic. There will be more fights to come between the BMA and the politicians, and more within the NHS itself as it tries to adapt to the modern patient – and others (including the patients themselves) resist that change. Alan Milburn used to say that every day as Health Secretary he had an argument. Even the more pacific of his fellow ministers over the past seventy-five years would struggle to disagree with that.

But the fighting in recent years has become pettier and Lilliputian in comparison to the scale of the challenges facing the health service. Protect the NHS? Yes, that's the real war that the public still want politicians to fight, but the politicians couldn't even define that in the pandemic, let alone in the longer lifetime of the health service. Instead, we have a reorganisation of the train set here, and forty 'new hospitals' there. At election time, everyone parades their commitment to 'our NHS', but without either the honesty about what will be necessary to make it thrive for another seventy-five years, or the vision for how to achieve that. Lists of thousands more nurses and so many billions more in spending pledges won't cut it.

Our health landscape today is returning to the two tiers of the pre-NHS days, where people who were rich could get excellent treatment, and the rest had to hope for the best. Now, to get treatment for many conditions, you either have to be rich so you can go private, or face languishing on a waiting list. It is not clear when the health service will be able to overcome its backlog. In some disciplines, it may never.

What the NHS now needs is someone – or several someones, as was the case by the time it was founded in 1948 – to create a new vision for it. That will be a health service that answers the needs of the future, rather than pays tribute to the problems it solved three-quarters of a century ago. There has been enough lovebombing from politicians too fearful or lazy to confront the truth about the state of the service and what it needs. Now, it needs someone who knows what they are really fighting for. Depending on how well they fight, it could be either the latest or the last battle of the NHS's long struggle to exist in place of fear.

Acknowledgements

The NHS is the size of a small country, and a similarly large group of people have ensured that this book exists. Tom Killingbeck had the wonderful idea of writing a history of the health service for its seventy-fifth anniversary – and as I was giving birth when he approached me about it, I was of insufficiently sound mind to turn it down. I am grateful for his enthusiasm and encouragement in the early half of the project. Alpana Sajip has been a truly wonderful editor and helped me prune my way out of various thickets of NHS complexity, as well as patiently waiting for the latest political explosion to subside as I tried to complete the manuscript. Once again, my agent Andrew Gordon has given me so much advice and support throughout this project, and I am so grateful for the way he has guided me as a writer. My researcher Lucia Henwood has been brilliant in finding interviewees, old articles and organisations for me. I am in awe of how young and talented she is.

A huge number of people within the health world have been extraordinarily generous with their time and wisdom. Nigel Edwards at the Nuffield Trust not only helped me understand so much but also kindly read through the book in its early stages, as did Andy Cowper of Health Policy Insight. The King's Fund opened their archive for me and suggested documents; and the Health Foundation advised me repeatedly. Geoffrey Rivett, the wonderful and detailed historian of the health service who himself worked within it in its early years, has been kind with his time and advice. The staff in the Sound Archive at the British Library have opened up recordings that were previously inaccessible and suggested ones I hadn't even thought of. They then had to put up with the unnecessarily loud sound of my furious typing, which led a number of disgusted fellow readers to move away from me in the reading rooms at St Pancras.

I am thanking my husband John for enabling me to write a book for the third time – with each manuscript there have been different challenges in terms of time and health, and he has risen to them all magnificently, whether it be spending the entire week home alone with our chicken-poxy toddler, or listening to me burble on about what I found at the National Archives. My *Spectator* colleagues have given me the freedom to disappear into an archive for a week – and to emerge talking non-stop about the NHS.

Finally, I am grateful to the many people who took the time to speak to me about their times in the NHS. As I write in this book, almost all of us have our own NHS stories, but for some of my interviewees the memories I asked them to recall were painful ones, either of terrible loss and suffering or of working in intolerable conditions. Thanks to their courage in being able to talk, we have a clearer understanding of how many fights there have been in the life of the health service.

Notes

Abbreviations

BMJ	*British Medical Journal*
CAB	The Cabinet Papers
HC Deb	House of Commons debate (Hansard)
HL Deb	House of Lords debate (Hansard)
MH	Ministry of Health
PREM	Prime Minister's Office

Chapter 1: Holding on for something new

1. Aneira Thomas, *Hold On Edna!: The Heart-Warming True Story of the First Baby Born on the NHS*, Mirror Books, eBook, 2020, p. 9.
2. Ibid., p. 116.
3. Party Political Broadcast for the Labour Party, first broadcast by the BBC on Saturday, 3 April 1948, at 21.15 on BBC Home Service Basic.
4. Charles W. Brook, 'Making Medical History', 24 March 1946, https://www.sochealth.co.uk/national-health-service/the-sma-and-the-foundation-of-the-national-health-service-dr-leslie-hilliard-1980/making-medical-history-charles-w-brook-1946/.
5. Ibid.
6. Charles W. Brook, 'Problems of the Post War Practitioner', *Medicine Today and Tomorrow*, June 1940, https://www.sochealth.co.uk/the-socialist-health-association/socialism-and-health/medicine-today-and-tomorrow/problems-of-the-post-war-practitioner/.
7. HC Deb, 17 October 1940, vol. 365, col. 852.
8. José Harris, *William Beveridge: A Biography*, Clarendon Press, 1997, pp. 1–2.
9. Nicholas Timmins, *The Five Giants: A Biography of the Welfare State*, 3rd edition, HarperCollins Publishers, 2017.

10. 'Social Insurance: General Considerations', CAB 87/76.

11. 'Heads of a Scheme for Social Security', 11 December 1941, CAB 87/76.

12. *The Times*, 17 March 1942, p. 5.

13. *The Times*, 15 July 1942, p. 5.

14. Timmins, *Five Giants*.

15. *Nine O'Clock News,* BBC, 2 December 1942.

16. William Beveridge, *Social Insurance and Allied Services* (Beveridge Report), Command Paper 6404, 1942, p. 7.

17. *Daily Telegraph*, 2 December 1942, pp. 1, 6.

18. *The Times*, 2 December 1942, p. 5.

19. *Tribune*, 4 December 1942.

20. Nicklaus Thomas-Symonds, *Nye: The Political Life of Aneurin Bevan*, Bloomsbury Publishing, 2014, p. 97.

21. Ibid., p. 251.

22. Published in 1937, *The Citadel* was – like the Beveridge Report a few years later – a bestseller. It also won awards and, according to a poll by Gallup, 'impressed' more people than any other book except the Bible.

23. Gallup poll, February 1939.

24. Minutes of Tredegar Working Men's Medical Aid Society, MH 49/27.

25. Timmins, *Five Giants*.

26. HL Deb, 24 February 1943, vol. 126, col. 268.

27. Social Insurance and Allied Services Debate, 18 February 1943, vol. 386.

28. Ibid.

29. The Labour Party, *National Service for Health: The Labour Party's Post-War Policy*, London: Labour Party, April 1943.

30. *The Times*, 27 July 1914.

31. *The Times*, 20 March 1838.

32. *BMJ*, vol. 1, 1943, p. 193.

33. First broadcast Friday, 5 February 1943 at 21.20 on BBC Home Service Basic.

34. Ministry of Health, Department of Health for Scotland. *A National Health Service* [White Paper], His Majesty's Stationery Office, 1944.

35. CAB 124/244, 10 February 1944.

36. John Pater, *The Making of the National Health Service*, King Edward's Hospital Fund for London, 1981, pp. 103–4.

37. Timmins, *Five Giants*.

38. This and other quotes that follow are from various Cabinet minutes and memos.
39. Michael Foot, *Aneurin Bevan: A Biography; Volume 2: 1945–1960*, Davis-Poynter, 1973, p. 134.
40. CAB 129/5.
41. CAB 129/6.
42. National Health Service Bill Debate, 30 April 1946, vol. 422.
43. *BMJ*, vol. 1, 1946, p. 461.
44. Ibid., p. 489.
45. Ibid., p. 541.
46. Ibid., p. 583.
47. *BMJ*, vol. 2, 1946, p. 27.
48. Cabinet Paper 48/23, 19 January 1948, CAB 129/23.

Chapter 2: Bills, bills, bills

1. *Hull Daily Mail*, 3 July 1948, p. 3.
2. *Western Morning News*, 5 July 1948, p. 2.
3. *Daily Herald*, 7 July 1948, p. 2.
4. *Manchester Evening News*, 5 July 1948, p. 3.
5. 4 July 1948, BBC Home Service.
6. *BMJ*, vol. 2, 3 July 1948.
7. 'Bevan's speech to the Manchester Labour rally, 4 July 1948', https://www.sochealth.co.uk/national-health-service/the-sma-and-the-foundation-of-the-national-health-service-dr-leslie-hilliard-1980/aneurin-bevan-and-the-foundation-of-the-nhs/bevans-speech-to-the-manchester-labour-rally-4-july-1948/.
8. Thomas-Symonds, *Nye*, p. 73.
9. *Sunday Dispatch*, 11 July 1948, p. 1.
10. *National Health Stories*, first broadcast on BBC Radio 4, https://www.bbc.co.uk/programmes/b0b7mxnq/episodes/player.
11. *Guardian*, 12 July 1948, p. 3.
12. Interview with author.
13. *Montreal Star*, May 1951, p. 33.
14. *National Health Stories*, 22 June 2018.

15. Timmins, *Five Giants*.
16. *Birmingham Post*, 4 July 2008.
17. *Liverpool Echo,* 13 July 1948, p. 2.
18. Broadcast on BBC Home Service, 6 October 1949.
19. Herbert Morrison, *An Autobiography*, Odhams Press, 2006, p. 267.
20. Foot, *Aneurin Bevan*, p. 292.
21. Thomas-Symonds, *Nye*, p. 181.
22. CAB 128/21.
23. Ibid.
24. Ibid.
25. Ibid.
26. HC Deb, 27 March 1952, vol. 498, cols. 880–96.
27. *Birmingham Post*, 2 May 1951, p. 3.
28. *BMJ*, vol. 317, no. 7150, July 1998, pp. 37–40.
29. Iain Macleod, *The Future of the Welfare State*, 1958.
30. Rudolf Klein, *The New Politics of the NHS*, 7th edition, Radcliffe Publishing Ltd., eBook, 2019, p. 23.
31. Charles Webster, *The National Health Service: A Political History*, Oxford University Press, 2002, pp. 32–3.
32. John Hopewell, *The Early History of the Treatment of Renal Failure*, British Transplantation Society, n.d., https://bts.org.uk/wp-content/uploads/2016/09/BTS_EarlyHistoryRenalFailure-1.pdf.
33. *National Health Stories*, 26 June 2018.
34. Ibid.
35. Ibid.
36. Virginia Berridge, *Demons: Our Changing Attitude to Alcohol, Tobacco and Drugs*, Oxford University Press, eBook, 2013, p. 145.
37. Harold Macmillan, entry for 19 April 1956, *The Macmillan Diaries: The Cabinet Years, 1950–1957*, ed. P. Catterall, Macmillan, 2003, p. 551.
38. Berridge, *Demons*, p. 146.
39. Interview, Oxford Brookes University, The Royal College of Physicians, 1984.
40. Ibid.
41. Berridge, *Demons*, p. 146.
42. Scottish Health Education Group, 1980.

Chapter 3: Making the modern health service

1. The Hospital Plan, HL Deb, 14 February 1962, vol. 237, cols. 472–581.

2. *Supplement to the BMJ*, 4 April 1959, https://www.bmj.com/content/1/5126/S109.

3. *National Health Stories*, 'Modern Hospital', 28 June 2018.

4. 'Zena Edmund-Charles', QniHeritage, https://qniheritage.org.uk/stories/zena-edmund-charles-mbe-nee-josephs/.

5. Ministry of Health, Central Health Services Council, 'The Pattern of the In-Patient's Day', Her Majesty's Stationery Office, 1961.

6. *Desert Island Discs*, 19 February 1989.

7. Simon Heffer, *Like the Roman: The Life of Enoch Powell*, Faber and Faber, eBook, 2014.

8. Enoch Powell, interview with Margot Jefferys, 11 July 1991.

9. *Daily Express*, 2 February 1961.

10. Heffer, *Like the Roman*.

11. CAB 129/102.

12. National Health Service (Increased Charges and Contributions), HC Deb, 1 February 1961, vol. 633.

13. Interview with Margot Jeffreys.

14. Sir George Godber, interview with Sir Christopher Booth, 13 January 1994, https://radar.brookes.ac.uk/radar/file/42415f8c-c725-4d4c-9e23-9d6a498f471f/1/Godber%2CG.pdf.

15. Ibid.

16. *BMJ*, vol. 2, 1958, p. S1.

17. Sir George Godber, *Change in Medicine*, Nuffield Provincial Hospitals Trust, 1975, p. 2.

18. *Studies in the Function and Design of Hospitals*, Nuffield Provincial Hospitals Trust, 1955, https://www.nuffieldtrust.org.uk/files/2017-01/functions-and-design-of-hospitals-web-final.pdf.

19. Interview with Margot Jeffreys.

20. Ministry of Health, *A Hospital Plan for England and Wales*, Command Paper 1604, 1962.

21. Alistair Horne, *Macmillan: The Official Biography*, Pan Macmillan, eBook, 2012.

22. *The Times*, 11 October 1962, p. 13.

23. Interview with Margot Jeffreys.

24. *Architectural Review*, 'Health and Hospitals: A Special Issue', vol. 820, June 1965, p. 417.

25. 'Wasting Disease', *Building*, 7 February 1992, https://www.building.co.uk/our-history-170-years-of-building/this-week-in-1997/5086164.article.

26. 'From Showpiece to Scrapheap', *HSJ*, 18 March 1998, https://www.hsj.co.uk/home/from-showpiece-to-scrap-heap/32683.article.

27. Michael Webb, 'A Hospital on an Expansive Plan', *Country Life*, 9 February 1967, pp. 276–7.

28. Nigel Crisp, *24 Hours to Save the NHS: The Chief Executive's Account of Reform 2000 to 2006*, Oxford University Press, eBook, 2011, p. 19.

29. Timmins, *Five Giants*, p. 210.

30. *The Speeches of John Enoch Powell, November 1957–September 1965*, 2011, File 5, 1962–1963, http://enochpowell.info/wp-content/uploads/Speeches/1962-1963.pdf.

31. Ibid., File 6, 1957–1961, http://enochpowell.info/wp-content/uploads/Speeches/1957-1961.pdf.

32. Ibid.

33. Timmins, *Five Giants*.

34. Paul Bridgen and Jane Lewis, *Elderly People and the Boundary between Health and Social Care, 1946-91: Whose Responsibility?*, Nuffield Trust Grant Report No. 1, 1999, https://www.nuffieldtrust.org.uk/files/2017-01/elderly-people-boundary-health-social-care-web-final.pdf.

35. PREM 19/5761.

36. *Desert Island Discs*, 19 February 1989.

37. Interview with Margot Jeffreys.

38. Stephanie Snow and Emma Jones, *Immigration and the National Health Service: Putting History to the Forefront* [policy paper], 8 March 2011, https://www.historyandpolicy.org/policy-papers/papers/immigration-and-the-national-health-service-putting-history-to-the-forefront.

39. HC Deb, 16 June 1971, vol. 819, cols. 547–72.

40. Heffer, *Like the Roman*.

41. HC Deb, 8 May 1963, vol. 377, cols. 439–559.

42. *Daily Herald*, 3 March 1955.

43. *Birmingham Daily Post*, 12 January 1961.

44. British Library, Sound and Moving Image Catalogue, Overseas Trained South Asian Geriatrician Interviews.

45. *Black Nurses: The Women Who Saved the NHS* [documentary], BBC, 2016.

46. *Reading Evening Post*, 23 December 1965.

47. Lord Howard of Rising, *Enoch at 100: A Re-evaluation of the Life, Politics and Philosophy of Enoch Powell*, Biteback Publishing, eBook, 2014.

Chapter 4: The fight for rights

1. 'Consuming Interest', *Spectator,* 22 November 1963, p. 29.

2. J. McN. Dodgson, 'A Survey of English Folk Medicine', https://bjgp.org/content/bjgp/6/3/462.full.pdf.

3. *The Times*, 12 July 1957, p. 9.

4. Lara Marks, *Sexual Chemistry: A History of the Contraceptive Pill*, Yale University Press, 2001, p. 109.

5. Birth Control Pills, HC Deb, 4 December 1961, vol. 650, cols. 922–3.

6. MH 135/108.

7. Ibid.

8. *The Times*, 2 June 1961.

9. *National Health Stories*, 'Sexual Health Service', 29 June 2018.

10. *Aberdeen Evening Express*, 30 July 1965.

11. Obituary by Sally Sheard, *Guardian*, December 2013.

12. Barbara Seaman, *The Doctors' Case Against the Pill*, Doubleday, 1980, p. 12.

13. Marks, *Sexual Chemistry*, p. 186.

14. Harold Evans, *My Paper Chase: True Stories of Vanished Times*, Little, Brown, eBook, 2009.

15. Abortion (Inter-Departmental Committee), HC Deb, 24 May 1937, vol. 324, cols.18–9.

16. MH 71/23.

17. Greta Barnes, *Scissors, Nurse, Scissors!* Obelisk Books, 2009, p. 45.

18. *The Times*, 10 February 1966, p. 6.

19. *The Times*, 15 July 1966.

20. Medical Termination of Pregnancy Bill, HC Deb, 22 July 1966, vol. 732, cols. 1067–1165.

21. *Independent*, 26 October 2017.
22. T. L. Lewis, 'The Abortion Act', *BMJ*, 25 January 1969.
23. Webster, *The National Health Service*, p. 135.
24. Klein, *The New Politics of the NHS*, p. 63.
25. DHSC, 'Abortion: Statistics, England and Wales: 2019', https:// assets.publishing.service.gov.uk/government/uploads/system/uploads/ attachment_data/file/891405/abortion-statistics-commentary-2019.pdf.
26. Professor Gordon Harold, oral evidence to the Joint Committee on Human Rights, *The Right to Family Life: Adoption of Children of Unmarried Women 1949–1976*, HC 748, 15 December 2021, https://committees. parliament.uk/oralevidence/3219/pdf/.
27. Interview with author.
28. *If You Love Your Baby . . . The Story of Forced Adoptions* [documentary], first broadcast on BBC News, 31 May 2021.
29. 'Editorials: The Report of the Maternity Services Committee', *British Journal of General Practice*, vol. 2, no. 113, 1959, https://www.ncbi.nlm. nih.gov/pmc/articles/PMC1890186/pdf/rcgpresnews00010-0009.pdf.
30. A. Susan Williams, *Women and Childbirth in the Twentieth Century*, Alan Sutton Publishing, 1997, p. 199.
31. A. A. Woodman, *Sunday Express Baby Book: Prenatal to Six Years*, London Express, n.d., p. 31.
32. Ibid., p. 32.
33. https://warwick.ac.uk/fac/arts/history/chm/outreach/hiding_in_the_ pub/memories/.
34. 'Listen with Mother', *AIMS Journal*, vol. 19, no. 2, 2007, https://www. aims.org.uk/journal/item/listen-with-mother.
35. Jessica Dick-Read and Prunella Briance, *What Every Woman Should Know About Childbirth*, William Heinemann Medical Books, 1965.
36. *BMJ*, 29 December 1956, https://www.bmj.com/content/2/5008/1545.4.
37. *BMJ*, 13 April 1957, https://www.bmj.com/content/bmj/1/5023/882.4. full.pdf.
38. D. L. Muirhead, '40 Years Hard Labour', *Ulster Medical Journal*, vol. 77, no. 2, 2008, pp. 79–85.

Chapter 5: Forwards and backwards

1. E. M. Tansey and L. A. Reynolds (eds), *Wellcome Witnesses to Twentieth Century Medicine*, vol. 3: *Early Heart Transplant Surgery in the UK*, Wellcome Trust, 1997, http://www.histmodbiomed.org/sites/default/files/44825.pdf.
2. Ibid.
3. Ibid.
4. Ibid.
5. *BMJ*, 11 May 1968.
6. *BMJ*, vol. 2, 1968, p. 558.
7. *Private Eye,* 5 July 1968.
8. *Aberdeen Evening Express*, 12 September 1969, p. 1.
9. Terence English, *Follow Your Star: From Mining to Heart Transplants*, AuthorHouse, 2011, p. 90.
10. Ibid., p. 91.
11. Interview with author.
12. English, p. 99.
13. *Evening Standard*, 13 March 1981, p. 13.
14. *Evening Standard*, 3 July 1985, p. 5.
15. Donald Longmore, *The Rise and Fall of the NHS*, ShieldCrest, 2012, p. 102.
16. Ibid., p. 103.
17. Interview with author.
18. *The Times*, 4 May 1982, p. 10.
19. *National Health Stories*, 4 July 2018.
20. *Observer*, 17 July 1978, p. 2.
21. *Observer*, 23 March 1980, p. 46.
22. '25 July 1978: A Very Special Night and a Very Special Baby Girl', Care Fertility, 17 July 2018, https://www.carefertility.com/blog/25-july-1978-a-very-special-night-and-a-very-special-baby-girl/.
23. *National Health Stories*, 4 July 2018.
24. Churchill Archives Centre, Cambridge, GBR/0014/EDWS.
25. *Daily Mirror*, 28 August 1978, p. 6.
26. M. Warnock, *Report of the Committee of Inquiry into Human Fertilisation and Embryology*, Command Report 9314, 1984.

27. *Observer*, 18 August 1985, p. 3.

28. William L. Ledger et al., 'Fertility and Assisted Reproduction: The Costs to the NHS of Multiple Births after IVF Treatment in the UK', *BJOG*, vol. 113, no. 1, January 2006, p. 21–5.

29. P. N. T. Wells, 'Sir Godfrey Newbold Hounsfield KT CBE: 28 August 1919 – 12 August 2004', *Biographical Memoirs of Fellows of the Royal Society*, vol. 51, 2005, pp. 221–35.

30. Ibid.

31. MH 99/127.

32. *The Times*, 6 July 1974, p. 1.

33. *Desert Island Discs*, 11 November 1990.

34. Wilfred De'Ath, *Barbara Castle: A Portrait from Life*, Clifton Books, 1970, p. 21.

35. Ibid., p. 41.

36. Anne Perkins, *Red Queen: The Authorized Biography of Barbara Castle*, Pan Macmillan, 2004, p. 393.

37. *The Times*, 5 July 1974, p. 4.

38. *The Times*, 6 July 1974, p. 1.

39. Perkins, *Red Queen*.

40. MH 150/786.

41. PREM 16/568.

42. Barbara Castle, *The Castle Diaries, 1964–1976*, Trans-Atlantic, 1990, p. 344.

43. MH 150/786.

44. *Castle Diaries*, p. 372.

45. Ibid., pp. 574–6.

46. *Reading Evening Post*, 12 December 1975, p. 4.

47. *Evening Standard*, 5 December 1975, p. 6.

48. *Castle Diaries*, p. 725.

49. Timmins, *Five Giants*.

Chapter 6: A Big Bang or a whimper?

1. Charles Moore, *Margaret Thatcher*, Penguin Books, eBook, 2013, p. 79.

2. Ibid., p. 88.

3. Interview with author.

4. Thatcher Archive, CCOPR 481/87.

5. Interview with author.

6. Timmins, *Five Giants*.

7. Nigel Lawson, *Memoirs of a Tory Radical*, Biteback Publishing, eBook, 2011.

8. Moore, *Margaret Thatcher*, p. 28.

9. T 639/88.

10. PREM 19/1091.

11. *The Times*, 15 November 1983, p. 2.

12. *The Times*, 4 February 1983, p. 2.

13. Timmins, *Wellcome Witnesses*.

14. PREM 19/1091.

15. Ibid.

16. Richard Crossman, *A Politician's View of Health Service Planning*, University of Glasgow, 1972, p. 10.

17. Sir Michael Bett in Martin Gorsky (ed.), *The Griffiths NHS Management Inquiry: Its Origins, Nature and Impact*, Centre for History in Public Health, London School of Hygiene and Tropical Medicine, January 2010, p. 27, https://www.lshtm.ac.uk/media/31881.

18. E. R. Griffiths, *NHS Management Inquiry: Griffiths Report on NHS*, October 1983, https://www.sochealth.co.uk/national-health-service/griffiths-report-october-1983/.

19. *Health Service Journal*, 3 July 2008, NHS60 anniversary supplement, p. 7.

20. Ibid., p. 70.

21. *BMJ (Clinical Research Ed)*, vol. 288, 1984, p. 255.

22. *Health Service Journal*, 3 July 2008, NHS60 anniversary supplement, p. 10.

23. Interview with author.

24. *Wellcome Witnesses*.

25. Interview with author.

26. *Sevenoaks Focus*, 22 October 1987, p. 39.

27. *Evening Standard*, 26 June 1987, p. 10.

28. *Birmingham Daily News*, 26 November 1987, p. 1.

29. Oral Answers to Questions, HC Deb, 26 November 1987, vol. 123, col. 364.

30. PREM 19/2335.

31. Sir Raymond Hoffenberg, Sir Ian Todd and Sir George Pinker, 'Crisis in the NHS', 1987.
32. *Daily Telegraph*, 18 January 1988, p. 2.
33. *Aberdeen Press and Journal*, 9 October 1987, p. 11.
34. PREM 19/2335.
35. Alain Enthoven, *Reflections on the Management of the National Health Service*, Nuffield Trust, 4 October 1985, https://www.nuffieldtrust.org.uk/research/reflections-on-the-management-of-the-national-health-service.
36. PREM 19/2335.
37. T 640/1335.
38. Moore, *Margaret Thatcher*, p. 88.
39. Nicholas Timmins, *Window Breakers and Glaziers: The Role of the Secretary of State for Health in Their Own Words*, The Health Foundation, 2015, p. 91.
40. Timmins, *Five Giants*.
41. Timmins, *Glaziers and Window Breakers*, p. 94.
42. Alain Enthoven, *In Pursuit of an Improving National Health Service*, Nuffield Trust, 1999, p. 91.
43. Ken Clarke in Eleanor MacKillop et al. (eds), *The NHS Internal Market: Witness Seminar*, Department of Public Health and Policy, University of Liverpool, 2018, p. 44.
44. Interview with author.
45. Ken Clarke in *NHS Internal Market: Witness Seminar*, p. 51.
46. Marshall Marinker in *NHS Internal Market: Witness Seminar*, p. 51.
47. Interview with author.
48. PREM 19/3496.
49. Julian Le Grand et al. (eds), *Learning from the NHS Internal Market: A Review of the Evidence*, King's Fund, 1998.
50. Interview with author.
51. 'Should the NHS Abolish the Purchaser-Provider Split?', *BMJ*, vol. 354, 2016, i3825.
52. Timmins, *Glaziers and Window Breakers*, p. 28.
53. Interview with author.
54. Timmins, *Five Giants*.
55. Interview with author.
56. Interview with author.
57. *Wellcome Witnesses*, p. 29.

58. Sir Bernard Tomlinson, *Report of the Inquiry into London's Health Service Medical Education and Research* (Tomlinson Report), Her Majesty's Stationery Office, October 1992, https://www.sochealth.co.uk/national-health-service/hospitals/tomlinson-report-1992/.

59. *Aberdeen Press and Journal*, 23 October 1992, p. 16.

60. *Aberdeen Press and Journal*, 24 October 1992, p. 5.

61. Interview with author.

62. Prayers, HC Deb, 23 October 1992, vol. 212.

63. *Pinner Observer*, 4 March 1993, p. 10.

64. *Guardian*, 22 October 1993, p. 2.

65. *Richmond and Twickenham Informer*, 5 November 1993.

66. 14 December 1993, PREM 19/4851.

67. 10 December 1993, PREM 19/4851.

68. Interview with author.

69. Dr Barbara Bonner-Morgan, *The Great Battle to Save Barts Hospital London: The Battle Between the Two London Hospital Giants*, Kindle eBook, 2018.

70. *BMJ*, vol. 335, no. 7619, 15 September 2007, p. 535.

Chapter 7: Infected

1. *Searching for 'Patient Zero': Britain's AIDS Tragedy*, first broadcast 11 November 2021 on ITV at 19.30.

2. *The Lancet*, 12 December 1981.

3. BBC Witness, 30 November 2018, https://www.bbc.co.uk/news/av/stories-46363059.

4. Interview with author.

5. *TV Eye*, 'AIDS: The Victims', first broadcast 28 February 1985, https://player.bfi.org.uk/free/film/watch-aids-the-victims-1985-online.

6. *Guardian*, 25 September 1985, p. 3.

7. Interview with author.

8. Maddy Mussen, ' "It Angered Me": Nurse Shares What Life Was Like on the Wards during the 80s AIDS Crisis', *The Tab*, 26 January 2016, https://thetab.com/uk/2021/01/26/it-angered-me-nurse-shares-what-life-was-like-on-the-wards-during-the-80s-aids-crisis-191978.

9. 'AIDS: The Victims'.

10. PREM 19/2775.

11. ITN, 9 April 1987.

12. BBC Witness, 2017.

13. *Birmingham Daily News*, 10 April 1987, p. 5.

14. *Searching for 'Patient Zero'*.

15. PREM 19/1863.

16. Interview with author.

17. PREM 19/1863.

18. Ibid.

19. Interview with Tim Jonze, *Guardian*, 4 September 2017, https://www.theguardian.com/culture/2017/sep/04/how-we-made-dont-die-of-ignorance-aids-campaign.

20. Interview with author.

21. PREM 19/2775.

22. Ibid.

23. Klein, *New Politics of the NHS*.

24. PREM 19/1863.

25. *Daily Mirror*, 19 November 1984, p. 16.

26. Gareth Lewis, interview with Krista Woodley, 23, 24 September and 23 October 2004.

27. Sian Edwards, interview with Haydn Lewis, Haemophilia and HIV Life History Project, 4–5 October 2005.

28. Diana Johnson, interview with author.

29. Interview with author.

30. *BMJ*, 1958, p. 607.

31. *Wellcome Witnesses*.

32. Dr Joe Selkon, in L. A. Reynolds and E. M. Tansey (eds), *Superbugs and Superdrugs: A History of MRSA* [transcript], 11 July 2006, p. 37.

33. *National Health Stories*.

34. Dinah Gould, 'The Fall and Rise of Cleanliness in British Healthcare and the Nursing Contribution', *Journal of Research in Nursing*, vol. 10, no. 5, September 2005, p. 15.

35. *National Health Stories*.

36. 'Full text: Michael Howard's MRSA Speech', *Guardian*, 2 September 2004, https://www.theguardian.com/politics/2004/sep/02/conservatives.uk.

37. *Investigation into Outbreaks of Clostridium difficile at Maidstone and*

Tunbridge Wells NHS Trust, https://www.whittington.nhs.uk/docu ment.ashx?id=1169.

38. Veronica Toffolutti et al., 'Outsourcing Cleaning Services Increases MRSA Incidence: Evidence from 126 English Acute Trusts', *Social Science and Medicine*, vol. 174, 2017, pp. 64–9.

Chapter 8: Control freaks

1. *Guardian*, 2 June 2000, p. 5.
2. Interview with author.
3. Interview with author.
4. *Guardian*, 14 April 1995.
5. Party Political Broadcast, April 1997.
6. *New Labour Because Britain Deserves Better*, Labour Party Manifesto, 1997, http://www.labour-party.org.uk/manifestos/1997/1997-labour-manifesto.shtml.
7. Interview with author.
8. Tony Blair, *A Journey*, Random House, eBook, 2010.
9. Timmins, *Glaziers and Window Breakers*, p. 125.
10. PREM 49/142.
11. Ibid.
12. NHS England, *NHS Identity Research: Phase One and Two Combined Research Report*, June 2016, https://www.england.nhs.uk/nhsidentity/wp-content/uploads/sites/38/2016/08/NHS-Identity-Research-phase-one-and-two.pdf.
13. Alastair Campbell, *The Alastair Campbell Diaries, Volume Two: Power and the People*, Random House, eBook, 2011, p. 268.
14. National Archives release.
15. PREM 49/141.
16. *CHC News*, January/February 1999, https://www.achcew.org/uploads/6/6/0/6/6606397/issue_027_jan_feb-99_copy.pdf.
17. Interview with author.
18. Timmins, *Five Giants*.
19. Interview with author.
20. Crisp, *24 Hours to Save the NHS*, p. 1.

21. *New Statesman*, 17 January 2000, pp. 14–15.
22. *Alastair Campbell Diaries, Volume Three: Power and Responsibility.*
23. *Breakfast with Frost*, 16 January 2000.
24. Andrew Rawnsley, *Servants of the People: The Inside Story of New Labour*, Hamish Hamilton, 2000, p. 338.
25. Interview with author.
26. *The NHS Plan*, Command Paper 4818-I, July 2000, https://webarchive.nationalarchives.gov.uk/ukgwa/20130107105354/http://www.dh.gov.uk/prod_consum_dh/groups/dh_digitalassets/@dh/@en/@ps/documents/digitalasset/dh_118522.pdf.
27. Interview with author.
28. Crisp, *24 Hours to Save the NHS*, p. 35.
29. Interview with author.
30. Simon Stevens, 'Reform Strategies for the English NHS', *Health Affairs*, vo. 23, 2004, pp. 37–44.
31. Interview with author.
32. Crisp, *24 Hours to Save the NHS*, p. 48.
33. Quotes in the next few paragraphs are taken from various interviews with author.
34. Timmins, *Glaziers and Window Breakers*, p. 155.
35. Evidence to House of Commons Health Select Committee, 6 February 2007   https://publications.parliament.uk/pa/cm200607/cmselect/cmliaisn/300/7020604.htm.
36. Timmins, *Five Giants*.
37. Interview with author.
38. Interview with author.
39. Michael Barber, *How to Run a Government*, Penguin Books, eBook, 2015, p. 13.
40. 'Speech by the Secretary of State for Health, Alan Milburn, 2002', 14 January 2002, https://www.nuffieldtrust.org.uk/health-and-social-care-explained/the-history-of-the-nhs/speech-by-the-secretary-of-state-for-health-alan-milburn-2002#speech-by-rt-hon-alan-milburn-mp-secretary-of-state-for-health-to-the-new-health-network.
41. *Health Committee: Evidence*, 2006, https://publications.parliament.uk/pa/cm200506/cmselect/cmhealth/934/934we.pdf.
42. Stevens, 'Reform Strategies for the English NHS'.

43. Interview with author.
44. *BMJ*, vol. 332, 2006, p. 614.
45. Stevens, 'Reform Strategies for the English NHS'.
46. Interview with author.
47. Interview with author.
48. NHS Foundation Trusts, HC Deb, 19 November 2003, vol. 413.
49. Health and Social Care, HC Deb, 7 May 2003.
50. Klein, *New Politics of the NHS*, p. 202.
51. ' "Evil and Orwellian" – America's Right Turns Its Fire on NHS', *Guardian*, 11 August 2009, https://www.theguardian.com/world/2009/aug/11/nhs-united-states-republican-health.
52. *BMJ*, vol. 32, 2000, p. 644.
53. National Archives, 'Speech by Patricia Hewitt', 25 October 2005, https://webarchive.nationalarchives.gov.uk/ukgwa/20070305230135/http://www.dh.gov.uk/NewsHome/Speeches/SpeechesList/SpeechesArticle/fs/en?CONTENT_ID=4121929&chk=AEiAHr.
54. BBC *Panorama*, 5 February 2006.
55. Timmins, *Five Giants*.
56. 'PFI Hospitals Design "Disaster"', BBC News, 23 October 2001, http://news.bbc.co.uk/1/hi/health/1615004.stm.
57. David Price et al., *'The Only Game in Town?': A Report on the Cumberland Infirmary*, UNISON, December 1999, https://allysonpollock.com/wp-content/uploads/2013/04/UNISON_1999_Price_Cumberland.pdf.
58. J. Appleby, 'Making sense of PFI', Nuffield Trust, 2017, www.nuffieldtrust.org.uk/resource/making-sense-of-pfi.
59. Richard Murray et al., *Financial Failure in the NHS: What Causes It and How Best to Manage It*, King's Fund, October 2014.
60. Timmins, *Five Giants*.
61. Dr Geoffrey Rivett, '1998–2007: Labour's Decade', Nuffield Trust, https://www.nuffieldtrust.org.uk/chapter/1998-2007-labour-s-decade#general-practice-and-primary-health-care.
62. *The Times*, 12 November 2009.
63. Matt Weaver, 'Nurses Barrack Embattled Hewitt', *Guardian*, 26 April 2006, https://www.theguardian.com/politics/2006/apr/26/publicservices.uk.
64. Timmins, *Five Giants*.

65. Timmins, *Glaziers and Window Breakers*, p. 145.

66. Ibid., p. 148.

67. Polyclinics, HC Deb, 17 June 2008, vol. 477.

68. John Carvel, 'Virgin Team Highlights NHS Shambles', *Guardian*, 22 July 2000, https://www.theguardian.com/society/2000/jul/22/future ofthenhs.health.

69. Jeremy Corbyn, Twitter, 30 July 2019, https://twitter.com/jeremycor byn/status/1156133063484723200.

70. Table 38 to the Department of Health and Social Care annual report and accounts 2019/20.

71. Interview with author.

Chapter 9: The biggest train set on Whitehall

1. Interview with author.

2. Interview with the *Spectator*, 8 July 2006, https://www.spectator. co.uk/article/-the-stroke-could-have-killed-me-.

3. Interview with author.

4. *Financial Times*, 18 June 2010.

5. Interview with author.

6. Andrew Lansley, 'The Future of Health and Public Service Regulation' [speech], 9 July 2005.

7. Interviews with author.

8. Nicholas Timmins, *Never Again? The Story of the Health and Social Care Act 2012*, Institute for Government/King's Fund, 2012, p. 36.

9. Speech, 4 January 2006.

10. Conservative Party, *Invitation to Join the Government of Britain: The Conservative Manifesto 2010*, Pureprint Group, 2020.

11. BBC News, *First Prime Ministerial Debate 15 April 2010* [transcript], http://news.bbc.co.uk/1/shared/bsp/hi/pdfs/16_04_10_firstdebate.pdf.

12. Denis Campbell, 'Doctors Warned to Expect Unrest over NHS', *Guardian*, 19 November 2010, https://www.theguardian.com/society/ 2010/nov/19/doctors-warned-expect-unrest-reforms.

13. Interview with author.

14. Interview with the *Independent*, 2005, https://www.independent.

co.uk/news/uk/politics/frontbencher-calls-for-nhs-to-be-broken-up-313546.html.

15. Interview with author.

16. Quotes from Lansley and Cameron are from interviews with author.

17. Suzanne Heywood, *What Does Jeremy Think?*, HarperCollins, eBook, 2020, p. 341.

18. NHS Reform, HC Deb, 4 April 2011, vol. 526.

19. Stefano Ambrogi, 'Lansley Says Sorry to Nurses Over Health Reforms', Reuters, 13 April 2011, https://www.reuters.com/article/uk-britain-nurses-lansley-idUKTRE73C22Q20110413.

20. 'Editor's Blog', Health Policy Insight, 10 June 2011, https://www.healthpolicyinsight.com/editors-blog-friday-10-june-2011--health-policy-intelligence-11--strongman-camerons-j-turn-on-nhs-reform-out-now/.

21. Health and Social Care Act 2012, https://www.legislation.gov.uk/ukpga/2012/7/contents/enacted.

22. 'NHS Reforms: Clegg Says Bill "Better" Despite Defeat', BBC News, 11 March 2012, https://www.bbc.co.uk/news/uk-politics-17330939.

23. Denis Campbell and Juliette Jowett, 'Scrap the Health Bill, GP Urges David Cameron', *Guardian*, 28 February 2012, https://www.theguardian.com/society/2012/feb/28/scrap-health-bill-doctor-warns.

24. Timmins, *Never Again?*.

25. Quotes from Everington, Morgan and Cameron are from interviews with author.

26. Interview with author.

Chapter 10: The fight for safety

1. Julie Bailey, *From Ward to Whitehall: The Disaster at Mid Staffs Hospital*, eBook, 2013.

2. Ibid.

3. *Independent Inquiry into Care Provided by Mid Staffordshire NHS Foundation Trust January 2005 – March 2009: Volume I*, Chaired by Robert Francis QC, The Stationery Office, 24 February 2010, https://assets.publishing.service.gov.uk/government/uploads/system/uploads/attachment_data/file/279109/0375_i.pdf.

4. Interview with author.

5. Interview with author.

6. 'Stafford Hospital Inquiry: Senior Doctor "Ignored" ', BBC News, 16 February 2011, https://www.bbc.co.uk/news/uk-england-stoke-staffordshire-12488859.

7. Interview with author.

8. Peter Walker, 'Alan Johnson Moves to "Close This Regrettable Chapter in Hospital's Past" ', *Guardian*, 17 March 2009, https://www.theguardian.com/society/2009/mar/17/alan-johnson-mid-staffordshire-nhs-trust.

9. Timmins, *Glaziers and Window Breakers*, p. 49.

10. Interviews with author.

11. Iain Martin, 'The Night I Saw Jeremy Hunt Hide Behind a Tree before Dinner with James Murdoch', Capx, 26 February 2016, https://capx.co/the-night-i-saw-jeremy-hunt-hide-behind-a-tree/.

12. This and other quotes from Hunt in this chapter are from interview with author.

13. This and other quotes from Oliver in this chapter are from interview with author.

14. Interview with author.

15. Mid Staffordshire NHS Foundation Trust Inquiry, HL Deb, 6 February 2013, vol. 743.

16. This and other quotes from Burnham in this chapter are from interview with author.

17. This and other quotes from Nicholson in this chapter are from interview with author.

18. Interview with author.

19. James Titcombe, *Joshua's Story: Uncovering the Morecambe Bay NHS Scandal*, Anderson Wallace Publishing, eBook, 2015.

20. Professor Dame Pauline Fielding et al., *Review of Maternity Services in University Hospitals of Morecambe Bay NHS Trust* (Fielding Report), 31 March 2010.

21. Titcombe, *Joshua's Story*.

22. Dr Bill Kirkup, *The Report of the Morecambe Bay Investigation*, The Stationery Office, March 2015, p. 5 https://assets.publishing.service.gov.uk/government/uploads/system/uploads/attachment_data/file/408480/47487_MBI_Accessible_vo.1.pdf.

23. *The Times*, 18 March 2013.

24. Interview with author.

25. David Cameron, 'PM on Plans for a Seven Day NHS' [speech], 18 May 2015, https://www.gov.uk/government/speeches/pm-on-plans-for-a-seven-day-nhs.

26. Conservative Party, *A Brighter, More Secure Future for England: The Conservative Party Manifesto 2015*, https://www.theresavilliers.co.uk/sites/www.theresavilliers.co.uk/files/conservativemanifesto2015.pdf.

27. Interview with author.

28. Rowena Mason, 'Jeremy Hunt Angers Junior Doctors by Saying Some Are Paid "Danger Money"', *Guardian*, 30 October 2015, https://www.theguardian.com/society/2015/oct/30/jeremy-hunt-angers-junior-doctors-by-saying-some-are-paid-danger-money.

29. Interviews with author.

30. Shaun Lintern, 'Huge Leak Reveals BMA Plan to "Draw Out" Junior Doctors Dispute', *HSJ*, 26 May 2016, https://www.hsj.co.uk/workforce/exclusive-huge-leak-reveals-bma-plan-to-draw-out-junior-doctors-dispute/7005113.article.

31. Rachel Clarke, *Your Life in My Hands: A Junior Doctor's Story*, John Blake, eBook, 2017, p. 131.

32. 'Junior Doctor Contract Negotiations', BMA, 17 January 2020, https://beta-qa.bma.org.uk/pay-and-contracts/contracts/junior-doctor-contract/junior-doctor-contract-negotiations.

Chapter 11: Fighting to breathe

1. Interview with author.

2. Tim Shipman, *All Out War: The Full Story of How Brexit Sank Britain's Political Class*, HarperCollins, eBook, 2016.

3. Ibid.

4. Interview with author.

5. 'Boris Johnson Got a "Complete Bitch Slap" from Theresa May after Breaking Ranks with Calls for Extra HNS Funding', ITV News, 23 January 2018, https://www.itv.com/news/2018-01-23/boris-johnson-breit-nhs.

6. Interview with author.

7. *Peston on Sunday*, ITV, 25 March 2018.

8. Interview with author.

9. Interview with author.

10. Interview with author.

11. *Spectator*, 15 September 2012.

12. World Health Organization, 'COVID-19: China', 5 January 2020, https://www.who.int/emergencies/disease-outbreak-news/item/2020-DON229.

13. Interview with author.

14. Department of Health and Social Care, 'CMO for England Statement on the Wuhan Novel Coronavirus', 24 January 2020, https://www.gov.uk/government/news/cmo-for-england-statement-on-the-wuhan-novel-coronavirus.

15. Public Health England, *Exercise Cygnus Report*, 2017, https://assets.publishing.service.gov.uk/government/uploads/system/uploads/attachment_data/file/927770/exercise-cygnus-report.pdf.

16. Bill Gardner and Paul Nuki, 'Exercise Cygnus Warned the NHS Could Not Cope with Pandemic Three Years Ago but "Terrifying" Results Were Kept Secret', *Telegraph*, 28 March 2020, https://www.telegraph.co.uk/news/2020/03/28/exclusive-ministers-warned-nhs-could-not-cope-pandemic-three/.

17. *Nature*, vol. 580, no. 9, 2020.

18. Jonathan Calvert and George Arbuthnott, *Failures of State: The Inside Story of Britain's Battle with Coronavirus*, HarperCollins, eBook, 2022, p. 92.

19. *Telegraph*, 13 November 2020.

20. Interview with author.

21. 'Coronavirus: 10 Days of Hospital Building in 60 Seconds', BBC News, 2 February 2020, https://www.bbc.co.uk/news/av/world-asia-china-51348297.

22. *Spectator*, 28 November 2020.

23. Simons Stevens and Amanda Pritchard, 'Next Steps on NHS Response to COVID-19' [letter], 17 March 2020, https://www.england.nhs.uk/coronavirus/wp-content/uploads/sites/52/2020/03/urgent-next-steps-on-nhs-response-to-covid-19-letter-simon-stevens.pdf.

24. Health and Social Care Committee and Science and Technology Committee, 'Oral evidence: Coronavirus: Lessons Learnt', HC 95, 26 May 2021, https://committees.parliament.uk/oralevidence/2249/html/.

25. *Gardner and Harris v. Secretary of State for Health and Social Care*, 2022, https://www.bailii.org/ew/cases/EWHC/Admin/2022/967.html.

26. https://www.judiciary.uk/wp-content/uploads/2022/07/Gardner-Harris-v-DHSC-judgment-270422.pdf.

27. A. G. Proudfoot et al., 'Rapid Establishment of a COVID-19 Critical Care Unit in a Convention Centre: The Nightingale Hospital London Experience', *Intensive Care Med*, vol. 47, 2021, pp. 349–51.

28. 'Regulation 28: To Prevent Further Deaths', July 2021, https://www.judiciary.uk/wp-content/uploads/2021/07/Kishorkumar-Patel-and-Kofi-Aning-2021-0233-Redacted.pdf.

29. Peter Blackburn, 'Inside the Nightingales', BMA, 5 May 2020, https://www.bma.org.uk/news-and-opinion/inside-the-nightingales.

30. *Health Service Journal*, 2 April 2020.

31. 'Was Building the NHS Nightingale Hospitals Worth the Money?', King's Fund, 5 May 2021, https://www.kingsfund.org.uk/blog/2021/04/nhs-nightingale-hospitals-worth-money.

32. *Health Service Journal*, 7 May 2020.

33. National Audit Office, *Readying the NHS and Adult Social Care in England for COVID-19*, HC 367, 12 June 2020, https://www.nao.org.uk/wp-content/uploads/2020/06/Readying-the-NHS-and-adult-social-care-in-England-for-COVID-19.pdf.

34. Lauren Turner, 'Covid: Nurse Who Cared for PM Resigns from NHS', BBC News, 18 May 2021, https://www.bbc.co.uk/news/uk-57162428.

35. *Evidence to Joint Session of the Commons Science and Technology Committee and the Health and Social Care Committee*, 10 June 2021.

36. Downing Street Covid briefing, 1 May 2020.

37. Calvert and Arbuthnott, *Failures of State*, p. 254.

38. Jeremy Hunt, *Zero: Eliminating Preventable Harm and Tragedy in the NHS*, Swift Press, 2022, p. 92.

39. Committee of Public Accounts, *Test and Trace Update: Twenty-Third Report of Session 2021–22*, 27 October 2021, https://publications.parliament.uk/pa/cm5802/cmselect/cmpubacc/182/report.html.

40. 'Coronavirus Contract Tracer "Paid to Watch Netflix"', BBC News, 3 June 2020, https://www.bbc.co.uk/news/uk-52904433.

41. NHS Staff Pay, HC Deb, 8 March 2021, vol. 690.

42. Interview with author.

43. Interviews with author.

44. *BMJ*, vol. 369, 2020, m1658.

45. Interview with author.

46. HCSA/Every Doctor, *Never Again: COVID from the Frontlines*, March 2022, p. 28, https://actionnetwork.org/user_files/user_files/000/076/914/original/Never-Again-final-edits-v23-print-3mmbleed.pdf.

47. Claire Press, 'Coronavirus: The NHS Workers Wearing Bin Bags as Protection', BBC News, 5 April 2020, https://www.bbc.co.uk/news/health-52145140.

48. Downing Street Covid briefing, 10 April 2020.

49. Interview with author.

50. Interview with author.

51. Interview with author.

52. Interview with author.

53. Nicholas Timmins and Beccy Baird, *The Covid-19 Vaccination Programme: Trials, Tribulations and Successes*, King's Fund, January 2022, p. 19, https://www.kingsfund.org.uk/publications/covid-19-vaccination-programme.

54. Interview with author.

55. Public Accounts Committee, *Oral Evidence: DHSC Annual Report and Accounts 2020-21*, HC 1115, 7 March 2022.

56. Kate Bingham and Tim Hames, *The Long Shot*, Oneworld Publications, eBook, 2022, p. 119.

57. Quote to author.

58. *BMJ*, vol. 370, 2020, m2670.

59. Emily Townsend, 'Ambulance Service Will Collapse by August, Predicts Its Nursing Director', *HSJ*, 25 May 2022, https://www.hsj.co.uk/west-midlands/exclusive-ambulance-service-will-collapse-by-august-predicts-its-nursing-director/7032502.article.

60. Rhys Blakely and Henry Zefferman, 'A&E Delays "Killing up to 500 People a Week"', *The Times*, 2 January 2023, https://www.thetimes.co.uk/article/a-e-delays-killing-up-to-500-people-a-week-g5kpxdpd6.

61. *The Times*, 28 May 2022.

Chapter 12: The last battle?

1. Nigel Lawson, *The View from No. 11: Memoirs of a Tory Radical*, Transworld Publishers, 1993, p. 613.
2. Health Services Bill, HC Deb, 27 April 1976, vol. 910.
3. *Hartlepool Mail*, 9 September 2004.
4. The Commonwealth Fund, 'Health Care System Performance Rankings', https://www.commonwealthfund.org/sites/default/files/2021-07/PDF_Schneider_Mirror_Mirror_2021_exhibits.pdf.
5. Parliamentary and Health Service Ombudsman, 'Missed Opportunities', https://www.ombudsman.org.uk/publications/missed-opportunities-what-lessons-can-be-learned-failings-north-essex/our-recommendations.
6. *Essex Chronicle*, 31 March 2022, p. 5.
7. Aneurin Bevan, *In Place of Fear*, Lume Books, eBook, 2020.
8. Health and Social Care Committee, *Oral Evidence: Clearing the Backlog after the Pandemic*, HC 599, 19 October 2021, https://committees.parliament.uk/oralevidence/2817/html/.
9. Interview with author.

Index